HEAL YOUR HEART

The New Rice Diet Program for
Reversing Heart Disease Through Nutrition,
Exercise, and Spiritual Renewal

Kitty Gurkin Rosati

John Wiley & Sons, Inc.

New York • Chichester • Brisbane • Toronto • Singapore • Weinheim

Copyright © 1997 by Kitty Gurkin Rosati

Published by John Wiley & Sons, Inc.

Library of Congress Cataloging-in-Publication Data
Rosati, Kitty Gurkin
    Heal your heart :   the new rice diet program for reversing heart
disease through nutrition, exercise, and spiritual renewal / Kitty
Gurkin Rosati.
        p.   cm.
    Includes index.
    ISBN 0-471-15702-3
    1. Heart—Diseases—Diet therapy. 2. Heart—Diseases—Patients—
Rehabilitation. 3. Cookery (Rice) 4. High-carbohydrate diet.
5. Salt-free diet.   I. Title
RC684.D5R67 1997
616.1'20654—dc20   96-42087

Printed in the United States of America

10 9 8 7 6 5 4 3 2

CONTENTS

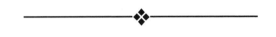

PART ONE
LIVING A HEART-HEALTHY LIFE

PART TWO

YOUR PERSONAL HEAL YOUR HEART PROGRAM

Chapter 5

Chapter 6

PART THREE

HEALING YOUR HEART

Chapter 7

Chapter 8

Chapter 9

Chapter 10

PART FOUR

HEAL YOUR HEART FOODS AND RECIPES

Chapter 11

Chapter 12

Chapter 13

Chapter 14

Appendix A

Appendix B

FOREWORD

❖

Your health is your most important asset. Never has it been clearer that you have the ability to prevent or reverse many of the chronic diseases that afflict most of us. Coronary heart disease and its risk factors—high blood sugar, high cholesterol, high blood pressure, diabetes, and obesity—have received the most attention; others include arthritis, kidney failure, sleep apnea, and psoriasis.

In 400 B.C., Hippocrates advocated building health through diet. In the twelfth century, Maimonides said that no disease which could be treated by diet should be treated by any other means. And, as the present century began, Thomas Edison predicted that the doctor of the future would use no medicines but would instruct his patients in diet, and so on. Now, as the century comes to a close, we know that the Rice Diet—a low-fat, low-salt diet used since the 1940s to treat high blood pressure, kidney disease, diabetes, and heart disease—is the diet of choice. The diet is uniquely appealing for physicians as well, because it allows them to tell if their patients are following it by measuring the amount of sodium in their urine.

Nowhere on earth can you experience a diet that more dramatically alleviates a greater variety of illnesses. And now the "going home" plan is available to those who cannot find a way to come and enjoy it first-hand. At last here is a book that combines low fat with low salt and makes it taste good. No one can deny the importance of low fat, because heart disease is the number one cause of death in the United States. In our experience, low salt is equally important. Eighty percent of our patients with high blood pressure can stop their medications and have lower blood pressures than they did on medication. Another 10 percent are able to decrease their medications with lower blood pressures. Even patients with normal blood pressures benefit from low salt. They have lower blood pressures and therefore lower cardiovascular risk, they feel better and they eat less, since there is so little salt to stimulate their appetites.

I first met Kitty in 1985 when she was a dietitian at Duke University's cardiac rehabilitation program. I had heard she was a vegetarian, so I asked her if she knew that tofu had as much or more fat than hamburger. She said she didn't, but would check it out. And she did. She knew about low fat, but was skeptical about low salt, so she tried it, with the beneficial effects that she will describe herself. This interest and willingness to continue to observe and to learn have put her in a unique position as a therapeutic nutritionist. The depth and breadth of her knowledge of nutrition are evident in the pages which follow.

The essentials of good health are proper diet, exercise, and rest. These elements are thoroughly and entertainingly presented with many interesting stories of actual patients. The composition, rationale for and results of the low-fat, low-salt diet are carefully described. The recipes are delicious and can easily be prepared by novice cooks like you and me.

—Robert Rosati, M.D.
Medical Director
The Rice Diet Program

INTRODUCTION

❖

My goal in writing this book is three-fold. First, to provide you with practical nutritional information for implementing and embracing a very low fat, no-salt-added nutrition plan for reversing heart disease—or even better, preventing it from occurring in the first place. Second, to share the benefits of exercise and get you started on a healthy regimen. Third, to provide some emotional and spiritual pathways that can not only improve the quality of your life but can greatly enhance your odds of adhering to the physical challenges of this plan for the long haul. As I, and many of those whom I have counseled, have discovered, our physical problems often have emotional and spiritual underpinnings. So I wanted to share my practical learning experiences with those of you who are struggling with heart disease and those who want to prevent it.

From this three-part mission, the Heal Your Heart Program was born. All three components are essential to the success of this program. The physical aspects, such as diet and exercise, and the emotional and spiritual needs, such as meditation, prayer, and community, can be equally important for maintaining or pursuing health.

This book has had a long gestational period: it has been in process for approximately half of my life. My interest in heart disease began during my freshman year in college when my father died of a heart attack at age 50. His death was a shock to me and was a pivotal point in my life. Like many who die prematurely of heart disease, he had "never been sick a day in his life." Yet he worked all the time, rarely took a vacation, smoked cigarettes, ate a typical American diet high in protein, fat, and salt, never exercised, and was going through a divorce. Although my mother was a registered nurse, she succeeded in getting him to a doctor only once. He did not like what the doctor said or did, so he canceled his follow-up appointment. Although I now know his body was waving many red flags, back then few people were talking about their cholesterol levels, and fewer still were sharing from their broken hearts in divorce support groups . . . and he seemed so "normal."

It was then that I developed an aversion to settling for "normal" health. A friend introduced me to vegetarianism, and as I began to learn more about how an animal-based diet sets us up for heart disease and other chronic diseases, it seemed sensible to avoid eating meat. At first I quit eating red meat. Then, after my housemate, Chris, undercooked some chicken one night, I quit poultry, too. I also began to exercise vigorously, determined to avoid my father's fate. Of course, the physical healing I was pursuing via my vegetarian, athletic lifestyle was far more obvious to me than the emotional and spiritual healing I was unconsciously seeking.

Soon after earning a graduate degree in nutrition, I gained experience consulting on nutrition for a wide variety of people and conditions. Although my work ranged from teaching university students to IBM executives, I always preferred counseling cardiac rehabilitation and alcohol and drug rehabilitation patients. It became increasingly obvious to me that those who really took my dietary recommendations seriously and showed up faithfully for the sessions were improving far more quickly than those who did not. What took me longer to realize was *why* some had the strength to change their unhealthy lifestyles while others lacked that strength.

I was immersed in the cardiac and addiction arenas for a long time before I had a conscious awareness of how God was leading me to work in the areas where I was in need of healing my own personal pain. It finally happened when I awoke nine days before my thirty-fifth birthday and found myself crippled from head to toe. When a vegetarian tri-athlete overnight becomes unable to walk stairs, even on massive amounts of anti-inflammatory drugs, words like humbled, terrified, and outraged are all understatements. Although I had faith that I would eventually be healed, and suspected that my symptoms were due to unresolved feelings of resentment, it was still a long and lonely period. But as I emerged from this crippling pain, I learned that emotional and spiritual growth were as important for my pursuit of health and physical healing as a low-fat vegetarian diet could have been for my father.

The Rice Diet Program Approach to Heart Disease

Duke University's Rice Diet Program was created over fifty years ago by Dr. Walter Kempner. It offered a revolutionary diet plan to patients with high blood pressure and kidney disease. It has since become world-renowned for helping all heart disease patients as well as those with other health problems. This expanded mission is reflected in its official name: Duke

University's Rice Diet Program and Heart Disease Reversal Clinic. But we still call it the Rice Diet Program for short.

Through my years of experience as the Nutrition Director of the Rice Diet Program, I can assure you that the risk factors and symptoms of heart disease can be quickly and effectively reversed by lifestyle choices. The lifestyle choices I will challenge you to embrace include an aggressive nutrition plan, a moderate exercise program, and a renewed emotional and spiritual journey on a path of your choice.

At the Rice Diet Program, I have witnessed the power of these three elements to dramatically reverse risk factors of heart disease. It has been this experience that inspired the Heal Your Heart Program that I outline in this book.

Like the Rice Diet, the Heal Your Heart nutrition plan, which I developed for our participants to follow when they go home, advocates a diet with very low fat and no added salt. The lower fat and sodium recommendations are more ambitious than the standard cardiac diet, but for good reason. The Rice Diet Program has proven that there is no faster, more effective, or safer way to lower the risk factors of heart disease.

As for the exercise component of the Program, my philosophy is simple: commit to an hour of moderate exercise per day, doing whatever exercise that you will stick to. The majority of you will prefer to walk, as it is usually the most readily available exercise.

The third component of the Heal Your Heart Program involves your emotional and spiritual consciousness. I will recommend a variety of avenues toward healing, and will share testimonials from participants who have enjoyed inner transformations that have led to lasting physical changes.

You may by this point be thinking it would take a miracle for you to make all the changes the Heal Your Heart Program recommends. But I want to encourage you to try it for a month. I convinced myself by living this plan as I am challenging you to do. You will only know whether the effort is worth it if you try. If you are not impressed enough with your results to continue after a month, at least you will have made a conscious, educated choice.

My hope for you is that your emotional and spiritual growth will inspire and undergird your enthusiasm for the nutrition and exercise guidelines, as well as your pleasurable pursuit of other life-fulfilling goals. If you would like more information about the Rice Diet Program, call me at 888 RICE DIET.

ACKNOWLEDGEMENTS

———————◆———————

A very special thanks to the many who have made this book possible. In previous years Kathy Nunemaker encouraged me to expand this book; her encouragement came through her enthusiasm for its truth and her editing skills. It is rare when you find someone who can share constructive criticism on your writing in a way that can be heard, much less enjoyed! God surely was exercising a profound sense of humor when I was led to her, a hospital chaplain with an editing background.

Thanks to my peers and the many patients and their spouses who have contributed to this book. Foremost to Kam Miller, a clinical exercise physiologist at Georgetown University's Cardiac Rehabilitation Program, who contributed the very instructive exercise advice. A woman of many talents, she also shared her computer/graphics expertise to make the allowances, menus, and forms more reader friendly. It was fun working with such a friend, someone with a passion to create, and a generous desire to assist another so afflicted. Thanks also to my colleagues Andrea Beckeley, Anne Gravitte-Sims, and Annie King for their invaluable support. Their community spirit was much appreciated, as was the team effort of those who contributed recipes: Lan Tan, Joy Nelson, Maria Zagorianos, Rhoda Harris, Lorraine Deieso, Alan Sukert, Carol Ericcson, Robert Rosati, Olga Mangiagalli, Camille Denti, Judy Ladner, May Segal, Joan Zipnick, Chahine Levine, and Farida Gindi.

Many thanks also to the people at John Wiley & Sons, especially my editor Judith McCarthy, who shared my vision for the book to be spiritually developed, and my belief that the book could be published by winter 1997. This year we have not only succeeded at birthing the book we envisioned, but were also both blessed with our first births. And as anyone who has experienced either knows, major miracles are required for both; an author and an editor birthing two boys and a book within one year is a close second to Moses parting the Red Sea! And thanks to Robbie (Judith's son) and Chess (my son) for their model behavior in utero and as newborns!

There are a number of people who have helped me on my emotional and spiritual road to recovery and who have assisted me in getting to know God in a very personal way. Special thanks to Frances Klass, who led me to a realization that God is as real today as ever and that my beliefs were not just due to early, successful programming as I had feared. Thanks to Tommy Tyson, my spiritual mentor and founder of The Aqueduct Retreat Center, who has guided me toward some of the most gifted spiritual teachers I have known. To have a community where you can seek refuge and healing among lovers of God like Waldemar Purcell, Keith Miller, and Morton Kelsey, is one of the greatest gifts on earth. Thank you Tommy, thank you, thank you, thank you.

And, of course, last but not least is a heart-felt thanks to my husband and mother who have both given up a lot of the time I would have spent with them. To my husband, Bob, goes grateful thanks for the many, many ways he offered his support. And, many will be thankful for his wonderful recipes which were developed during the times when I was on the computer rather than in the kitchen! And, to my Mom, for teaching me that I can do anything that I truly want. Without such early advice and confidence building, this book would not have been possible.

PART ONE

❖ ❖ ❖

LIVING A HEART-HEALTHY LIFE

❖ ❖ ❖

1

Reversing the Risks of Heart Disease

If you or someone you love has suffered from heart disease, you know how frightening it can be. And you probably know that you are far from alone. Approximately 42 percent of all deaths in the United States are due to heart disease. And, except for 1918 (the year of the great influenza epidemic), heart disease has been the number one killer every year since 1900. While significant progress has been made in treating heart disease, it still remains the number one killer of both men and women. However, you can improve your odds of having a healthy heart, even if you already have heart disease, by living a healthier lifestyle in general, with a focus on three elements: eating a diet that is very low in fat and salt, making sure that you have regular exercise, and taking care of your emotional and spiritual needs.

Through my own life experiences and work with thousands of heart disease patients, I have come to appreciate the strong connection between our emotional and spiritual health and our physical health. I firmly believe in treating the whole person and the root causes of their problems. Why mop the floor beneath an overflowing sink instead of turning off the faucet? We can aggressively attend to the root causes of heart disease—your risk factors.

I feel strongly about the redeeming powers of this three-part approach to healing the whole person because I have seen it work. Through my work at the Rice Diet Program at Duke University and elsewhere, I have helped thousands of heart disease patients reclaim their health and their lives. So, the Heal Your Heart Program I offer here includes all three of these components: nutrition, exercise, and inner healing. Why is this program effective at treating heart disease? Because it helps you control the things that gave you heart disease in the first place—your risk factors.

WHAT ARE YOUR RISK FACTORS?

There are several known factors that increase your odds of having heart disease. These are commonly called risk factors and they fall into two categories: nonmodifiable and modifiable. The nonmodifiable risk factors are those you can do nothing about; they include age and family history of heart disease. The modifiable risk factors are those that you can act on, so those are the ones that this program will help you improve. Modifiable risk factors include a high cholesterol level in the blood, high low-density lipoprotein (LDL), low high-density lipoprotein (HDL), high blood pressure (hypertension), high triglyceride (if cholesterol is high) high blood sugar (diabetes), cigarette smoking, and excess weight. Each of these modifiable risk factors is important, but they are of even greater concern if you have two or more of them. Of course, another risk factor is the actual signs and symptoms of heart disease, but this, too, can be reversed by following the Heal Your Heart Program and the advice of your doctor.

It is difficult—if not impossible—to say which risk factors are most important to you because each one can affect your other risk factors. But a high cholesterol level is the most highly respected predictor of heart disease. And although it affects fewer people, diabetes, especially in women, gives you a much greater risk of having heart disease. Hypertension is also a strong risk factor for heart disease, but even more so for strokes. And, although obesity was the last to be officially recognized as a major risk factor for heart disease, its importance cannot be overemphasized because (except for smoking) being overweight can cause all the other modifiable risk factors to worsen. So rather than being distracted by risk factors you can't control, such as your family history or your age, let's stay focused on the bottom line truth. You *can* reverse or control all your modifiable risk factors of heart disease. The Heal Your Heart Program will show you how.

HOW THE RICE DIET PROGRAM REVERSES RISK FACTORS

At the Rice Diet Program at Duke University we help people prevent and reverse heart disease risk factors. Many of the people who come to the Rice Diet do so because they are overweight, which is a risk factor not only for heart disease, but for many other diseases as well. We help them learn to eat right and to "re-educate" their eating habits so that they can lose the extra pounds and learn to maintain a healthy weight and lifestyle.

The Rice Diet Program was started in 1939 by Dr. Walter Kempner, who was the first to clinically research and practice the therapeutic effect of very low sodium, fat, and protein intake. Well before it was fashionable to acknowledge that cholesterol levels were important, Dr. Kempner started his own laboratory to check his patient's levels.

In 1954, he reported that of 800 patients with high cholesterol, 93 percent experienced a significant reduction in their cholesterols after an average of 124 days on the Rice Diet. Before the Rice Diet, their average cholesterol was 283, and after the Rice Diet their average dropped to 205! And the Rice Diet has consistently shown such results, proving that diet can have an enormously beneficial effect on cholesterol levels—without medication.

At the Rice Diet Program, patients are introduced to the diet in two phases. During Phase One, historically called the Rice and Fruit phase, patients eat only grains and fruits, with rice encouraged as a choice at least daily. This phase is very strict, containing less than 50 milligrams of sodium and 700 calories per day. Rice and Fruit was initially the dietary prescription used by Dr. Kempner for the treatment of kidney disease, congestive heart failure, and hypertension because it produced the quickest and most impressive results, and was the diet lowest in sodium, fat, and protein that could sustain health for long periods of time. In 1939, when the use of this dietary treatment began, diuretics, other hypertensive medications, and dialysis machines had not yet been invented. So patients with very sodium-sensitive disorders either embraced this very-low-sodium prescription or died, usually within a few months or years. At the Rice Diet Program, after fifty-five years of clinical experience with the diet, we still view the diet as the preferred and primary therapy, and respect the Rice and Fruit phase as the most powerful diuretic available. After years of experience with different maladies, this low-sodium, low-fat, and low-protein diet proved effective in treating all the other modifiable risk factors of heart disease, including high cholesterol, diabetes, and obesity, and offered relief as well to many with arthritis, allergies, and a host of other problems.

> **It is important to note that we do *not* recommend that you follow Phase One, eating only rice and fruit, on your own. This phase of the diet must be carefully monitored by the experienced staff at the Rice Diet Program, because the sudden drop in sodium can cause electrolyte imbalances that can lead to dizziness, fainting, and other problems.**

Phase One of the Rice Diet lasts as long as necessary for each patient, but usually two to three weeks. Phase Two of the Rice Diet includes all grains, beans, fruits, and vegetables, and provides up to 250 milligrams of sodium and 1,000 calories. Phase Two allows slightly more sodium because vegetables contain more natural sodium than do fruits, and it allows more calories because of the addition of the calorically dense starches, such as sweet potatoes and dried beans and peas. Neither Phase One nor Phase Two contains added fat or sodium.

Some patients move on to Phase Three, which includes all of the Phase Two vegetarian choices plus fish or chicken. We recommend that all patients stay on Phase Two until they have reached their health goals. Not only will they reach their goals faster, but the odds that they will achieve them are much greater in Phase Two. Because of this, Phase Three is infrequently approved, and we rarely serve meat at the Rice Diet Program.

The nutrition portion of the Heal Your Heart Program was inspired in part by Phases Two and Three of the Rice Diet, and is the basis for the Going Home Nutrition Plan I teach participants before they leave our center. It allows approximately 250 additional milligrams of sodium, which is enough to avoid electrolyte imbalances and dizziness problems. In addition to a safety margin, this extra 250 milligrams of sodium offers some flexibility and freedom to choose from a greater variety of foods, such as nonfat dairy products, seafood, or even bagels.

Although the foundation and focus at the Rice Diet Program has always been the dietary therapy, good exercise habits and the importance of inner healing is also emphasized. We have found that an inner healing of our emotional and spiritual selves is a key component in achieving and maintaining the nutritional and exercise components, thus our overall health.

THE HEAL YOUR HEART PROGRAM

I have developed the Heal Your Heart Program of nutrition, exercise, and inner healing through my years of working with cardiac patients, both at Duke University and elsewhere. It is a challenging program, but one that will help you achieve real results in reversing your risk factors through natural means—with few or no drugs. As a nutritionist, I focus on eating well. You'll find information on the latest nutrition research as well as tips and recipes for making a very low-fat, low-sodium diet not only bearable, but enjoyable. And, since exercise is also key to recovery, this program includes specifics on how to start and maintain a healthy exercise regimen. However, diet and exercise are only part of the story. Through my work with patients and in my own life, I have come to believe that we can only be truly healed if we look within and develop our spirituality. So, the Heal Your Heart Program involves all three of these elements to give you a well-rounded approach to your own healing.

In the next three chapters I'll describe how this program can help you reverse your major risk factors for heart disease. I recommend you read all three chapters because the risk factors are so closely related, but if you know you have high cholesterol, give special attention to Chapter 2. If you are overweight or have diabetes, read Chapter 3 more closely. If you have high blood pressure, be sure to read Chapter 4 carefully.

Part Two helps you design your personal version of the Heal Your Heart Program, and Part Three offers practical guidelines and tips for making the program part of your life. Part Four contains recipes for delicious dishes that you can enjoy in good conscience!

Here is a general overview of each component of the Heal Your Heart Program and why each is important to your good health.

Healing Your Heart Through Nutrition

The nutrition component of the Heal Your Heart Program calls for a diet that is *very* low in sodium, fat, and cholesterol, and high in fiber. In addition, the Heal Your Heart Program includes only foods that have no sodium added, and minimal amounts of caffeine and alcohol.

Here are the general daily guidelines of the nutrition plan:

❖ *Calories:* 1,000–2,000, depending on your need for weight loss

❖ *Total fat:* less than 10 percent of total calories to reverse heart disease; less than 20 percent for preventing heart disease

❖ *Saturated fat:* less than 5 percent of your total calories

❖ *Cholesterol:* less than 100 milligrams (mgs.)

❖ *Sodium:* less than 500 milligrams

❖ *Fiber:* more than 30 grams

Many people are surprised by how low the sodium and fat levels in the plan are. This is largely because most of us have been taught that low-sodium diets are only for people with high blood pressure. I used to think that, too. It was not until I began working at the Rice Diet Program that I had the opportunity to follow all participants (high blood pressure or not) consuming a diet that was very low in fat, but also very low in sodium. I was hired as a dietitian for the Rice Diet Program even after I admitted that although I was interested in teaching diets of less than 10 percent fat, I was not convinced that "no salt" was worth the effort except for patients with high blood pressure and congestive heart failure and kidney disease. I'm grateful that I insisted on trying the Rice Diet for a month as an incoming participant would, eating vegetarian foods without added fat and sodium. Much to my amazement, my arthritis-like joint pain and swelling decreased markedly! I would never have believed that lowering my sodium could cause such an improvement in my joints. Since then I have also seen patients who do not have high blood pressure swear by our no-salt-added diet for weight loss, arthritic pain, psoriasis, and general good health.

The allowance of less than 10 to 20 percent of calories from fat may also sound particularly strict if you have heard that the American Heart Association recommends less than 30 percent of calories from fat. Why the sharp difference? The most respected regression studies have shown that a diet containing 25 to 30 percent of calories from fat produces only a 4 to 14 percent reduction in cholesterol levels, which is not enough to reverse plaque formation in the majority of arteries examined. In fact, all of the studies that have used this amount of fat in the participants' diets, and assessed their arteries with arteriograms (a high-tech method for quantifying arterial change), have found the AHA-type diet inspires a progression of plaque in the majority of people consuming it.

While the most beneficial level can be debated, I recommend 10 to 20 percent of calories from fat if your goal is preventing heart disease, and less than 10 percent of calories from fat if you have heart disease and are seeking to reverse it. Dr. Kempner and Dr. Dean Ornish have shown that people on diets containing less than 10 percent fat reduce their cholesterol levels as much as those receiving cholesterol-lowering medication. In fact, when Dr. J.E. Roussouw and associates analyzed seven regression studies (*New England Journal of Medicine,* 1990) they found dietary interventions to be more effective at reversing plaque in the arteries than cholesterol-lowering drug therapy, despite similar cholesterol reductions.

The Lifestyle Heart Trial, conducted by Dr. Dean Ornish, was one of the most exciting and empowering research efforts so far on our ability to reverse plaque in the arteries through a very-low-fat diet and other lifestyle changes. It was the first "high-tech" evidence that lifestyle changes alone—no drugs, no surgery—could reverse atherosclerosis in just one year. The twenty-eight patients in the experimental group consumed less than 10 percent of calories from fat, less than 5 milligrams of cholesterol, and less than 2 units of alcohol per day. They were also asked to practice stress management techniques for at least one hour per day, including stretching exercises, breathing techniques, meditation, progressive relaxation, and imagery. Their exercise regimen involved a minimum of three hours per week, for a minimum of thirty minutes per session. The participants also attended two four-hour sessions each week where they shared food, exercise, group discussions, and practiced the stress management techniques. The twenty patients in the control group made only moderate changes in lifestyle that were consistent with the more conventional recommendations.

Dr. Ornish's results were impressive. Overall, 82 percent of the experimental group's patients experienced a regression of atherosclerosis, whereas the control group showed a *progression* of plaque in 53 percent! In other words, the majority of the group following traditional recommendations (AHA-like dietary guidelines and moderate exercise) found a worsening of their arteries within one year. On the other hand, in the experimental group severe blockages were more likely to regress than milder ones. This is good news for those of you who already have heart disease, because the severely blocked arteries are the ones more likely to cause future problems. In fact, it is heartening to know that one of the patients with the most blocked arteries and highest cholesterol enjoyed one of the most impressive reversals of plaque.

So why, given these impressive findings, are most physicians still more likely to prescribe medication than a very-low-fat-diet? There are three main reasons: (1) that is what they have been trained to do (2) most have not worked in an environment where very-low-fat diets were taught and dramatic results realized, and (3) most physicians do not believe their patients will maintain a very-low-fat diet.

During my fourteen years of counseling heart patients, I have not only seen that a diet very low in fat and sodium (especially one low in saturated fat) lowers cholesterol, weight, blood pressure, blood sugars, and other heart disease symptoms, but I've also found that, with the help of the information and recipes provided in this book, patients *are* able to maintain this plan and even discover that it can be quite delicious!

This is not only true of the very motivated patients I encounter at Duke's Rice Diet Program, but elsewhere as well. I served as the consulting nutritionists on a project in East Texas with a population of cardiac patients that traditionally consumed a diet very high in fat and sodium. Within the year and a half that I worked with them, Mother Francis Hospital's cardiac diet became dramatically lower in fat, cholesterol, and sodium, and patient acceptance of the cardiac diet actually improved. So it *is* possible for you to live happily on the Heal Your Heart nutritional plan.

Healing Your Heart Through Exercise

Exercise and nutrition are closely connected, since exercise has long been associated with eating. Our ancestors, some not so distant, had to expend a great deal of effort to get the nourishment they needed. They hunted, gathered, planted, and harvested. Unfortunately, it doesn't take much effort to hunt and gather at the neighborhood supermarket, so we don't always burn off what we eat.

Our bodies thrive when we are active. We are designed to use the food we eat. When we are not active, our bodies suffer the consequences: increased weight, blood pressure, cholesterol, triglyceride, and blood sugar levels.

Obviously, heart disease and its risk factors have causes other than lack of regular exercise, but exercise has a strong influence on the heart's health, and is therefore an important component of the Heal Your Heart Program. Regular aerobic exercise, like walking, provides the greatest benefits for your heart. Here are some of the most obvious health benefits of exercise:

❖ *Losing weight.* Your body will adjust to whatever you demand of it. If you start exercising regularly, your body will adjust by reducing fat weight. You perform the activity better if your are closer to your body's optimal weight; your body knows this and tries to help you make it easy on yourself.

❖ *Cardiac risk factor reduction.* Once you are exercising regularly, you'll likely see a reduction in other risk factors, such as high blood pressure, an increase in your body's ability to use insulin (thus lower blood sugars), an increase in your good cholesterol (HDL) and a reduction in the desire to use tobacco products.

❖ *Sleep, sex, and self-confidence.* People who exercise also report a more regular and satisfying sleep pattern, increased libido, more energy, and more self-confidence. Also, studies suggest that continuing to exercise as you grow older can help maintain your brain's reaction time and information processing abilities.

Healing Your Heart From Within

Although not everyone with heart disease is ready to become a vegetarian, an athlete, and passionately pursue their path to inner healing, my mission for this component of the Heal Your Heart Program is to encourage you to do the most that you can for yourself and to realize that you are well worth the effort to improve your health. It is exciting to see a growing number of people reclaiming not only their responsibility to maintain their physical well being through healthy diet and exercise practices, but also renewing their desire for emotional and spiritual health and wholeness. I believe this inner healing will not only enhance your ability to discover and actualize your true purpose in life, but will also empower you to accomplish your more specific goals, such as weight loss, cholesterol reductions, and commitment to exercise. Attending to your emotional and spiritual needs can give you the focus, sense of purpose, energy, and desire to swim against the self-destructive currents that surround us.

The Rice Diet Program has long advocated inner healing. Its founder, Dr. Kempner, would insist that each able participant take a daily walk and think about themselves. In later years, patients seen using Walkman headsets were told of the importance of being alone with their thoughts and feelings, rather than being constantly distracted. A special sense of spirit and community has always been a key part of the Rice Diet Program. As people share their health challenges and life circumstances with others while walking and dining together, inner healing happens.

I've not only seen this with patients, but have personally experienced the need for inner healing. Over the years I've seen many patients who used food as an emotional comforter rather than as a source of nutrients. But it was not until I was thirty-seven years old, recently hired as the Rice Diet Program's nutrition director, that I realized that I, too, had a habit of "feeding" my emotions. Although I had attended numerous eating disorder conferences in my ten years of professional practice and read most of the "it is not what you are eating, but what is eating you" books, I did not think I ate for emotional reasons. My experience at the Rice Diet Program taught me otherwise. Is it possible that you, too, may be eating unhealthily for deeper reasons than "it tastes good?"

Satisfying Our Emotional Hunger

When I first accepted my position at the Rice Diet Clinic and chose to experience the dietary regime as a patient would, I began with Phase One, eating rice and fruit only. Three weeks into the diet, I found myself halfway through a "health food bakery" brownie before I realized it was not rice and fruit. I saw that I was eating the brownie in an effort to feel good; someone had just hurt my feelings. For the first time in my life, I truly understood the difficulties some people have with food.

Since then I have become much more aware of which feelings turn on that deep desire for chocolate and have become much more adept at admitting and facing those feelings through meditation and journalizing about my dreams, thoughts, and feelings. I honestly have found that I crave chocolate less often. This emotional and spiritual prevention is much healthier for my body and my psyche than covering up those feelings with chocolate. I am now convinced that this kind of inner work is absolutely crucial if overeaters and unhealthy eaters are to make significant and permanent lifestyle changes.

Many experts in the field of addiction believe that most of us are addicts of some form or fashion or are co-dependents who support another's addiction. It is thought that the addict and the co-dependent are trying to fill a perceived "hole in their soul" with something, whether it be food, alcohol, cigarettes, or drugs. They use these things in place of the unconditional love of their Higher Power, which is indeed the only thing that can fill a hole in the soul.

But addictive behaviors do not always involve consumption of substances. One can also be addicted to work, sex, or controlling others. An addiction to such behaviors, while less obvious than an addiction to a substance, can be just as unhealthy and deadly. In the past decade of working with thousands of people, I cannot remember one who had a heart attack before age forty who was *not* struggling with work, sex, or control addictions—usually it was all three.

Stephen was a typical younger heart patient who worked sixty hours per week and seemed always to be "looking for love in all the wrong places." For years he had suffered through a marriage that was filled with power struggles and affairs until it ended in a painful divorce. His heart, indeed, was broken. Until his heart attack nearly took his life, he was unaware that he had been acting out the same drama his parents had lived through. Once he began therapy he realized that he had picked a wife who, like his mother, was a perfectionist who never thought what he had done was quite good enough. She controlled and manipulated him with what, in our society, is considered a very normal, *conditional* kind of love. He also began to see that his addiction to work and sex in response to this absence of unconditional love had been like his father's. His unhealthy and excessive reliance on material success and futile affairs was an attempt to find something or someone who could fill the "hole in his soul."

Unfortunately, this has become a way of life for many of us. Unhealthy family patterns, obsessions, and addictions are often unconsciously passed on to the next generation. We act out these patterns without any awareness that they are unhealthy until a crisis brings us to a deeper understanding of our lives. There is nothing like a heart attack to shatter one's denial and to catapult a person into a new orbit of self-understanding.

I understand addictive behaviors because I have struggled with them myself. My personal crisis, resulting in a new understanding and purpose, came via a subtle form of control addiction. Despite my years of commitment to taking care of my body with a regimen of vegetarianism and tri-athletic training (running, swimming, and cycling), I woke one morning in great pain. I was paralyzed and unable to walk without massive doses of anti-inflammatory medications. My healthy eating and exercise habits had not accounted for the devastating health effects of wanting to control others and resenting them when I failed. Although I knew on the first day of my pain that resentment was the culprit, it took nine months of emotional, spiritual, and physical work before I was totally, physically healed. So I know firsthand that inner healing is extraordinarily important to healing your whole self.

YOU *CAN* FIND HEALING

Al Bennison, a recent Rice Diet participant, is living proof that the three components of the Heal Your Heart Program can work. After two years of participation in a cardiac rehabilitation program in which he exercised for fifty minutes three times a week and was taught the traditional cardiac diet of 30 percent fat and 200 mgs. cholesterol, Al was still taking medication that cost $1,220.90 a month to control his symptoms of diabetes, high cholesterol, high blood pressure, and other problems associated with heart disease. After two by-pass surgeries and eight years of depending on insulin to reduce his elevated blood sugar, his prognosis was not looking any brighter. But, inspired by the successful lifestyle changes accomplished by a friend who had attended Duke University's Rice Diet Program, he began again to believe that he, too, could improve his quality of life.

Al came to the Rice Diet Program to insure that he would have the medical supervision needed to confidently make the changes that would restore his health. He followed the strict parameters of the Heal Your Heart Program. One month later he had lost thirty pounds and had achieved normal blood pressure, cholesterol and blood sugar levels, while at the same time discontinuing eight medications and saving $1,146.81 monthly. He became happier, healthier, and more vibrant. And he is now a true believer in the program, who inspires others to follow his lead toward good health.

Anyone hearing Al's story cannot help but feel hopeful that they too can make such life-transforming changes. The following letter from his daughter may also give you a sense of how noticeably he has changed, and what these lifestyle changes mean to someone who loves him.

> Dad, who recently finished a month-long stay at the Rice Diet, is doing just great. He lost 30 pounds, but even more important, he was able to discontinue taking insulin, his blood pressure medication, and some heart medications. This is nothing short of a miracle! I had been very worried about his health in recent years, but I feel more confident that he'll be around for a long time to come. Please pass along my gratitude to the Rice Diet staff.
>
> Thanks for giving me back my Dad.
>
> —Carol Goodman

❖ Table 1.1   Alan's Medication Savings ❖

MEDICATION	COST PER MONTH		
	BEFORE 2ND BYPASS	AFTER BYPASS	AFTER RICE DIET
Allopurinol	16.19	16.19	0
Beta carotene	0	0	4.55
Coumadin	169.00	169.00	0
Aspirin	0	0	8.55
Fish oil caps	8.99	8.99	0
Glucotrol	59.44	59.44	32.81
Lanoxin	11.24	12.09	15.33
Lopid	348.06	348.06	0
Lopressor	42.16	42.16	0
Novolin	168.41	176.00	0
Prep pad	3.59	3.59	0
Synthroid	16.73	16.73	0
Syringe	35.99	35.99	0
Tambocor	112.33	142.06	0
Trental	178.02	178.02	0
Vitamin B-100	12.58	12.58	0
Vitamin E	0	0	6.55
Total Cost	$1182.73	$1220.90	$74.00

If Al's life-transforming experience and his daughter's thank-you letter do not fill your heart with hope for your own transformation, maybe the data on his medication savings, shown in Table 1.1, will!

The aggressive, three-part Heal Your Heart Program described in this book does work. It is not easy to make the radical lifestyle changes recommended, but I hope you will realize that your life and good health are well worth it. Try to give each part of the program your best effort. They work synergically together; each aspect of the program fuels your desire and willingness to do the other parts.

2

Lowering Your Risk of High Cholesterol

While there are now many factors associated with an increased risk of heart disease, high cholesterol is still considered one of the most serious. There are of course other culprits as well, such as being overweight or having high blood pressure, but if you have high cholesterol, lowering it is probably the single most proven way to reduce your risk of heart disease.

Cholesterol and Your Heart

Cholesterol, a white, fatlike substance produced by the liver, is present in all animals. It is essential for our survival, as it is used in our cell walls, bile acids, and sex hormones. Unfortunately, excessive cholesterol can also cause plaque to build up and clog arteries. This is the underlying cause of most heart disease.

You can have your blood cholesterol level determined by a simple blood test. When you are tested, request that your doctor or lab do a full lipid panel, which means they will determine the total cholesterol, generally just called cholesterol, as well as your HDL or "good cholesterol," your LDL or "bad cholesterol," and your triglycerides. Triglycerides are the main component of fats and are only considered a risk factor of heart disease if they are high in addition to a high cholesterol level.

Although the National Cholesterol Education Program (NCEP) suggests that a blood cholesterol level of 200 milligrams per deciliter (mg./dl.) is a

15

good national goal, a more ambitious one would be 150. There are few guarantees in life, but having a blood cholesterol level of less than 150 is probably the closest you can get to a guarantee that you will not be troubled with heart disease. The Framingham Heart Study has provided us with some of the best epidemiological evidence ever collected on the relationship of diet to heart disease. In 1948, half of the town's 20,000 residents were studied to determine risk factors for heart disease, and these same residents have been examined every two years since. One of the more interesting findings from the Framingham Heart Study is that no one in the history of the study has ever had a heart attack whose blood cholesterol level was less than 150! Their years of data have also shown that for every 1 percent that cholesterol rises, the chance of heart disease deaths increases by 1 percent. (*Journal of American Medical Association,* 1987) In fact, 35 percent of people in the study who have heart attacks have cholesterol levels between 150 and 200. So this zone is far from being exempt. So it would seem that if you want to do everything within your power to prevent or reverse heart disease, you should strive for a cholesterol level of less than 150. If you can get your cholesterol under 150 you don't even have to concern yourself with the further breakdown of "good" and "bad" cholesterol analysis.

"Good" and "Bad" Cholesterol

Your total cholesterol, though, is only part of the story. Your total cholesterol includes various fatty components, including low-density lipoproteins (LDL), known as "bad" cholesterol, and high-density lipoproteins (HDL), known as "good" cholesterol. Cholesterol, like fat, will not mix with water. But, if cholesterol is wrapped in a protein, known as a lipoprotein, it can move through the body with ease. HDLs and LDLs are thought to be the most important lipoproteins. It is easy to remember which is good and which is bad: the *HDLs* you want in *high* amounts, and the *LDLs* you want in *low* amounts, to reduce your risk of heart disease.

Lowering Your Total Cholesterol and LDL

LDLs are referred to as "bad" cholesterol because it is found in high amounts in those with heart disease. LDLs are thought to deposit the cholesterol in artery walls, thus it is a key culprit in the plaque-forming (or atherosclerosis) process. When plaque forms, it narrows the artery. Obviously, the smaller the diameter of the artery, the more limited the blood flow to the heart.

The American Heart Association recommends that your LDL number be less than 130. But, follow a stricter guideline if you want to increase your odds for reversing heart disease. The lower your LDL number the better, but a goal of less than 90 would be appropriate to inspire a regression of atherosclerosis.

The three most important things you can do to help lower your cholesterol and LDL are to reach and maintain your ideal body weight, eat less saturated fat, and eat less dietary cholesterol.

Raising Your HDL

HDLs are the "good" cholesterol that your body makes. It is said to be good because people with high HDL readings have lower than average incidences of heart disease. The most important function of HDLs seems to be that of taking the cholesterol from the arteries and returning it to the liver, presumably to do something constructive such as making cell walls or sex hormones.

The AHA reports that the average HDL reading ranges from 40 to 50 for men and from 50 to 60 for women. The AHA considers an HDL reading of less than 35 to be a risk factor for heart disease. But if the average person has heart disease by retirement age, why accept a "normal" HDL? The higher your HDL reading the better. I recommend you try for an HDL reading of at least 55 for men and 65 for women. Women naturally tend to average a higher HDL, which may be part of the reason why they have less heart disease than men and experience it later in life.

The four main things you can do to increase your HDLs are: exercise regularly, reach and maintain your ideal body weight, stop smoking, and (less important but still beneficial) increase your consumption of olive oil, fish, garlic, and onion.

Since increasing your HDL (good) cholesterol may be almost as important as lowering your total and LDL (bad) cholesterol, and may be even more important for women, it's important to note that eating more olive oil, fish, garlic, and onions may help increase your HDL. Through years of counseling ambitious heart patients who were truly adhering to very-low-fat diets, I have observed that while total cholesterol and LDL levels plummet, HDL levels can sometimes be sacrificed at the same time. I have also seen patients achieve impressive recoveries of their HDLs, without subsequent raises in their total cholesterol or LDLs when they increased their intake of these foods. If your HDL reading is lower than the previously stated optimal goals (55 for men, and 65 for women) after one or two months on this program, try increasing your olive oil intake by two teaspoons per day, and garlic and onion intake as much as you'd like. In another month or so have your total cholesterol, LDL and HDL retested at the same lab. If you have maintained low total cholesterol and LDL levels and raised your HDL, continue to enjoy your olive oil. If your HDL is still lower than you'd like, try increasing your fish intake.

Although alcohol has been shown to raise HDLs in some studies, there is still debate as to whether it is the same HDL fraction that is linked to reducing our risk of heart disease. And despite the final verdict, since excessive alcohol intake can lead to problems far greater than a less-than-optimal HDL, I would not recommend that you start drinking if you do not already. But, for those of you who presently do enjoy moderate amounts (less than ten alcoholic beverages per week), the evidence is fairly strong for the benefits of red wine over other alcoholic beverages. But, teetotalers take heart; one of the beneficial substances in red wine, resveratrol, is also found in grapes and grape juice! Those of you trying to lose weight should abstain until you reach your goal; "empty calories," which are exemplified by alcohol and sugar, are difficult to justify when your caloric intake is being limited for weight loss reasons.

While this book is mainly concerned with how diet, exercise, and spirituality can help heal you, I can't overemphasize the importance of quitting smoking if you are a smoker. Dr. Richard Pollin, director of the National Institute on Drug Abuse, is succinct in his summary that smoking is "the foremost preventable cause of excess death in the United States." Most people associate smoking with various forms of lung disease, but it actually kills more people with heart disease than any other disease. In the United States approximately 30 percent of the deaths from heart disease, or 170,000 deaths each year, are attributable to smoking. But, from a cardiac prevention and rehabilitation perspective, the most sobering statistic is that those who smoke at least a pack of cigarettes a day have two and a half times the risk of a heart attack as nonsmokers. When *you* are ready to quit, remember that the following groups offer programs that can help you do so: American Lung Association, American Cancer Society, American Heart Association, Smokers Anonymous, YMCAs, hospitals, and private companies such as Smokenders or Schick. To help locate some of these supportive organizations please see Appendix B: Sources for More Information.

Lowering Your Triglycerides
Many do not consider elevated triglycerides a risk factor for heart disease unless the cholesterol is also high. Ideally your triglyceride number will be under 150, but if your cholesterol number is below 150, the triglycerides are definitely of less concern.

Triglycerides usually increase if you are overweight, or are consuming too much fat, sugar, or alcohol. Often when people switch from a meat- and fat-based diet to one much higher in carbohydrate, their triglycerides will elevate, then quickly normalize. But, even if the triglycerides remain high, there is rarely a problem for vegetarians, who have a very low incidence of heart disease despite their typically low HDLs and relatively high triglycerides.

So the best bet is to get your cholesterol under 150, your weight ideal, and limit your refined sugar and alcohol intake. Then, if your triglyceride number is still over 250, consult with your doctor.

Lowering Your Cholesterol/HDL Ratio

Although all of these risk factors of heart disease are worth respecting, the ratio of cholesterol to HDL outpredicts all other cholesterol numbers. The AHA and National Cholesterol Education Program consider a ratio of 4 to 1 or less to mean you probably have enough "good" HDL on board to usher out the "bad." But a ratio less than 3 to 1 obviously would afford you more protection since it reflects a higher percentage of HDL to cholesterol. In fact, it has been suggested that a cholesterol/HDL ratio under 3 to 1 offers protection similar to that of having a blood cholesterol level below 150. Again, as with all of the risk factors, the lower it is, the better for reducing your risk of heart disease.

FAT AND YOUR CHOLESTEROL LEVELS

There are three types of fat: saturated, monounsaturated, and polyunsaturated. While all should be kept to a minimum, their effect on your cholesterol levels vary.

In chemical terms, "saturated" refers to the number of hydrogen atoms that are attached to the carbon chain, which is the backbone of a fat molecule. A saturated fatty acid has all carbons (except the end ones) saturated with hydrogens, whereas a monounsaturated fatty acid has one double bond—thus two hydrogen atoms missing—and a polyunsaturated fatty acid has two or more double bonds—thus four or more hydrogen atoms missing.

Saturated Fat—Your Body's Number 1 Enemy

Saturated fat is found in all fats to some degree, but is especially high in animal fats (except seafood), milk products (butterfat), coconut oil, palm kernel oil and palm oil.

Eating high amounts of saturated fat is the most proven cause of high cholesterol and heart disease. In fact, eating too much of this kind of fat actually raises the blood cholesterol level more than does eating cholesterol itself. The cholesterol in food, known as "dietary cholesterol," does not raise most people's blood cholesterol levels, while saturated fats basically raise everyone's.

So avoiding saturated fat is of the utmost importance in lowering your cholesterol, since it raises blood cholesterol more predictably than *any* other substance. Although many variables contribute to high cholesterol (such as obesity and stress), generally speaking, the higher your saturated fat intake, the higher your blood cholesterol and risk of heart disease.

Kromhout and fellow researchers exploring the twenty-five-year follow-up data of the Seven Countries Study (*Preventive Medicine,* 1995) reported that saturated fat intake was by far the major determinant of differences in heart disease death rates. They reported that the intakes of saturated fatty acids, lauric acid, myristic acid, palmitic acid, and stearic acid were the most strongly correlated to higher cholesterols. Verschuren and associates (*Journal of American Medical Association,* 1995), in their examination of the twenty-five-year follow-up data from the Seven Countries Study, emphasized that the higher saturated fat intake and corresponding higher cholesterols of northern Europeans and Americans over Mediterraneans, while important, only explains part of their differences in heart disease deaths. They encouraged further exploration into the beneficial effects of the Mediterranean diets' higher content of monounsaturated rich olive oil and antioxidants.

Monounsaturated Fat

Generally speaking, when monounsaturated fats are used to replace saturated fats, blood cholesterol levels will decrease. But, some monounsaturated fats seem to be more advantageous than others. For instance, although peanut oil is rich in monounsaturated fats, it is one of the most atherogenic, or plaque-promoting, vegetable oils. On the other hand, olive oil and canola oil (rapeseed oil) are the oils richest in monounsaturated fat and are probably the two healthiest oil choices we can make.

Dr. Grundy and associates (*American Journal of Clinical Nutrition,* 1987 and 1988) and Drs. Mensink and Katan (*The Lancet,* 1987) demonstrated that when olive oil is used in place of a saturated fat, cholesterols lower without a corresponding lowering of HDL. Research led by Drs. Renaud, McDonald, Weaver, and associates (*American Journal of Clinical Nutrition,* 1986, 1989, and 1990) also found that canola oil increased HDL, as well as antithrombotic effects (which inspires less blood clots). The ability of both olive oil and canola oil to lower cholesterol without lowering HDL, as polyunsaturated fats tend to do, improves your cholesterol to HDL ratio. This clinical evidence, as well as the low incidence of heart disease and long life expectancies in populations consuming olive and canola oils, are why these oils are used almost exclusively in the recipes in this book.

The widespread interest in olive oil, and in the Mediterranean diet that uses it as the primary oil, stems directly from the results of the Seven Countries Study by Keys and his colleagues (*Circulation,* 1970, and *Journal of Preventive Medicine,* 1984), which demonstrated (after 5 to fifteen years follow-up) that the death rate from heart disease in southern Europe was two- to three-fold lower than in northern Europe or the United States. This study also showed that deaths in Crete, from heart disease and all other causes, was much lower than among the nine other cohorts from southern Europe. The authors found that the population of Crete had the greatest life expectancy in the Western world, despite cholesterols that were similar to those in the rest of the Mediterranean region.

Dr. Walter Willett and others, from the 1993 International Conference on the Diets of the Mediterranean, summarized the following reasons why olive oil may be preferable to other fats:

❖ It is high in oleic acid, which is considered to be antithrombotic (prevents clot formation) compared with saturated fats.

❖ Olive oil is less likely than the polyunsaturated-rich oils to be involved in the oxidation of LDLs, a process which is thought key to the development of atherosclerosis and heart disease.

❖ Substitution of olive oil for carbohydrates in some studies has shown increases in HDLs without increases in LDLs, which would reduce our risk of heart disease.

❖ Mediterranean people have used olive oil as their principle fat for thousands of years with no adverse effects; long-term effects of the more recent widespread use of polyunsaturated oils are unknown.

❖ Olive oil inspires the consumption of large amounts of vegetables and legumes throughout the Mediterranean region by enhancing the taste.

With all these beneficial effects of olive oil, you may be asking yourself if it is really worth insuring a less-than-20-percent-fat diet if olive oil is your only or primary oil used. This is an important question, which is yet to be conclusively answered. But it is worth further investigation considering that in the early 1960s, when the Cretan-Mediterranean diets were inspiring 90 percent lower death rates from heart disease than in America and the highest life expectancy in the world, the Cretan diet was 40 percent fat! In women, breast cancer rates were less than half that of those in the United States, and overall rates of several other chronic diseases were lower than those in northern and central Europe. Although this appears to suggest that 40-percent-fat diets promote health as much as the very-low-fat Asian diets (if the primary oil consumed is olive oil) other lifestyle factors must be considered.

Realize that it is basically impossible to factor for the health advantages of many of the Mediterranean practices: a strong commitment to religious and spiritual discipline and practice; the social support and sense of community that accompanies the sharing of food with family and friends; lengthy meals that provide relaxation from daily stress—complete with postlunch naps; and carefully prepared, delicious meals, made from the freshest ingredients, that really stimulate enjoyment of healthy vegetarian-based meals. So when patients ask whether they could receive the same health benefits of a low-fat diet with a high-fat, olive-oil-only vegetarian diet, I usually say that they probably would *if* they loved their spouse, were fulfilled by their work, and practiced the Mediterranean lifestyle habits just described!

The Mediterranean diet is characterized by a high proportion of calories from cereals, vegetables, and fruits; less meat consumption than in northern Europe and the United States; and a greater reliance on vegetable rather than animal fats. But, unfortunately during the past thirty years, the intake of the Mediterranean countries (belonging to the European Union) has become much more like northern Europe and the United States with significant increases in meat and fat intake and reductions in cereal intake. Fat intake in the Mediterranean area during the past generation has increased from 15 to 30 percent in the early 1960s to 15 to 40 percent in the late 1980s, with an accompanying increase in saturated fats from meat and processed foods.

In 1989, France was the country in southern Europe that demonstrated the lowest deaths from heart disease. In fact people in southern France, especially women, have a death rate from heart disease and all other causes much closer to that for Japan (where women have the greatest life expectancy in the world) than for other Western countries. As you might expect, the diet in southern France contains more bread, vegetables, fruits, vegetable fat, and wine—and less butter—than the diet in northern France.

Polyunsaturated Fats

Most of the attention to the benefits of the Mediterranean diet in preventing heart disease has focused on the effect of olive oil reducing the oxidation of LDL cholesterol, but, the Cretan diet also includes a high intake of the polyunsaturated fat, alpha-linolenic acid (18:3n-3). In Crete, a high intake of alpha-linolenic acid is found in purslane (a dark green leafy vegetable) and nuts, and is thought to offer impressive health advantages. And, in southern France, the alpha-linolenic acid intake is supplied mostly by walnuts and canola oil. The probable role of 18:3n-3 in the prevention of heart disease is also supported by observations of Japanese from Kohama Island. They consume high amounts of alpha-linolenic acid while enjoying the longest life expectancy in the world, as well as the lowest heart disease death rates. Their dietary sources are mainly canola and soybean oils. Thus, the two populations documented to have the greatest life expectancies both have high intakes of 18:3n-3.

The Lyon intervention trial demonstrated that the Cretan Mediterranean diet is far more effective than the general prudent cardiac diet, which emphasizes reductions in saturated fat and cholesterol but does not emphasize the benefits of olive oil and the 18:3n-3-rich oils. Although the specific factors that contribute to the protective effects of the Cretan diet need further investigation, the use of olive oil and 18:3n-3 rich oils were thought by the Lyon investigators (Renaud, et. al.; *American Journal of Clinical Nutrition,* 1995) to be of utmost importance. Olive oil because of its effects on reducing the oxidation of LDL cholesterol, and the n-3 fatty acids for their major benefits in reducing blood clots and arrhythmias (irregular heart beats). Interestingly enough, the study participants enjoyed protective effects within a few months, without significant differences in their cholesterols and associated factors (lipids profiles). Those consuming the Cretan diet had 70 to 80 percent reductions in heart attacks, deaths from heart attacks, angina, heart failure, stroke and thromboembolisms (throwing clots) compared to the groups consuming the traditional cardiac diets.

The positive effect of linolenic acid is primarily attributed to its conversion to an omega-3 fatty acid, which is a type of polyunsaturated fat thought to be beneficial for preventing heart disease and its risk factors. Some studies show that omega-3 fatty acids lower cholesterol, but generally they seem to produce more impressive reductions in blood pressure and triglycerides. Omega-3 fatty acids also help prevent blood clots and coronary artery spasms, which are two underlying causes of heart attacks. High amounts of omega-3 fatty acids are found in the oilier fish, such as mackerel, salmon, trout, bluefish, and tuna. Even though some of these fish may be high in fat, they are still good choices, as this kind of fat can reduce your risk of heart disease rather than promote it, as other animal fats do. Burr and his associates (*The Lancet,* 1989) found that men after heart attacks reduced their death rates by 29 percent by consuming at least two weekly portions (200 to 400 grams) of fatty fish. Other groups consuming small increases in fiber and decreases in fat did not produce the significant findings created by these relatively modest increases in fatty fish intake. Although the research on the benefits of the omega-3 fatty acids from fish is growing, no one really knows whether the inclusion of seafood is better or worse for your heart than a strict vegetarian diet. But, it is safe to say that fish is indisputably the healthiest meat choice. The only animal fat than can really be justified for a heart patient is that found in fish.

Although linolenic and omega-3 fatty acids are powerful deterrants for heart disease, not all polyunsaturated fats are equal. In general, when polyunsaturated fats are used in place of saturated fats, blood cholesterol decreases. But this does not mean that large amounts are good for you, because all fats contain some saturated fatty acids, and some polyunsaturated fats have been shown to lower HDL levels as well as LDL levels. In fact, large amounts of polyunsaturated fats are thought to increase the risk of cancer, heart disease, and many problems with immune system functions. Walnuts, almonds, and sesame seeds are a few examples of other polyunsaturated fats that you can enjoy in small amounts.

Don't Be Fooled by Hydrogenated Fats

Hydrogenated fats are oils that have had hydrogen added to them to create a smoother, creamier product with a longer shelf life. Unfortunately, it also creates a more saturated fat, known as "trans fatty acids," or "trans fats," which can also raise your cholesterol and LDL, and lower your HDL. The most commonly eaten hydrogenated fats include shortening, margarine, and the added fat in most processed grain products (such as cookies, crackers, cereals, and breads) and condiments (such as spreads, dressings, and sauces). Because their effects on the human body are not yet fully understood, I recommend that you avoid hydrogenated fats as much as possible.

It is essential to read beyond the "No cholesterol, 100% vegetable oil" claim emblazoned on food packages, because not only do saturated fats raise cholesterol more than dietary cholesterol itself, but the "trans fats" created by the hydrogenation process are not calculated into the saturated fat analysis. Olive, canola, sesame, and almond oils are the preferred oils, rather than manufactured "plasticized fats," such as "shortening" or any type of "partially hydrogenated vegetable oil." Trans fatty acids now contribute between 5 and 6 percent of the total dietary fat intake in the United States. Ironically, many people turned to hydrogenated products such as margarine to reduce their saturated fat and cholesterol intake from the natural alternative butter. But there are now growing questions on the effectiveness of such products.

Two other studies have confirmed Mensink, and Katan, findings (*New England Journal of Medicine,* 1990) which demonstrated that trans fatty acids increase LDL cholesterol to a similar degree as do saturated fats. Trans fatty acids also decreased HDL cholesterol, thus the increase in the ratio of total cholesterol to HDL from trans fatty acids was approximately double that for saturated fats. Unlike other fats, trans fatty acids were found to increase lipoprotein (a), another risk factor for heart disease, in two of three studies.

Several epidemiological studies have observed positive associations between intake of trans fatty acids and heart disease. Kromhout and associates recently examined dietary fat intake and twenty-five-year heart disease death rate from the Seven Countries Study (*Preventive Medicine,* 1995). In this well-respected long-term study of 12,763 men, they found a strong positive association between heart disease death rate and not only saturated fat and cholesterol, but trans fatty acid intake as well. And, Thomas and associates (*Journal of Epidemiological Community Health,* 1983) found higher levels of trans fatty acids in the fat tissue of those dying of heart attacks than in the tissue of those dying from other causes. In a prospective study of 85,095 women (without diagnosed heart disease, stroke, diabetes, or high cholesterol), Dr. Willett and associates (*The Lancet,* 1993) found their intake of trans fats was directly related to their risk of heart disease. Although the percentage of United States heart disease deaths attributable to intake of trans fatty acids is still unclear, Dr. Willett and associates suggest that "more than 30,000 deaths per year may be due to consumption of partially hydrogenated vegetable fat."

Although we do not have fully conclusive evidence that trans fatty acids cause heart disease, the clinical and epidemiological evidence is substantial. It is obvious that synthetic and harmful substances added to our food supply should be kept to a minimum. Although it would seem logical that proving the safety and health advantages of new products should be the responsibility of the manufacturer, it is not. So until the FDA changes its agenda and requires companies to prove nutritional benefits of new products, it is our responsibility to be proactive, label-reading health advocates and avoid processed food ingredients, especially partially hydrogenated fats containing trans fatty acids.

In my experience, the best way to control your cholesterol levels is a three-prong approach, including good nutrition, exercise, and an awareness of the connection between the health of your mind and the health of your body. This last part is important in that being strongly "centered" can help you maintain the healthy diet and exercise regimens needed to heal yourself.

You may notice that I have not mentioned cholesterol-lowering medications as part of your solution. While I do believe that you can lower your cholesterol dramatically through lifestyle changes alone, I am *not* suggesting that you alter your current medication doses without consulting your physician. Instead, I hope to inspire you to make changes in your life that will prove to yourself *and* to your physician that you do not need medication, or at least that you do not need as much, to achieve an acceptable cholesterol level.

NUTRITION AND YOUR CHOLESTEROL

The Heal Your Heart nutrition plan will be outlined in detail in Part Two of this book, but it is important to know that for cholesterol-lowering purposes, your best bet is to eat a vegetarian diet that is very low in fat (especially saturated fat), and high in soluble fiber and in certain substances called antioxidants.

Why a Vegetarian Diet?

Since saturated fat is the worst thing possible for your cholesterol levels, your first step is to limit it as much as possible from your diet. The best way to do this is to eat a vegetarian diet. That means avoiding *all* animal products, including dairy products, until your cholesterol levels are less than 150. Then, if you want to, you can start enjoying fish and nonfat dairy products as long as your cholesterol levels remain at this ideal.

Although we do not know whether a strict vegetarian diet is superior to one with added fish and nonfat dairy, we do know that a vegetarian diet lowers cholesterol more than does a diet that includes poultry (even skinned chicken breast). Since chicken is relatively low in saturated fat, most people think it is good for preventing heart disease, but it is not for those seeking the most dramatic results.

Numerous studies have now shown that a vegetarian diet can help reduce your cholesterol, as well as your chances of developing osteoporosis, certain cancers, heart disease, and its risk factors: obesity, hypertension and diabetes. Despite this, some people are still concerned that a vegetarian diet is not "complete" enough to be healthy. Specific concerns are that vegetarians do not get enough protein, calcium, iron, or other nutrients. These concerns need not worry you.

How Much Protein?

The Recommended Dietary Allowances (RDA) for protein for the average adult is 63 grams per day for men and 50 grams per day for women, but this is far more than most people actually need. Dr. Walter Kempner and others have found that patients stayed in positive nitrogen balance (the most widely accepted test for protein adequacy) on only 20 to 25 grams of protein. But, either way you look at it, it is hard *not* to get enough protein. Protein is found in plentiful amounts in grains, legumes (beans and peas), vegetables, nuts, and seeds; whereas, fruits, fats, and alcohol contain negligible amounts. You would have to eat primarily from the latter group to get a protein deficiency. This would be a strange diet and would also provide inadequate amounts of many other nutrients. By far, the largest number of people in the world suffering from protein deficiencies do so because of a lack of calories or availability of food, not because they don't eat meat.

Although Frances Moore Lappe's *Diet for A Small Planet* (Ballantine Books, 1971) was one of the best books ever written on vegetarianism, we now know that the combinations of foods recommended in the earlier editions of the book are not necessary. (The strategy outlined how certain high-protein vegetable food groups had to be eaten at the same meal with other food groups to provide all the essential amino acids your body needs.)

While it is true that certain food groups are low or "limiting" in specific amino acids, this does not create a problem as long as you eat a varied diet. For example, grains are low in the amino acids lysine and threonine, but beans and peas are high in these. While the legumes are low in methionine and tryptophan, these amino acids are plentiful in grains. No problem: there is an amino acid pool in your body that allows the essential amino acids from today's lunch of bean soup to complement the essential amino acids from tonight's stir-fried vegetables and rice. As an American Dietetic Association position paper on vegetarian diets states, "A mixture of plant proteins throughout the day will provide enough essential amino acids."

In fact, too much protein is more likely our problem. Evidence to support this is coming out of China (where many people eat vegetarian diets), from the most comprehensive study ever undertaken on diet and health. This study, which was a joint effort involving Cornell University, the Chinese Academies of Preventive Medicine and Medical Sciences, and Oxford University in England, gathered information from more than 6,500 adults living in 65 representative counties of China. Dr. Colin Campbell, the study's principal American investigator, states that the data coming out of the study will challenge many of our beliefs about protein, cholesterol, and calcium. He has reported that protein intake correlated with an increased risk of heart disease even more than did fat intake. He stated, "We now know from human and animal studies that animal protein increases serum cholesterol even apart from the known effects of saturated fat." (*American Health,* September 1989) In short, more of us need to be concerned about animal protein excesses than deficiencies.

The Advantages of Soy Protein over Animal Protein

The cholesterol-lowering effect of soy protein as compared to animal protein was recognized in animals more than eighty years ago. But more recently, Dr. James Anderson and associates (*New England Journal of Medicine,* 1995) conducted a meta-analysis of thirty-eight controlled clinical trials on the effect of soy protein on cholesterol in humans. They found that with an average daily intake of 47 grams of soy protein (about half the total protein intake), subjects experienced a 9 percent reduction in cholesterol, 13 percent reduction in LDL, and 11 percent reduction in triglyceride more than did those on the control diets. The higher the subjects' cholesterols the more dramatic was the corresponding drop in cholesterol from the soy protein. Although 47 grams of soy protein would be easy for most Asian populations, most Westerners would find the two to four servings of soy products a challenge (one serving = 4 ounces of tofu or 3 ounces of meat analog). The studies have proven that the soy protein itself is a powerful factor in the cholesterol-lowering response, but they also emphasize isoflavones, which are structurally similar to estrogen. Isoflavones have been shown to partially stimulate estrogen receptors, which is advantageous since elevated estrogen concentrations are thought to be largely responsible for the lower risk of heart disease in premenopausal women. Since soybean protein is preferable to animal protein with respect to cholesterol response, and since soybeans are one of the few sources of isoflavones found in Western diets, be sure to try recipes and products containing soy.

Avoiding High Homocysteine: Other Benefits of Beans over Meat
The effect of animal protein on raising homocysteine levels may be causing us more problems than its elevating effect on cholesterol and blood pressure. Epidemiologic studies have shown that elevated plasma homocysteine is an independent risk factor for heart disease. This means the relationship between high homocysteine levels and high rates of heart disease remains after adjusting for other risk factors, including age, cigarette smoking, hypertension, cholesterol, sedentary lifestyle, body mass index, and diabetes.

Homocysteine is formed in our bodies when animal protein is broken down. So the more meat you eat the more likely you are to have high levels of homocysteine in your blood. On the other hand, eating a diet rich in folic acid and vitamins B_6 and B_{12} appears to lower homocysteine. Foods rich in these vitamins include beans and peas, whole grains, vegetables (especially spinach, collard greens, broccoli, sweet potatoes, and cauliflower), yeast, eggs, dairy, and fish. For years the lower risk of heart disease in vegetarians was attributed to the lack of animal fat and cholesterol in their diets, but an alternate and more accurate explanation might be their low intakes of animal protein and high intakes of folic acid and vitamin B_6, which lead to lower levels of homocysteine.

Effective metabolism of homocysteine requires an adequate supply of vitamin B_6, vitamin B_{12}, and folic acid. Considerable vitamin B_6 and folic acid are lost during food processing. Folic acid is sensitive to heat, with approximately 98 percent of it potentially destroyed during cooking. Folic acid absorption can also be impaired as a result of bile acid sequestrants or niacin therapy, or as a secondary condition in impaired kidney function. Vitamin B_6 losses of 10 to 50 percent have been reported during processing and storage of foods. Vitamin B_{12} deficiencies may occur in people consuming largely or exclusively vegetarian diets, or can be produced by certain drug treatments or clinical conditions. Dr. Lindenbaum and his associates (*American Journal of Clinical Nutrition,* 1994) found vitamin B_{12} deficiency was so common in the Framingham population that they recommended its supplementation along with folic acid and vitamin B_6, especially among the elderly. Dr. Ubbink and his associates (*American Journal of Clinical Nutrition,* 1993) found with a daily vitamin supplement (10 mg. vitamin B_6, 1 mg. folic acid, and .4 mg. vitamin B_{12}), high plasma homocysteine levels normalized within six weeks. So, they proposed such supplementation to be both an efficient and cost-effective way to reduce homocysteine levels, and thus heart disease.

Although vitamin B_6, vitamin B_{12}, and folic acid are all needed to convert homocysteine into other things, thus maintain healthy low levels, more research is needed on what amounts of these vitamins are optimal. Some interesting research in South Africa, led by Dr. J.B. Ubbink (*Journal of Nutrition,* 1994) tested each of the three vitamins on a group of 100 men with high homocysteine and found folic acid to have the most powerful influence. Folic acid and vitamin B_{12} supplementation reduced plasma homocysteine concentrations by 42 percent and 15 percent, respectively, while vitamin B_6 did not inspire a change at all.

Since it has been shown that the majority of people with high homocysteine levels have insufficient levels of folic acid and vitamins B_{12} or B_6, and that innocuous amounts of these vitamins supplemented will lower moderately elevated homocysteine levels to the normal range, your need to supplement should be considered. See details on supplementation recommendations in Chapter 7.

Getting Enough Calcium

When told to temporarily eliminate dairy products from their diets, many patients fear they will develop osteoporosis if they don't have at least two cups of milk a day. The recommended amount of calcium needed to fend off osteoporosis varies widely, depending upon whom you ask. The U.S. RDA for adults is 800 milligrams; the international recommendation is half that amount. This major difference of opinion can largely be explained by the fact that the more protein and sodium you eat, the more calcium your body loses through your urine. Thus, the average American who consumes excessive amounts of animal products two or three times a day needs far more calcium than the typical vegetarian. Studies have shown that one's average calcium loss on a diet of 142 grams of protein would be three times the average loss on a 95-gram protein diet. Since protein and sodium cause us to lose calcium, it doesn't seem efficient to try to prevent osteoporosis by recommending milk, which is high in protein and sodium. In fact, Dr. D.M. Hegsted has reported in the *Journal of Nutrition* (1986) that fractures of the hip (a common site of osteoporosis) actually occur more frequently in populations that consume higher levels of calcium that were derived mainly from dairy products! And do not expect calcium supplements to compensate for high animal-protein diets. Another study, conducted by Dr.

❖ TABLE 2.1   OSTEOPOROSIS AND SELECTED NUTRIENTS ❖

LOCATION	HIP FRACTURES RATE/100,000	DAIRY INTAKE GRAMS/DAY/PERSON	PROTEIN INTAKE GRAMS/DAY/PERSON	
			TOTAL	ANIMAL
United States	98	462	106	72
Sweden	70	502	89	59
Israel	59	315	105	57
Finland	44	711	93	61
United Kingdom	43	455	90	54
Hong Kong	32	95	82	50
Singapore	20	113	82	39
South Africa/Black townships	6	10	55	11

Lindsay H. Allen and associates (*The American Journal of Clinical Nutrition,* 1979), showed that six men on a high-protein diet for four months remained in negative calcium balance even though they were ingesting high levels of calcium supplements.

Table 2.1 shows that the populations with the highest rates of hip fractures are also the ones that have higher intakes of protein. Furthermore, a high consumption of dairy products seems to offer little protection for the bones, since the countries with the highest dairy intakes—the United States, Sweden, Israel, Finland, and the United Kingdom—also have the highest rates of osteoporosis-related hip fractures. On the other hand, low intakes of dairy products do not appear to harm the bones, as the countries with the lowest dairy intakes—Hong Kong, Singapore, and rural South Africa—have the lowest rates of osteoporosis. (All numbers have been rounded off to whole numbers, and figures for hip fractures from some countries may be from the population of a large city within that country.)

Whether protein or sodium excesses are more to blame for the high incidence of osteoporosis in the United States is debatable, but the evidence against both is growing. Although scientists have known for decades that increasing our sodium intake increases the calcium lost in the urine, they have now demonstrated that this sodium-induced loss of calcium in the urine does translate into loss of bone density. Researchers at the University of

---

Table 2.1 Osteoporosis and Selected Nutrients Source: Printed with permission from John McDougall, M.D. for exerpt from McDougall's Medicine: A Challenging Second Opinion, *(Clinton, NJ: New Win Publishing, Inc.)*

Western Australia (*American Journal of Clinical Nutrition,* 1995) followed more than 100 postmenopausal women for two years and found that those who consumed the most sodium lost the most bone in their hips and ankles. Specifically, women who averaged about 3,000 milligrams of sodium a day needed to consume about 1,700 milligrams of calcium to prevent any bone loss. On the other hand, women who consumed only 2,300 milligrams of sodium needed only 1,200 milligrams of calcium to maintain their bones. Unfortunately, the effect of significantly lower sodium intakes was not reported. But, Bess Dawson-Hughes, M.D., chief of the Calcium and Bone Metabolism Laboratory at Tufts University, stated, "All the studies are coming to the same conclusion. They're all showing a high impact on calcium retention from sodium restriction." (*Tufts University Diet and Nutrition Letter,* 1996)

Numerous other dietary factors may alter our calcium balance, thus increasing our risk of osteoporosis. High dietary phosphate, found in meat and sodas, causes increased fecal losses of calcium. And high intakes of caffeine-containing beverages cause increased urinary calcium losses. The Framingham data (*American Journal of Epidemiology,* 1990) showed that caffeine use increased the risk of osteoporosis; consumption of three or more cups of coffee a day increased the risk of hip fractures by 53 percent. In a prospective study on middle-aged women (*American Journal of Clinical Nutrition,* 1991), high caffeine users had three times the hip fractures of non-caffeine users, and those consuming 1 ounce of alcohol a day had more than double the risk of nondrinkers for hip fractures.

Fortunately, research has also shown that vegetarians absorb and retain more calcium from foods than do nonvegetarians. So the answer seems to be to get your calcium from nonmeat, nondairy sources, and minimize your other modifiable risk factors: exercise regularly, don't smoke, and don't consume many sodas (high in phosphates), caffeinated and alcoholic beverages, animal products (because of high protein and phosphates), and sodium-rich foods. See Table 7.5 for a list of healthy calcium-rich foods.

Is Iron Deficiency a Problem?

Although iron deficiency is reportedly the most common nutritional deficiency in the United States, a vegetarian diet does not have to be the cause. Chapter 7 will tell you how to enhance your iron intake and absorption to prevent or alleviate this problem.

While it is a good idea to enhance your absorption of available iron (rather than taking iron supplements, which often lead to constipation), you do not really have to worry about having "iron-poor blood." In fact, there is growing evidence that a high iron level could increase your risk of heart attacks. A 1992 study of Finnish men showed a positive association between the risk of heart attacks and high amounts of iron in the blood. Thus, typical vegetarian iron levels, which are a little on the low side, are likely one more benefit of a vegetarian diet and its ability to prevent and reverse heart disease.

Getting Other Nutrients

Some fear that vegetarians don't get enough vitamin D and vitamin B_{12} and that high-fiber vegetarian diets can make their bodies less efficient at using minerals such as zinc, copper, magnesium, manganese, and selenium. A little information can alleviate a lot of needless fear here. Of all the foods we eat, vitamin D is only found naturally in egg yolks and fish oil, so it is added to milk to increase its nutritional value. But because our bodies are able to synthesize vitamin D through exposure to sunshine, all you need to do is get ten to fifteen minutes of sunshine two to three times per week. If you cannot insure this minimal amount of outdoor time and do not want to eat egg yolks, fish oil, or milk, a supplement is advisable. Vitamin B_{12} is also found largely from animal sources, with the exception of unpredictable amounts of tempeh, sea vegetables, and algae. Fortified foods such as specific brands of nutritional yeasts, some breakfast cereals, soy milks, and meat analogs, or a vitamin B_{12} supplement (which is generally included in multivitamin/mineral pills) is recommended if you choose a strict vegetarian diet.

As for getting enough of the minerals zinc, copper, magnesium, manganese, and selenium, research has shown that vegetarian diets rarely cause deficiencies of these nutrients. In fact, many studies have shown vegetarians actually have higher amounts of these in their bodies than do meat eaters. Probably the most noteworthy of this group is zinc, which is important for the immune system to perform optimally. It is found in high levels in seafood; whole grains and legumes also contain substantial amounts.

How Fiber Can Help Lower Your Cholesterol

Fiber helps combat heart disease in many ways, but one of the most important is by reducing cholesterol. Other conditions lessened or prevented by a high-fiber diet are hiatal hernia, hemorrhoids, diverticular disease, irritable bowel syndrome, constipation, and gallbladder disease.

There are two different types of fiber, insoluble and soluble, and each is helpful to us in its own way. Insoluble fiber is composed of cellulose, lignin, and hemicellulose. Soluble fiber is composed of gum and pectin. Although these categorizations refer to their solubility in water, neither is literally soluble as fiber is defined as the nondigestible part of food. All grains, beans, fruits, and vegetables contain varying degrees of both types of fiber, depending upon the variety of the plant, where it is grown, and what processing (such as milling or cooking) it has experienced.

The Benefits of Insoluble Fiber

In general, most grains (especially the outer bran part, such as wheat bran) and vegetables are high in insoluble fiber. While it does not seem to directly affect your heart's health, insoluble fiber is beneficial for other reasons.

Insoluble fiber is generally thought to speed food through the intestines, but more accurately, it normalizes transit time. It has been found to have a laxative effect in people who are constipated, while it may also alleviate diarrhea and normalize laxation. If wheat bran is increased significantly, fluids should also be increased to prevent constipation. Insoluble fiber also helps reduce the risk of colon cancer.

Soluble Fiber and Your Heart's Health

Soluble fiber is found in high amounts in oats, beans, barley, and fruit. It is soluble fiber that is known to help reduce the most significant risk factors of heart disease, most notably by lowering cholesterol, especially LDL. It also helps lower triglycerides, blood pressure, and weight, as well as reduce insulin requirements and increase insulin sensitivity, thus improving diabetes control. Specifically, eating soluble fiber from oats, oat bran, psyllium, pectin, beans and peas, barley, rice bran (that has not been defatted), and selected gums (guar, acacia, locust bean, and karaya) has been shown to reduce serum cholesterol from 6 to 38 percent. The cholesterol-lowering effects of oat, bean, and barley products have provided the most impressive results so far in human studies. Rice bran has been much less studied, but it has exhibited a cholesterol-lowering effect in rats, some beneficial effects in men with mildly elevated cholesterol, and triglyceride reductions in healthy adults.

Dr. James Anderson, of the University of Kentucky in Lexington, is one of the leading researchers on the cholesterol-lowering benefits of oat bran. During his research he has seen significant reductions in cholesterol (19 percent reduction), and in LDL cholesterol (23 percent reduction), when people ate 50 grams of oat bran daily. Fifty grams is approximately a half cup of raw oat bran or three oat bran muffins. Interestingly, after his research subjects went home and continued to eat oat bran daily, their cholesterol levels fell even further—up to 24 percent. (Do *not* take this as advice to eat oat bran and then alter your current medication dose without consulting your physician. Consult your doctor before making *any* medication changes.)

Of course oat bran alone won't make you healthy. Most studies show that oat bran lowers cholesterol more if you are eating it as part of a low-fat diet. One study found no reductions in cholesterol when 30, 60, or 90 grams of oat bran were added to diets that were high in saturated fat. So beware of the common American tendency to seek a magic bullet. Oat bran and other soluble fibers will not dramatically lower your cholesterol unless you also lower the fat in your diet.

While oat bran has received much attention for its cholesterol-lowering abilities, there are other sources of soluble fiber that can also have a positive effect. So don't feel limited to oats. Beans, barley, most fruits, and some vegetables will give you fiber and allow some variety in your diet. In fact, beans and barley seem to reduce cholesterol almost as much as oat bran.

The Antioxidant Potential

Cutting down on your saturated fat and increasing your soluble fiber are likely the most important dietary changes you can make to prevent and reverse heart disease. But you should also know about the benefits of antioxidants, which are currently being extensively studied by researchers. While antioxidants have been associated with many health benefits including reductions in free radical damage (which seems to contribute to cancerous tumor growths), undesirable skin changes (such as wrinkling), cataracts, arthritis, and neuromuscular disorders, our major concern here is their effects on risk factors for heart disease.

"Antioxidant" is a name given to certain substances such as vitamins C, E, and beta-carotene (a precursor of vitamin A), because these prevent the oxidation of LDL (a major factor in the atherosclerosis process). What exactly do they do? It seems that antioxidants reduce our risk of heart disease by preventing the plaque formation process, but some studies have shown these substances may also preserve the function of our blood vessel linings, lower both LDL cholesterol levels and blood pressures, and reduce clotting tendencies.

Many studies show an impressive correlation between antioxidants and a reduction in heart disease. Dr. H. Esterbauer and others have found the positive effect of the antioxidants to be profound. In 1989, they reported that the major antioxidant in LDL is vitamin E and that oxidation of LDL only occurs if it is depleted of its vitamin E and beta-carotene.

All of the large epidemiological studies on antioxidants support this. They all found that high levels of vitamin E intake or supplementation were associated with a significant reduction in heart disease. One of these, the U.S. Nurses' Health Study, followed 87,245 female nurses, ages thirty-nine to fifty-nine, for an average of eight years. In this large study, the risk of heart disease among women who took vitamin E supplements was observed to be about 40 percent lower than in women who did not take these supplements. The findings showed that two years of vitamin E supplementation was necessary before significant reductions in risk were seen. Reduced risk was only seen with vitamin E supplementation of at least 100 IU (International Units) per day, and not with the amounts found in dietary intakes or multivitamin use, which provided only about 30 IU of vitamin E per day.

In 1991, Dr. R.A. Riemersma and his associates published (*The Lancet,* 1991) their study involving 6,000 men, ages thirty-five to fifty-four, of whom 110 had angina pectoris (the chest, back, or arm pain that occurs as a result of inadequate blood flow to the heart). They found that the men with angina had lower average blood levels of vitamins E, C, and beta-carotene than did a comparison group of 394 men without angina. In fact, the risk of having angina was more than double in men with the lowest antioxidant levels as compared with men who had the highest levels.

The Physicians' Health Study trial found that men with angina who were assigned to take beta-carotene had fewer heart attacks than did those taking the placebo. They also found that although beta-carotene intake was not associated with a lower risk of heart disease among those who had never smoked, it was found to be beneficial to current and former smokers. Although no one really knows for certain, it is likely that the increased oxidative stress brought on by smoking may increase the susceptibility of fats to become oxidized, thus increasing a smoker's need for antioxidants.

Dr. D.A. Street and his associates reported further evidence of beneficial effects of antioxidants in the *American Journal of Epidemiology* in 1991. The researchers collected blood from several thousand people and froze it for several years. After 125 of the participants had suffered heart attacks, the investigators retrieved the blood samples, measured the beta-carotene levels, and compared them with blood samples of an equal number of participants who had not had heart attacks. They found that those with the lowest beta-carotene levels had about twice the risk of having a heart attack as did those with the highest levels.

Are Antioxidants Too Good to Be True?

Those of us who have been following the studies on the benefits of antioxidants took two steps back on April 14, 1994. That day *The New England Journal of Medicine* published a well-designed study from Finland. It showed that not only did beta-carotene and vitamin E supplements fail to reduce the risk of lung cancer and heart disease in smokers, but they might have actually caused harm. In the study, the researchers randomly divided 29,000 Finnish male smokers into groups that got one of the following daily: a placebo, beta-carotene (33,333 IU), vitamin E (50 IU), or beta-carotene and vitamin E. After five to eight years, the beta-carotene users had an 18 percent higher incidence of lung cancer! There was even a suggestion that the beta-carotene supplements might have raised the risk of heart disease. Although this Finnish trial was inconclusive about vitamin E's previously reported ability to reduce the risk of heart disease, they only gave 50 milligrams a day, compared to earlier studies, which suggested that at least 100 milligrams a day may be needed to lower the risk. The vitamin E appeared to reduce the risk of prostate cancer, but increase the risk of hemorrhagic stroke.

Although one study can never be the final word on an issue, the Finnish study must be taken seriously. Most of the earlier studies observed lower cancer and heart disease rates among people who ate plenty of fruits and vegetables that were rich in beta-carotene rather than taking supplements. It may be that beta-carotene-rich fruits and vegetables exert many protective effects because of substances in them other than the beta-carotene. If this is true, beta-carotene supplements would not necessarily provide the desired benefits.

In addition to our not really knowing what all the potential beneficial aspects of beta-carotene-rich fruits and vegetables are, could an increase in the beta-carotene itself really have caused these problems? Yes. First of all, these studies have all examined beta-carotene despite the fact that beta-carotene only accounts for approximately 25 percent of the carotenoids in our blood. And as the National Cancer Institute's Regina Ziegler speculated in the June 1994 *Nutrition Action,* "It's conceivable that large amounts of a single form could interfere with the absorption, transport, or utilization of other forms of beta-carotene, other carotenoids, or other important compounds in fruits and vegetables." So we don't yet have the complete picture on how the major antioxidants can help us.

Phenolic Compounds and Alcohol
Phenolic compounds are some of the other substances found in fruits and vegetables that offer antioxidant benefits. They are found in red wine and many other vegetarian products, and have been shown to inhibit the oxidation of LDL, which is crucial for the plaque process to procede. They have also been shown to reduce thrombotic, or clot forming, tendencies. Dr. Bianca Fuhrman (*American Journal of Clinical Nutrition,* 1995) and associates found that moderate red wine consumption for two weeks resulted in a significant reduction in fat oxidation in the blood, whereas white wine consumption inspired a significant increase in the blood's propensity to undergo fat oxidation. The antioxidant response could not be explained by the vitamin E and beta-carotene levels, but did relate to the polyphenol concentration in the blood and LDL. They concluded that some phenolic substances (such as resveratrol) that exist in red wine, but not white wine, are absorbed, bind to LDL, and may be responsible for the antioxidant properties of red wine.

Phenolic compounds also impart an astringent or "puckery" mouthfeel to wine, tea, coffee, and cocoa. Phenolic compounds, which include both flavonoids and nonflavonoids, flavonols, anthocyanins, and soluble tannins, also contribute astringency and color to fruits and vegetables. So for those seeking to avoid or limit their wine consumption, plenty of naturally occurring polyphenols with impressive antioxidant power (such as quercetin) can be enjoyed in asparagus, onions, grapes, apples, citrus rind, and tea.

No one really yet knows what part antioxidants, and polyphenols in particular, play in the mystery of why the Mediterranean people enjoy such low rates of heart disease despite fat intakes comparable to populations with high rates of heart disease. Obviously their higher intake of olive oil is a major factor, but antioxidants are also being given more and more credit. The Mediterranean populations consume more antioxidants than those of many other countries through their large intake of fresh fruits and vegetables. They also traditionally consume more wine. Overwhelming epidemiologic data show that moderate alcohol consumption reduces the risk of heart attacks, with two drinks a day decreasing risk by 30 to 40 percent. Although many believe that this effect is largely due to antioxidants in red wine, similar protective effects for equivalent amounts of alcohol have been seen for all kinds of alcoholic beverages.

On the other hand, similar amounts of alcohol have been positively associated with breast cancer incidence in almost thirty studies. The overall effect of alcohol appears beneficial up to two drinks a day unless you are a woman with a family or personal history of breast cancer. Considering the rising incidence of breast cancer, and the small but apparent increased risk of breast cancer with just one alcoholic drink per day, alcohol would not be the best source of antioxidants for women. Obviously this advice holds true for other circumstances and populations needing to avoid or limit alcohol intake, such as drivers, pregnant women, and those with a family or personal history of alcoholism. An intake of more than two drinks per day in men is associated with a greater risk of death from cancer, trauma, cirrhosis and other diseases.

Supplementing with Antioxidants

As the researchers debate the details on how antioxidants protect us, what should you do? It is difficult at this point to make a blanket recommendation. Of course, it would be safe for you to take supplements up to the U.S. RDA for these nutrients: 60 mg. of vitamin C, 30 IU of vitamin E, and 5,000 IU of beta-carotene (which would meet the U.S. RDA for vitamin A).

Dr. Walter Willett, a world-renowned nutrition epidemiologist in the Department of Nutrition at Harvard agreed with me that the evidence is strongest for the beneficial effects of vitamin E supplementation (200 IU), then vitamin C (500 mg.), with beta-carotene supplementation being the most questionable. It seems that until further evidence clears the cloud of concern over beta-carotene, it would be best to supplement with no more than a standard multivitamin/mineral and eat at least five servings of fresh fruits and vegetables a day, concentrating on the darker orange and green ones. The evidence is very strong that a higher dietary intake of these nutrients has a powerfully protective effect against heart disease.

The preferred source of all antioxidants—as well as all vitamins—is from the whole foods themselves, which also provide fiber and many known and yet-to-be-discovered beneficial substances. The antioxidant research lends further support to our belief that the ultimate nutritional solution to preventing or reversing heart disease lies in eating a well-balanced intake of grains, beans, fruits, and vegetables.

Exercise and Your Cholesterol

Although nutrition is probably the most important element in lowering your cholesterol and reducing your risk of heart disease, the benefits of exercise should not be overlooked. Regular exercise has been shown to help patients improve numerous heart disease risk factors, including obesity, hypertension, and HDLs. It also increases our level of physical activity and sense of well being. Research from twenty-two studies of cardiac rehabilitation programs have shown that exercise can decrease deaths after a heart attack by about 20 percent. Of course, heart patients should consult with their cardiologist before starting an exercise program.

Although many walkers are discouraged as joggers flash by them, extended studies of people with different exercise levels have shown that surprisingly low levels will increase longevity. A study of male Harvard graduates found that those regularly enjoying even simple activities like gardening, climbing stairs, and walking had fewer heart problems and lived on average two years longer than men who were more sedentary. A large research study known as MRFIT (Multiple Risk Factor Intervention Trial) also showed that men performing moderate activities, such as thirty minutes of daily walking, had 20 percent fewer overall deaths and 35 percent fewer heart disease deaths than did less-active men.

In addition to helping you achieve and maintain ideal body weight and blood pressure, a regular aerobic exercise program has been shown to increase your good cholesterol (HDL). Most studies suggest that the equivalent of twelve or more miles of brisk walking per week is required to increase our HDLs significantly. Although the beneficial responses to exercise have been more extensively investigated in men than women, the Cooper Institute for Aerobics Research in Dallas showed that walking offers women similar benefits. In their study, 102 previously sedentary women, ages twenty to forty, were randomly assigned to one of four groups. One group was the nonwalking control group; the other groups all averaged three miles of walking, five days a week. One group strolled at 3 m.p.h., one averaged a

4-m.p.h. brisk walk, and one a 5 m.p.h. more rapid "aerobic" walk. The good news for slow walkers was that both strollers and aerobic walkers realized a 6 percent increase in their good HDLs.

So remember when you are designing your exercise program to choose activities that you enjoy, and thus will do frequently, not necessarily intensely. Other aerobic activities that can benefit you include bicycling, rowing, jogging, low-impact aerobic dance, and swimming. High-impact aerobics (and other high-impact activities) are not generally recommended, but if you choose to do them, monitor yourself carefully for injuries, and be sure to cross-train.

I have personally seen the beneficial effect exercise has on HDLs many times. The program director at my first cardiac rehabilitation contract was one of those who taught me the power of the exercise component. She had been a marathon runner with HDL readings in the high 90s, but a month of inactivity while she concentrated on her doctoral thesis plunged her HDL reading into the 40s. Obviously, the lesson here is two-fold; while your HDL level can be very responsive to your exercise regimen, it is very unforgiving if you stop! You'll find specific recommendations on exercises in Part Three of this book.

SPIRITUALITY AND YOUR HEALTH

While most people assume that diet and exercise are more powerful deterrents of the progression of heart disease than is a pursuit of emotional and spiritual healing, the evidence for the preventive and healing power of the latter is growing. Not only does this evidence show physiological benefits from emotional and spiritual disciplines; it also shows that general attitudes and "sense of well being" improvements are reported. There is no doubt in my mind that being spiritually and emotionally healthy will give you the strength needed to maintain the diet and exercise components for lowering your cholesterol. Lifestyle changes are not easy, and I have seen many well-intentioned people fail at making these changes in part because they were not in touch with their inner selves.

My personal and professional experience has often shown that physical symptoms are emotionally and spiritually based. Since many of these words are our attempts to describe indefinable concepts, and many of us were raised with different belief systems, let me briefly summarize what I mean by them to enhance the odds that we stay on the same page.

I will be discussing the way our spiritual, emotional, and physical selves connect and affect each other through the terminology outlined in the model shown in Figure 2.1. The *physical self* is our body. The majority of this book addresses the best nutritional plan for your body's long-term health. The exercise advice also addresses the physical needs of your body.

You will note the word *soul* is used to include not only our emotions, but our mind, will, and subconscious. So if I use the words "emotional healing," I will not be simply describing the process of getting "in touch with" your feelings, but also will be referring to the healing or integration of this process with a healthier mental response. This includes a healthier "will," or desire to respond in the best way, and a deeper sense of peace in the subconscious—that area of ourselves that is deeper than we can really consciously understand.

Since we come from various spiritual disciplines and backgrounds, and wide differences in our acknowledgement of our spiritual selves in general, it is probably best if I describe *spirit* as our higher calling—that part of ourselves that seeks to understand our creation and purpose. It seems we are all serving something or someone. If it is not God, or some Higher Power

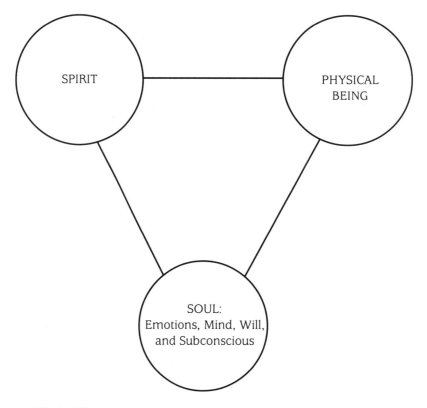

FIGURE 2.1   Our Whole Self

that we think created us and is in charge of the universe, then it is ourselves, money, or possibly some other object or substance of addiction. Some people insist they are *atheist* (denying the existence of God). However, all the participants who have ever identified themselves as such in the Inner Healing groups I offer at the Rice Diet Program have left saying that they meant they were *agnostic* (believing there is no definite proof of God, but not denying the possibility that God exists). I believe we are all born with a spiritual self, a large part of ourselves that yearns to know why we are here and wonders about the invisible forces that affect us. It is just that some are more aware and connected with this desire and feeling than are others.

The belief that healing needs to include these areas of ourselves is not a new one, nor did it arise from the holistic movement of the 1960s. The Gospel is an account of the most famous healer the world has ever know, Jesus Christ. Jesus' concern extended beyond "saving souls"; his redemptive concern encompassed the whole person, including the body. For example, in his mind there was no sharp cleavage between sickness and sin; the former belonged to the body and the latter to the soul. His ministry was focused on a total need, and thus a total healing. Unfortunately, in recent times the word "sin" has become loaded with judgment and guilt for many people. If we are habitually involved with sins—which I define as our thoughts, feelings, and actions that do not serve our Higher Power, or our spiritual selves—we may suffer on many levels, including physical dis-ease.

Through understanding my physical, emotional, and spiritual connected-ness, I began to understand how my emotional resentment, which was not serving my Higher Power or my spiritual self, had grown so exaggerated that I became physically impaired with a crippling joint disorder. I am not implying that all arthritis is due to overblown resentments; and this does not mean I am a bad, resentful person. It simply means that I am a human being who temporarily lost touch with my Higher Power or my loving spiritual self, allowed resentment to preoccupy my emotions, mind, and will, and consequently paid some physical consequences for it.

In a society that reveres allopathic medicine, which usually treats the symptoms rather than the cause, we usually find it much easier to claim that we inherited arthritis from our mama, or have a poorly functioning heart because daddy did, or are overweight because of an underactive thyroid, than to admit that our emotional responses may be the root cause. It is much easier to view physical illness as the result of fate or genetics; if it were the result of our emotions, then we would feel responsible for it. I am sharing this observation not to "lay blame" on people for their diseases, but to share from my own suffering and that of others in hope that it can empower you to pursue a total healing, not just a lower cholesterol. Again, I repeat, this is not to say that *all* physical diseases are due to emotional and spiritual dis-ease, but it is worth journeying inward to explore whether your problem has roots beyond the more obvious physical ones.

There are many ways that you can tune in to your spiritual self and learn to listen to your soul. Some of the ways that have been most beneficial to me and to many of the patients I've worked with are meditation, prayer and faith, community or group support, and journalizing.

Meditation

Meditation has been practiced throughout the world for centuries. But it became more accepted in mainstream medical circles when Dr. Herbert Benson, Associate Professor of Medicine at the Harvard Medical School and Director of the Hypertension Section of Boston's Beth Israel Hospital, reported the first respected scientific evidence that the "relaxation response" achieved during meditation had profound physiological benefits. He reported many beneficial effects on heart disease risk factors in his books *The Relaxation Response* (Avon Books, 1975) and *Beyond the Relaxation Response* (Berkley Publishing Corp., 1984). He found that our bodies' physiological responses to stress (aptly labeled "fight-or-flight" responses) were reversed during meditation. Whether the stress is due to a saber-toothed tiger chasing you or to someone cutting you off in traffic, your body's involuntary responses include increased blood pressure, heart rate, blood clotting time, and blood flow to the muscles; and a tendency toward arterial spasm and arrhythmias. Of course, these responses would help you if a tiger were actually pursuing you with lunch in mind, but far more often in today's world you are unable to run it off. Instead you are strapped into your car by your seat belt, your fists and jaws clenched, while your body's natural responses to stress are setting you up for a heart attack!

In *Beyond the Relaxation Response,* Dr. Benson states that "choles-terol levels can also be lowered by eliciting the relaxation response—especially if this phenomenon is combined with a person's deep personal beliefs." A study on this subject, conducted by Dr. Michael J. Cooper and Dr. Maurice M. Aygen, was reported in the *Journal of Human Stress,* 1979. They found that meditation, which elicits this relaxation response, was able to lower cholesterol significantly. In fact, some cholesterol levels dropped by as much as 35 percent, which rivals the response of the most powerful cholesterol lowering medications! On the other hand, the control group, which did not practice any meditative techniques, experienced no significant cholesterol changes.

Regular meditation can help you not only by reducing the feelings of stress, but by allowing you to take time to be alone, away from the distractions of life, and more able to get in touch with yourself, to simply *be*. During these times of simply being, you will enjoy more moments of connecting with your Higher Power, and more opportunities to really know yourself and what you want to do with your life that you aren't doing. Meditation also allows you the time to be mindful of unresolved issues, and enables you to bring them to your consciousness, which can facilitate your healing emotionally and spiritually before physical dis-ease is a problem, or more of a problem. Freud was keenly aware that "symptoms vanish with the acquisition of knowledge of their meaning." Although an inner journey can be initially painful, it is surely more farsighted to exercise preventive emotional and spiritual measures not only to prevent physical dis-ease, but to fulfill our individual human potential and maximize our joy.

Prayer and Faith as Fuels

Prayer is a path to spiritual development; it is communication with our Higher Power or Creator. One could view meditation as listening to God, and prayer as talking to God. Interestingly enough, Dr. Larry Dossey, whose book *Healing Words: The Power of Prayer and The Practice of Medicine* (Harper, 1993) summarizes the research that has been conducted on the efficacy of prayer, has found that prayer tends to "work" best if the prayer is general, rather than specific. For instance, rather than having a wish list of what we would like God to do for us next, Dr. Dossey's review of the research found that prayers, in general, tend to be more effective if they are seeking for "God's will to be done," rather than *our* will to be done. If you already believe in God you know God's will is for you to be healthy—physically, emotionally, and spiritually. Prayer could only assist and undergird you in your healing pursuits.

But, if you find it hard to believe that prayer can help you, or if you are simply interested in the world's increasing desire for spiritual knowledge, you can research the growing volume of scientific investigation of the effectiveness of prayer. A most impressive research experiment on the relationship between prayer and healing was conducted by Dr. Randolph Byrd, a practicing cardiologist, who followed 393 patients admitted to the coronary care unit at San Francisco General Hospital. The patients were divided into two groups. One group (192 patients) was prayed for by home prayer groups, and the other group (201 patients) was not.

The results were impressive. It was discovered that the patients who had been prayed for were:

- ❖ 5 times less likely to need antibiotics

- ❖ 3 times less likely to develop pulmonary edema

- ❖ not in need of endotracheal intubation (12 in the unremembered group needed this mechanical ventilatory support)

- ❖ less likely to die (13 compared to 17).

In *Healing Words: The Power of Prayer and The Practice of Medicine* Dr. Larry Dossey writes, "If the technique being studied had been a new drug or a surgical procedure instead of prayer, it would almost certainly have been heralded as some sort of breakthrough." He also states that Dr. William Nolan, who wrote a book debunking faith healing, acknowledged that Dr. Byrd's study will stand up to scrutiny. The *Chicago Sun-Times* (January 26, 1986) quoted Dr. Nolan "Maybe we doctors ought to be writing on our order sheets, 'Pray 3 times a day.' If it works, it works."

While some criticize Dr. Byrd's study, Dr. Dossey points out that you can continue to debate Dr. Byrd's study design, but you would not be likely to debate the statistical significance of the reduction in deaths if one of the fewer deaths was yours! Your spiritual, emotional, and physical health are worth giving it a try.

Dr. Dossey reports that prayer seems to "work" whether you *believe* it will or not. Although you could find evidence to support either argument, a group of researchers led by Dr. Thomas E. Oxman, a psychiatrist from Dartmouth Medical School, found convincing results to support the power of faith for heart patients. In the first-ever study on religion in heart surgery, Dr. Oxman found that belief (or lack of it) turned out to be a safety factor (or risk factor) on the operating table. He and his associates observed 232 patients, all over fifty-five years of age, for six months after their bypass or aortic valve replacement surgery. Of these, twenty-one died. The researchers examined the impact on survival of a number of biomedical, psychological, and social factors, as well as religious feeling and activity. Controlling for biomedical differences, Dr. Oxman found that patients who felt no comfort from religious beliefs were three times more likely to die than those comforted by their faith.

Dr. Oxman's data, first reported in 1995 in *Psychosomatic Medicine,* instantly inspired scientific skeptics to assume the observed benefit was due to the social support the people got in church. But, Dr. Oxman's data proves otherwise. While the social support was indeed found to be a strong survival factor (the people who did not participate in organized social activities, such as church suppers or local government were four times as likely to die as those in such supportive environments), faith's comfort was an independent factor almost as strong.

Numerous other research studies have shown the benefits of practicing one's faith and its prevention of heart disease or its risk factors. In Jerusalem, researchers at Hadassah University found that residents who described themselves as secular had four times the risk of suffering a heart attack than did residents who described themselves as religiously orthodox. These Hadassah scientists also noted higher cholesterol levels among seventeen- to eighteen-year-old secular residents compared to their religiously orthodox counterparts. The cholesterol differences could not be explained by differences in their dietary fat intake. In a large study done in Washington County, Maryland, those who reported attending church at least weekly were much less likely to die from heart disease than those who attended less frequently. And, this decreased risk held true even after adjustments were made for differences in the participants' smoking habits, water quality, and social class.

Dr. Morton Kelsey, a student of Carl Jung, professor at Notre Dame, Episcopalian priest, and author of over twenty-five published books, said in his 1932 talk to the Alsatian Pastoral Conference entitled ''Psychotherapists or the Clergy'':

> Among all my patients in the second half of life—that is to say, over thirty-five—there has not been one whose problem in the last resort was not that of finding a religious outlook on life. It is safe to say that every one of them fell ill because he had lost what the living religions of every age have given to their followers, and none of them has been really healed who did not regain his religious outlook.

Community and Group Support

If you do not find meditation, prayer, and faith right for you, do not be dissuaded. Everyone's path is different, and much of the adventure and fun in life is in finding your own. It is important to realize that spirituality is related to meaning and purpose in life, concern and caring for others, and commitment to a larger force. The commitment to a larger force can be found in many different ways, including group support.

Several studies have shown the importance of social support for reducing risks of death from a variety of causes, and heart disease in particular. For example, heart attack patients who lived alone or who had limited emotional support were at an increased risk for death after their heart attacks. In the *Annals of Internal Medicine* (Dec. 1992), Dr. Lisa Berkman and her associates reported that among those with heart attacks, individuals without a source of emotional support were twice as likely to die as those who had two or more sources of support. In-hospital death rates were 38 percent, 23 percent, and 12 percent for those with zero, one, and two or more sources of emotional support, respectively. Similarly, patients who were followed after coronary angiography (a test in which dye is injected into the arteries of the heart for assessment of blockages or health) or angina, who were not married and lacked a confidant, or who had limited emotional support were at increased risk for death.

In addition to traditional religious groups, such as churches and synogogues, many specialized groups have arisen in pursuit of healing. Most notable internationally are the many "anonymous" groups based on the healing successes of Alcoholics Anonymous. At the Rice Diet Clinic and Heart Disease Reversal Program we offer similar groups—safe, confidential gatherings where participants know they can come and share from their hearts. Here we try to practice unconditional love by truly listening to others without offering judgment or free advice. Most people find it very refreshing to be really heard. The healing power of simply sharing our stories—our truths, our fears and our faiths—is quite frankly beyond description. Many of these shared stories will be recounted throughout this book in hopes of passing on the healing that is also possible for you.

If you don't really think you are a "group" person, you may feel more comfortable trying one led by experts in the field of stress management, and after reading something written by them. In their book *Anger Kills* (Random House, 1993), Drs. Redford and Virginia Williams summarize the characteristics that are correlated to heart disease and offer many behavior modification techniques to remedy them. The Williamses also offer intensive retreats at the Rice Diet Program, where they teach these coping strategies, and guide participants in getting in touch with their feelings and communicating them more effectively. Since numerous studies have shown that heart attack patients who continue to lead stressful lives have two to three times the incidence of repeat heart attacks than survivors who learn to control their stress, it is worth exploring ways to perceive things differently.

Journalizing into Recovery

Like meditation, prayer, and group involvement, the practice of journalizing can also help us truly see ourselves and confront and embrace our feelings, leading to a healing of body, mind, and spirit. Putting your deepest thoughts and feelings into a journal can have a powerfully therapeutic effect even if they are never read by another human being.

Dr. James Pennebaker and Sandra Beall researched this therapeutic response by asking a group of student volunteers to write about either traumatic experiences or superficial topics. They asked some of those who were writing about traumas just to vent their emotions without recording facts, others to write down the facts only, and others to write about both facts and their emotions. The volunteers kept journals for four days, writing fifteen minutes a day.

The results were far more powerful than had been anticipated. Four months later, there was a 50 percent drop in the monthly visitation rate to the health center by those who wrote about both facts and feelings surrounding a traumatic event. Such a dramatic healing benefit was *not* enjoyed by those who wrote only about their emotions, or who wrote only about the facts, or who wrote only about superficial topics and avoided difficult subjects entirely.

To confirm these findings further, Dr. Pennebaker teamed up with Janice Kiecolt-Glaser, a clinical psychologist and her husband, Ronald Glaser, an immunologist, from Ohio State University College of Medicine in Columbus. The experiment they did together was similar to the previous one except this time responses in the immune system were measured. Those who wrote thoughtfully and emotionally about traumatic experiences showed heightened immune function compared with those who only wrote about superficial topics.

For those interested in pursuing more information and instruction on journalizing techniques available see Appendix B: Sources for More Information. Dr. Ira Progoff's *At a Journal Workshop* is the basic text and guide for using the Intensive Journal process that his associates teach internationally. I would highly recommend these weekend intensive journalizing workshops to anyone interested in embarking on or continuing an introspective walk.

The important thing to remember is that your healing must involve emotional or spiritual components, as well as the physical. After experiencing the power of the spiritual in my own life, as well as seeing it in many Rice Diet participants, I am convinced we need to honor the *whole* person. If we have not contemplated the true purpose of our lives, and our connectedness with self, others, and our Higher Power, we cannot be emotionally content and physical dis-ease usually follows.

We are fortunate that the interconnectedness of our spirit, soul, and body is currently being researched. Better understanding will open up greater numbers of paths on which to pursue healing. It is indeed a gift to live in a time in which we have access to prayer and support groups, and meditation classes, as well as facilities where all the components of healing are offered. The responsibility is now yours to incorporate them into your own healing process.

3

LOWERING YOUR RISK OF EXCESS WEIGHT AND DIABETES

If you are very overweight, you probably already know that you don't feel healthy. But many people don't realize that being even *slightly* overweight can also cause health problems, including heart disease. Excess weight is discussed along with diabetes in this chapter because the two can be very closely intertwined.

Excess weight is associated with every nutritionally related heart disease risk factor (high blood pressure, cholesterol, triglyceride, blood sugar), as well as other health problems such as sleep apnea (a condition in which people do not get enough oxygen to the brain and fall asleep uncontrollably throughout the day), gallbladder disease, gout, and some types of cancer. Obesity has also been blamed for the development of osteoarthritis of the weight-bearing joints. The incidence and severity of *all* of these problems are reduced by weight loss.

Dr. Kempner described obesity as a risk factor of heart disease over fifty years ago, and the Framingham Heart Study has since proven to the world that obesity is an independent, long-term predictor of heart disease.

As for diabetes, people with this condition are more likely to die of heart disease than of anything else. This is especially true for women. The risks for heart disease in diabetics is so much greater that some physicians think all diabetics should have cholesterol-lowering drugs as an automatic part of their treatment. This opinion was encouraged by a recent study, known as the Scandinavian Simvastatin Survival Study, which showed that drugs lowered the risk of heart attacks in diabetics by 50 percent. Although this is an impressive finding, I much prefer solving the problem at its root rather than resorting to drugs.

The majority of people who have diabetes have adult-onset, or Type II diabetes, which means that most of them would never need oral medicine, much less insulin, to enjoy a fasting blood sugar under 100 if they followed the Heal Your Heart Program and kept an ideal body weight.

Although diabetes cannot literally be *cured* by these natural means, the symptoms of diabetes, as well as the typical and undesirable side effects of diabetes (kidney and heart disease, and circulation problems which often lead to blindness and amputations), can be reversed or eliminated via the Heal Your Heart Program of nutrition, exercise, and inner healing. Weight loss is key because it will reduce the glucose the body makes, while improving the efficiency of the insulin, which decreases the insulin needed to move the glucose from the blood into the cells. This is of growing interest to many investigators who think that a high insulin should be considered a heart disease risk factor.

How Much Is Too Much Weight?

In 1995, new, stricter weight recommendations, courtesy of the U.S. Departments of Agriculture, and Health and Human Services, added to the numbers of people officially considered obese. But even under the old guidelines, the number of obese Americans was growing. Approximately a third of all Americans are overweight enough to be categorized as obese (more than 20 percent above ideal body weight)—up from a fourth of the population in the 1970s.

Many people weigh more than they would like, but feel that "a few extra pounds won't kill them." They may be wrong about that. The Framingham Study also showed that even being of "average" weight is not good enough. Men and women of average weight (weights of people in the study compare favorably with those in the general U.S. population, which were about 20 percent above the ideal weights recommended by the Metropolitan Life Insurance Company in 1959) had appreciably higher heart disease death rates than did those weighing less. The ratio of their actual weights to their desirable weights was a significant predictor of heart disease even after adjustments for other risk factors (which, of course, are effected by weight). Being of average weight, like being average with respect to the other risk factors of heart disease, is not an ambitious goal or proactive approach for those of us trying to prevent or reverse heart disease. Remember that in most developed nations the average person has heart disease in their sixties, so don't be consoled by assuming that average is anywhere close to optimal!

And that's not all. The Framingham Study, and other studies also showed that your risk of dying of heart disease depends on *how long* you're overweight. In other words, if you have been overweight since a young age, you have a higher risk of dying of heart disease than someone who put on the pounds more recently. So younger people who have excess weight are especially at risk. Unfortunately, many people don't realize how risky their weight is, because the consequences take many years to show up. This means that many don't take obesity as seriously as they do other heart disease risk factors.

There is strong medical evidence to support the importance of maintaining a low weight. For instance, a respected Harvard study, published in the September 1995 *New England Journal of Medicine,* found that women who had gained 20 to 40 pounds since the age of eighteen were two and a half times more likely to die of heart disease than those who had maintained their weight.

The new recommended weight ranges come from a number called the body mass index (BMI), which is an indirect measure of body fat. These were calculated by first looking at the research data on BMI and how it relates to relative risk of death. The BMIs associated with high death rates were noted and the range of healthy BMIs were determined. The research showed that healthy BMIs range from 19 to 25, 25 to 29 implied "moderate overweight," and any number higher signaled "severe obesity." Although some are still debating these categorizations, the bottom line on the Harvard study's findings was that a sharp rise in the risk of death occurred when the BMI reaches 27 and greater. Although we should all strive for a BMI in the healthy 19 to 25 range, this is of utmost importance if you have a family history of heart disease and cancer, and if you have high blood pressure, cholesterol and blood sugar (diabetes), or a high percentage of belly fat. Excessive fat in the abdominal area has been associated with an increased risk of heart disease and other problems.

Calculating Your Body Mass Index

To determine your BMI, follow this 4-step formula:

> **Step 1.** Multiply your weight in pounds by .45.
> > Example: 150 pounds $\times$ .45 = 67.5
> **Step 2.** Multiply your height in inches by .025.
> > Example: 5'9", or 69 inches $\times$ .025 = 1.725

Step 3. Multiply the answer from Step 2 by itself.
Example: $1.725 \times 1.725 = 2.976$
Step 4. Divide the answer from Step 1 by the answer from Step 3.

Example: $\dfrac{67.5}{2.976}$ = BMI of 22.7

If your answer is between 19 and 25, you are in the healthy range. If it is higher, you need to lose weight in order to improve your chances of good health.

Even if you are only slightly overweight, you owe it to your heart to lose the excess.

As with cholesterol, controlling your weight and diabetes is not simply a matter of "going on a diet." If you are overweight, you have probably tried several diets over the years that have either not worked or didn't last. I believe that to truly heal your heart, changing only a portion of your life won't work. Reaching and maintaining a healthy weight and control of diabetes involves permanently changing both nutrition and exercise habits and connecting with your inner self.

NUTRITION AND YOUR WEIGHT

The Heal Your Heart nutrition plan will help you lose weight as well as control many health concerns, such as diabetes. It is not the latest fad diet, but is instead a way of changing your whole approach to food—for good.

Your plan will include a low-calorie, low-fat, low-sugar and low-salt diet. What's left? Don't worry—there's lots! Your plan will be high in fiber and can include lots of delicious fruits, vegetables, grains and beans. It is healthy for diabetics as well as those who need to lose weight—and even those who have both health conditions.

The Calorie and Fat Connection

Calorie counting is an arduous chore and in my opinion, too much emphasis has been placed on it. When patients concentrate too much on calories, they often overlook good nutrition. A food with a low calorie count is not necessarily the best choice at all times. For example, patients who are overly focused on calories often insist that they want to eat the "lite" bread, at only 50 calories a slice, rather than a whole grain cereal such as oatmeal or barley, which would offer half again more calories. Unfortunately, these calorie-conscious types rarely look beyond the calorie information on the nutritional analysis to find that the lower-calorie "lite" bread is highly refined, and loaded with salt and cellulose—which is ground up pine trees! The bread's refined nature often inspires the desire for seconds or thirds, thus blowing the low-calorie justifications. The higher-calorie whole grains oats and barley, on the other hand, are loaded with nutrients and blood-sugar-stabilizing soluble fibers, so they are well worth every calorie they offer.

Fat, however, is a wise thing to concentrate on limiting. As you read in Chapter 2, fat, especially saturated fat, is a direct cause of high cholesterol levels. Eating excess fat also helps makes us fat. Let's look at the connection between fat and calories.

Calories are simply a measurement of energy. All calories from food come from fat, protein, and carbohydrate. However, each gram of fat has more calories (about 9) than does each gram of protein and carbohydrate (about 4). So it makes sense that if we reduce the grams of fat we eat, we are eating fewer calories than if we modified any other aspect of our diet. Unfortunately, a few decades ago, starchy foods got the unfounded reputation of being fattening. But it turns out the opposite is true; starchy vegetables, grains, and beans contain little fat and are easily utilized by your body. It is not the baked potato that adds to the hips, but the fatty butter, sour cream, and cheese toppings that most people use in excess.

On the other hand, it is almost impossible to overeat "whole foods" (unprocessed vegetarian foods) that grow from the ground: grains, beans, fruits, and vegetables. These foods contain little or no fat and are known as complex carbohydrates (versus simple, or refined carbohydrates such as sugar, honey, and syrups). As research by Dr. Dean Ornish and others has shown, when you eat primarily complex carbohydrates and eliminate animal protein and fat-rich foods from your diet, you will lose weight without counting calories. This is true for two primary reasons. One reason is that our bodies burn carbohydrate-rich "whole foods" very efficiently, while the fat we eat is much more easily converted into fat on our bodies. This is because it takes a lot more calories for our body to digest and metabolize complex carbohydrates than to process dietary fat. So we burn some calories just by eating carbohydrates! Studies by K.J. Acheson and others back this up, showing that very little of our complex carbohydrate intake is converted into body fat. The other reason we lose weight eating only whole foods is that they do not contain many of the "overeating triggers" that processed foods (such as refined chips, cookies, and crackers), animal products (such as meat and cheese), fried foods, or refined sugars, contain.

"Trigger foods" are those that inspire you to eat more than you had initially intended. If eating one slice of bread typically means you follow it with two or three more, bread is a "trigger food" for you. Not that bread is "bad," but it is typical of many processed foods in that you are much more likely to eat it in excess than you would a whole food alternative. For instance, you may find that one slice of a heavy whole-grained bread may be sufficient for you. However, if you find that *all* breads are difficult or impossible for you to eat in moderation, you may find it beneficial to avoid them until your weight or blood sugar goals are achieved.

So, if you can stick to eating carbohydrate-rich whole foods and avoid fat in your diet, you probably won't need to count calories. If you find that counting calories does work for you, that's fine. Part Two of this book will show you how to tailor the Heal Your Heart Program nutrition plan to your needs, with or without counting calories.

The Effect of Sugar and Other Processed Foods on Weight and Blood Sugars

Although we have discussed some advantages of complex carbohydrates over the more refined sugars and syrups, we need to also appreciate how counterproductive refined sugar intake can be for overeaters and diabetics. Most people struggling with overeating problems report that baked products and/or foods containing refined sugars are their primary food triggers. No one really understands all of the reasons for this but a few are obvious. Processed, refined products like flour and sugar have been milled or ground into much smaller particles, which become blood sugar much faster than does the original "whole" product. This is clearly a poor choice for a diabetic or hypoglycemic, who already suffers from extreme high or low blood sugar swings. Many diabetics and hypoglycemics are coached by their well meaning health professionals to consume diets high in animal protein and/or fat to help slow their absorptioin of sugar into the blood, but when heart disease will likely soon be their biggest problem, this dietary advice seems short-sighted and less than preventive. The Heal Your Heart Program nutrition plan, with its focus on complex carbohydrates—especially ones rich in soluble fiber, will produce better short- and long-term results for diabetics and hypoglycemics while preventing the future development of heart disease.

When you eat too much refined sugar your blood sugar will rocket skyward. This may produce a temporary energy boost or buzz, but it will rather quickly be followed by a crash—your blood sugar rebounding to a much lower level. Anyone, but especially a hypoglycemic or diabetic, could experience a headache, light-headedness, irritability, a spacey feeling, or a desire to eat a great deal of food immediately.

Although most sweeteners have just 16 calories per teaspoon, beware of foods that contain numerous teaspoons. Refined sugar calories can quickly add up and are nutritionless. This is especially true for the many no-fat desserts on the market now. Sure Entenmann's and Snackwell's sweets are fat-free as advertised, but the fine print shows that they are loaded with empty-calorie sugars, refined wheat flour, chemicals, and no significant nutritional value. If you are concerned with weight loss and blood sugar swings, you would not ruin your prognosis by *one* serving of these desserts (especially after a mixed meal, which slows the sugar absorption into the blood), but who can eat just one? Even the artificial sweeteners, which were supposed to be the big cure for obesity a few years back, have not been shown to facilitate long-term weight loss. In fact, I am convinced they feed the sugar or sweet addiction. Most everyone can relate to the *Cathy* comic strip that depicts her justifying a second piece of chocolate cake because she was drinking a diet drink. We all play games in our head about food and how we justify it, and refined products simply fuel this irrational flame.

Why Avoid Salt?

Many patients are surprised when we tell them that they should be avoiding salt even if they do not have high blood pressure. It's true that most heart diets allow much more salt than the Heal Your Heart Program does, but there are many good reasons that we should all avoid salt, blood pressure aside.

How Sodium Seduces Us into Overeating

Although Dr. Kempner did not at first set out to treat obesity with his original Rice Diet, he found that people following the diet lost weight quickly and effectively. There are several reasons for this, but followers of the diet strongly believe that the no-salt requirement helps them lose weight and keep it off.

Why is this? The reason is that salt inspires cravings and makes us think we're hungry when we're not. It may sound strange, but eliminating salt is the key to the Rice Diet's ability to tame the appetite and therefore control obesity. I have never experienced any nutrition plan that inspires a more dramatic shift in a person's relationship with food. When the true flavor of our food is not masked by salt, we begin to enjoy foods for the natural flavors, sustenance, and health they provide rather than expecting them to fulfill cravings. Even people with the most severe cases of food addiction agree that the low sodium Rice Diet almost immediately relieves both their desire for excessive portions and their cravings for "comfort" or "binge" foods. Within days almost all remark that they cannot believe how far food has moved from the center of their universe! Of course, salt elimination is only part of their treatment. As patients stay long enough for their other issues to surface, their inner healing journeys usually lead them to the roots of their overeating problems. We'll address that later in this chapter.

How Salt Affects Diabetes

Although the body can turn most foods into blood sugar (glucose), carbohydrate is the most common and rapid provider of blood sugar. Diabetes occurs when there is too much glucose in the blood and the body does not have enough insulin available (or there is too much ineffective insulin) to transport it into the body's cells to provide nourishment. Hypoglycemia is basically the opposite of diabetes in that it is characterized by low blood glucose levels. Fortunately, both conditions respond very favorably to this diet very low in fat and *sodium* and high in soluble fiber.

There is now evidence that if you eat something with salt you have a higher blood glucose rise, thus absorb more calories from it, than if you eat it without added salt. This was demonstrated by Dr. Anne Thorburn and associates (*British Medical Journal,* 1986) in research that showed that an increase in sodium intake significantly increased the glucose and insulin response after a meal. For those who care why, the two most probable ways that salt increases the plasma glucose and insulin responses are by accelerating the digestion of starch and accelerating the absorption of glucose.

Participants took four test meals randomly, which were equal caloric amounts of brown lentils or white bread, with and without 4.25 grams of added salt (one third the daily sodium intake of many people in Western countries). After the salted lentil and bread test meals were consumed, the amount of glucose found in the blood was significantly higher than after the unsalted meals. When there is a greater amount of glucose in the blood there are more potential calories to absorb. This suggests that adding salt to our meals is not advantageous to diabetics (who already have blood sugars that are too high) or to those trying to lose weight. In addition, the higher blood sugar response to the salted versus unsalted bread meal was followed by a hypoglycemic, or low blood sugar, response. The already unstable blood sugar responses of diabetics and hypoglycemics do not need the extra effects that added sodium seemed to inspire.

The plasma insulin concentrations, forty-five minutes after eating the salted lentils, were 22 percent higher than the insulin levels after eating the unsalted lentils. More dramatic was the insulin concentration difference after eating salted versus unsalted bread: an average of 39 percent greater over the three hours following the meals. Remember there is a growing concern among researchers regarding the correlation between high insulin levels and heart disease. The goal is to have relatively low amounts of *efficient* insulin, which produces relatively low and stable blood sugar levels. Efficient insulin keeps the glucose moving properly from the blood into our cells to nourish them.

Since high blood sugar (diabetes) is a risk factor for heart disease, and high insulin levels are thought by some to be, it would seem logical that adding sodium to foods does not help your heart from this sodium perspective either. And obesity, which is a risk factor for heart disease as well as many other undesirable conditions, is also not benefitted by adding salt to foods and creating more available calories. So limiting our sodium intake is desirable long before the "red flags" of hypertension and kidney disease are waving!

Fiber's Effects on Weight and Diabetes

So now for what you *can* eat—fiber, and lots of it. As we discussed in Chapter 2, increasing soluble fiber intake has been reported to lower cholesterol, especially the LDL—bad cholesterol. However, a high-fiber diet has other benefits, too. Fiber can actually help control your weight as well as reduce insulin requirements and increase your insulin sensitivity, thus improving diabetes control. The blood sugar stabilizing effects of oat, bean, and barley products have provided impressive results in human studies, while rice has been less studied in people but has shown strong results in animal studies.

How Fiber Helps You Lose Weight

There are many different ways that fiber can help prevent obesity and facilitate weight reduction when needed. One of the most obvious and potentially important effects of dietary fiber with respect to obesity is that foods with higher fiber content tend to be lower in calories than low-fiber foods. Fiber is the nondigestible part of food; it creates bulk or substance in a food, but you derive no calories from it. Another benefit of a fiber-rich diet is that it requires more chewing, so it increases the time required for the consumption of the meal. This additional time the food stays in your mouth, as well as the gut-filling properties of the bulky fiber itself, trigger signals that induce satiety or a sense of being satisfied or full. This is the main reason I usually eat a couple of servings of vegetables first—usually as two to three cups of salad or a cup or two of steamed vegetables—before enjoying pasta, seafood, or some higher-calorie choices. By the time you chew this much higher fiber, low-calorie food, you have less room and desire for excessive portions of food.

The effectiveness of fiber in treating obesity appears to vary depending on the type of fiber. Soluble fiber, found in high amounts of oats, beans, peas, and barley, has a slower transit time (from the time you eat it to the time you excrete it). So foods high in soluble fiber impart more of a sense of fullness per calorie eaten. Soluble fiber can also lead to a slight malabsorption of fats and bile acids (so you absorb less fat and cholesterol), and can improve your glucose tolerance and insulin sensitivity, which may influence centers in the brain that regulate your hunger. In other words, fiber helps us want to eat fewer calories, feel fuller on the calories we are eating, and thus lose weight without feeling deprived.

How Fiber Helps Control Diabetes

The fiber and diabetes connection is a bit more complicated. It seems that certain soluble-fiber-rich, high-carbohydrate foods, such as oats, beans, and barley, are more slowly absorbed than other carbohydrates and can therefore actually stabilize blood sugar and reduce insulin responses. So if you are a diabetic, which means you tend to have too high a blood sugar level, soluble fiber can be life transforming. You can improve your condition dramatically by focusing on eating soluble-fiber-rich foods at every meal. These foods really do become blood sugar more slowly than do carbohydrates that do not have much soluble fiber.

If you ate a cup of oats for breakfast, beans for lunch, and barley for supper, your blood sugar would rise slowly but surely over the next one to five hours, helping you feel nourished and energetic until the next meal. On the other hand, white toast for breakfast, a big bowl of potato soup for lunch, donuts for afternoon snack, and white bread, white rice, or some other processed grain for supper would send your blood sugar screaming up and down all day.

Refined carbohydrates are not recommended for anyone, but for diabetics they are among the worst food choices. And although meat and fat produce a slow blood sugar release, as do soluble-fiber-rich foods, they also add too much fat and sodium to your diet, increasing the already high risk of heart disease for diabetics. Thus, the best nutrition recommendation for diabetics is a diet high in carbohydrates *and fiber* and low in fat and sodium.

Unfortunately, the recommendations most diabetics receive rarely get more specific. But studies have shown that eating highly viscous soluble fibers, as well as cellulose, and certain insoluble fibers, can bring about impressive improvement in the symptoms of diabetics. Foods especially high in these fibers include beans, barley, oats, oat and rice bran, rye kernels (the whole kernels, not rye bread), pasta, and fresh fruits such as apples and oranges (rather than their juices).

Studies by Dr. James Anderson, Professor of Medicine and Clinical Nutrition at the University of Kentucky, have shown that high-fiber diets can actually reduce or even eliminate the need for insulin injections for some diabetics. In insulin-dependent patients, he reported a 38 percent reduction in insulin needs. Of twenty-five lean, non-insulin-dependent patients, twenty-four eliminated their need for insulin therapy with a high-fiber diet. If you are diabetic, you have a two to three-times higher risk for heart disease than do nondiabetics, so you should be especially careful to eat enough soluble fiber. It will not only improve your diabetes management by reducing your insulin (or blood-sugar-lowering medication) requirements, increasing your insulin sensitivity, and stabilizing your blood sugar, but will significantly reduce your other risk factors for heart disease such as high cholesterol, LDLs, triglycerides, and obesity.

The dramatic improvements that major dietary change can create make it of utmost importance to consult with your doctor, especially for those of you taking any medications. Please note that insulin and other medications should not be altered without your doctor's supervision.

EXERCISE AND YOUR WEIGHT

Exercise will help you lose fat weight—in fact, that is one of the signs that your body likes to exercise. If you start exercising regularly, your body will adjust to this new challenge by reducing fat weight. It does this because you perform the activity better if you are closer to your body's optimal weight; your body knows this and is trying to help you make it easy on yourself. In Part Three we'll discuss which exercises and intensities burn more fat than others, but here I'll explain why exercise is so important and go over the difference between aerobic and strength exercising.

Aerobic Exercise and Weight Loss

The word *aerobic* literally means "utilizing oxygen," so with respect to physical exercise, aerobics is a method for producing beneficial changes in the respiratory and circulatory systems by activities which require a modest increase in oxygen intake. Aerobic exercise is also the only type of exercise that uses fat as an energy source. If you want to lose fat weight, you need to do aerobic exercise such as walking, cycling, or swimming. You also need to pay attention to the duration of your exercise.

For the first 30 minutes of your aerobic exercise session, you will burn predominantly carbohydrates. You will also burn some fat calories, but not as many as you will after the 30-minute mark. After 30 minutes, you begin to burn predominantly fat.

Because of this, breaking through the 30-minute mark is key to losing fat weight. So, moderately paced aerobic workouts of 45 minutes to one hour are recommended for fat-weight loss. Completing these workouts at least five times a week greatly increases your fat-burning time.

Before you start your aerobic exercise program be sure to read Chapter 6: Designing Your Personal Heal Your Heart Program and Chapter 9: Healing

Your Heart Through Exercise for tips on getting started, safety, listening to your body, the advantages of warm-ups and cool-downs, and other important details. As with all forms of exercise, it is very important to ease into aerobics slowly, and listen to your body's feedback.

Strength Training and Weight Loss

Although aerobic exercise burns fat, strength training can also help you lose weight by increasing your caloric burn throughout the day. Strength training increases your muscle mass, which in turn increases your resting metabolic rate. This is the amount of energy required to sustain your body during a resting state. Increasing your muscle or active tissue thus increases the amount of energy required to sustain your body at rest. So you'll burn more calories when you are doing nothing! This increase is not huge, but it can burn several more calories per hour and every bit helps.

Furthermore, muscle can help improve your posture. When your muscles are strong, you can hold up your body better. Also, you will be able to do your normal daily activities with greater ease. Toned muscle is firm. Most people want firm, toned bodies when they are trying to lose fat weight.

If you want to include strength training in your weight loss regimen, start with your aerobic workouts and be sure you have made these part of your regular routine. Then add strength training. This allows you the chance to get into your program without feeling overwhelmed. It will also allow your body to become adjusted to the new exercise regime. After a couple of weeks of doing your aerobic exercise, you'll probably find it is nice to have something new to revitalize your workouts and you.

Exercise and Diabetes

It has been known for some time that regular exercise enhances the effectiveness of the insulin in our bodies. In fact, exercise functions very similarly to the oral medication for diabetics; it enhances insulin's receptivity. A simple analogy is that insulin is like a key that unlocks the cells in the body so that the blood sugar can enter them for nourishment, and with diabetics the key doesn't work that well. (In Type I diabetes there is an inadequate amount of insulin; in Type II diabetes the insulin is less than receptive and effective.) The majority of diabetics are Type II, and if they exercised at least every other day their insulin's receptiveness would improve just as if they had taken oral medication. **Again, do not discontinue or reduce your medication just because you have committed to a new exercise program. Consult your doctor regarding your plans for a significant lifestyle change and the follow-ups that will be needed to assess you.**

INNER HEALING FOR WEIGHT CONTROL AND DIABETES

I have rarely seen people who overeat simply because they are physically hungry. Our bodies tell us how much they need; it's when we are unable to listen to our true physical needs that we run into trouble. The problem many people have with food is that they are no longer able to "hear" what their bodies are telling them because they have become accustomed to using food as a replacement for something else. In Chapter 1, you read about how addictions keep us from living healthy lives. Overeating is an addiction, so simply being told to eat right and exercise won't be enough. You need to address the emotions that you are attempting to mask with your food addiction.

Stress and unresolved emotional issues can also affect diabetes management. So it is unfortunate that inner healing work is not encouraged to improve blood sugar control and as a preventive measure for diabetes as well as all diseases. I have counseled numerous diabetic patients who had unusual onsets of diabetes (such as contracting it in their late twenties), who, when questioned, admitted very stressful incidents just prior to their diagnosis. Since journalizing has been shown to reduce the need to visit doctors by 50 percent, and to heighten immune functions, why not try it for weight reduction, diabetes management, and the prevention of many other diseases?

Journalizing: From Food to Feelings

Chapter 2 covered some of the ways to get in touch with your inner self and begin to heal, including meditation, prayer, and journalizing. Keeping a journal about your eating habits is one of the most effective ways to address the overeating addiction and improve diabetes management.

There are many formats for journalizing, so experiment with a few until you find a style that suits you. For starters use the Food Journal with Feelings form, Appendix D. It inspires you to examine what feelings may be fueling your addictive or unhealthy consumption. This can help you break through any denial about how you use food and bring about a transformation in your relationship with food. In addition to documenting your food intake and feelings before, during, and after you eat, spend some time each day recording facts and feelings.

Progoff's Intensive Journal Process, the most internationally renowned journalizing course, is now offered periodically at the Rice Diet Program. Thus far, participants have said the course exceeded their expectations for helping them take a deeper look at their addiction. The course offers several different approaches or techniques for journalizing. One of the primary sections of the workshop is called the dialogue section. We usually think of dialogue as meaning "he said then she said," but in this journalizing process, each participant takes an area of his or her life from which energy flows and examines it. There are at least five of these basic areas: persons (living or dead), work (employment or "love work" that is your creative outlet), body, events and situations, and society or groups you are part of. This journalizing technique takes you out of the simple diary format and makes your journal an active agent for helping you process your life.

One of the participants, Pam, reported how effective the exercise of "dialogue with body" had been for her. She, as well as many other overweight participants, shared how she began to disassociate herself from her body as she grew larger, and reported how the technique of dialogue with body had been a profound means for re-integrating her body to her soul and spirit. Others have described how they only related to their face after their bodies reached a certain weight, and how helpful this technique had been for re-integrating parts of the body back to the whole. Another participant, Susan, found that the "dialogue with body" exercise helped her sleep better. This is how she tells it:

> By communicating with my brain I became refocused and tamed my obsessive-compulsive thought patterns by recognizing that my brain was a part of my body that was trying to take over. By focusing on the rest of my body, I found it easier to relax into sleep. My "dialogue with work" was also very beneficial for me. Writing on my work, which is being a mom, helped me regain the security and confidence again to go home and resume this mission. It helped me move through the guilt I was creating for myself. The "dialogue with person" has also helped me by facilitating my communication with difficult family members. It helped me further accept the reality that I cannot change anyone but myself.

Others have "Eureka" moments while journalizing on their dreams. This was by far the most powerful part of the course for me, as most of my more profound emotional and spiritual insights have been through dreams. This technique gave me the tools that I needed to be able to interpret my own dreams, rather than relying on others. Journalizing has helped many participants at the Rice Diet Program get to the root cause of their issues, rather than overeat or worsen their physical problems.

It *Can* Work This Time

Most overweight people have tried many diet plans and failed to keep weight off. But if you follow the three-pronged approach of the Heal Your Heart

Program, you *can* lose weight and keep it off. That is what many patients at the Rice Diet Program have found. Here are some of their stories. I hope they will inspire you to follow their lead.

Bert came to realize that he needed to make some serious changes after many years of ignoring his weight problem. His success is an inspiring testimony of how simple dietary and exercise changes, along with inner searching, can dramatically improve a very bleak prognosis, and he has become an advocate of these changes, eager to spread the good news. Here's his story:

> I've been overweight as long as I can remember. I was 350 pounds at my high school graduation, and at least 400 pounds for the previous five years. But, my weight was just part of my problem. Eight months prior to my coming to the Rice Diet Program, I was taking 18 medications, 3 times a day. I was in atrial fibrillation, left-ventricular dysfunction, and had a bad case of sleep apnea. In addition to the sleep apnea disrupting my nighttime sleep (due to lack of blood supply to the brain), I fell asleep frequently in less than optimal places. Unfortunately, I often fell asleep behind the wheel while driving. But, the weight and sleep apnea problems still were not enough to get my attention. You know when your parents say, "Don't eat so much or you'll explode?" Well, I did. My legs split open and fluid was just flowing out of me. This got me to the hospital, where I was in CCU [Critical Care Unit] for 12 days and ICU [Intensive Care Unit] for 9 days. I lost alot of weight, especially water weight—97 pounds in 27 days of hospitalization! You can't lose that much weight that fast without being real sick with congestive heart failure. My heart was no longer able to pump the fluid out of it.
>
> Forty-eight hours after my hospital discharge I walked into the Rice Diet Program. The Rice Diet Program and my new friend, Mike, saved my life. Mike, my walking mentor, pushed me to exercise when I hated it. Now I must admit I truly enjoy it. I am so grateful that I prioritized my life over my excuses, and stayed long enough to really realize that a salt-free, low-fat vegetarian diet is what I must eat for life. Literally, for life!
>
> I learned a lot about my eating addiction when I stopped taking the hotel shuttle to the Rice Diet Program and got my own car. Within the first week, I found myself turning into a Burger King, and later that same day into a McDonald's. I gained 5 pounds the next day, and 4 pounds the following day—9 pounds in 2 days! This made me really start to fully appreciate how important it is for me to stay conscious about my sodium

intake—talk about a trigger food! My only weakness now is for Chinese soup, which I make at home from very-low-sodium chicken bouillon, but I occasionally eat it in restaurants, as well. Although I know it is one of the saltiest things I could ever eat, I find that I am more successful with my program if I *sometimes* get what I really want. If I plan for it, I do not feel guilty, and the next day I return to my no-salt, low-fat, vegetarian lifestyle choices.

My future is bright. I have now lost 220 pounds in 10 months! I am very optimistic about my future success; I have a specific game plan. I plan to continue to lose 1 to 2 pounds per week, but I have made a promise to myself that I will return to the Rice Diet Program if I gain 10 pounds. My plan also includes returning here two times per year for the next 2 to 3 years. Although you may wonder why I don't just go "do it" rather than depend upon the Rice Diet Program, I realize I am facing a life-long addiction that has taken more of my time and money than this place will ever see. It takes a while for this level of healing, and re-energizing follow-ups are key to my game plan. I am dedicated to seeing my goals successfully realized.

Sally lost a phenomenal 185 pounds within 12 weeks at the Rice Diet Clinic. (But don't get too excited about this weight loss rate; it is important for you to know that no one loses this much weight, this fast, unless they are very sick, probably in severe right heart failure.) Sally understands that she nearly died of obesity, and proudly speaks about the miracle that has taken place:

For years I handled my job well, but took no time for myself. I was on automatic pilot and it got a little worse each year. Until one fateful day I found myself literally on the pavement after a fall in my office parking lot. At 608 pounds I could not get up. My sheer mass would not allow it. I was totally helpless. A few people who passed by could not help me either. Eventually a crowd gathered and I was so ashamed. Then somebody called the paramedics and they, with great difficulty, got me on my feet. They wanted to take me to the hospital, but I refused. It was only then that I knew that I was in big trouble, and I needed to make a radical change. I had to do something, and do it now. I decided to come to the Rice Diet Program. It was an intuitive or a spiritual thing that led me here. It was a gift and I was determined to make the most of it. Little did I know what I would find.

My prayer when I fell was, "God, I'll do anything. Please help me." I suppose I would have admitted I was Catholic had someone asked, but I had not stepped foot in a church in twenty years, so I was not calling out God's name out of familiarity or friendship. I only prayed under duress. It took me being flat on my face to admit I was out of control, and in need of Someone's help who was more in control than me. It was not until I was bedridden from my fall, and struggling to finish my "to do" list before leaving for the Rice Diet Program, that I even noticed my list included "priest." I didn't even remember writing it. Later, when my sister was trying to help me pack from my list, she asked me what "priest" meant. I told her I wasn't sure but that it seemed like since I was going to be leaving for so long, and I was so scared, it couldn't hurt to go to confession. When the priest she brought tried to anoint me with oil, I freaked because I thought that meant I was on my deathbed. He explained that since the early '60s at the Second Vatican Council, the anointing, called the Sacrament of the Sick, was made available for the sick to be healed as well. Later during my confession, I told him something I hadn't spoken out loud in twenty years. The release was incredible; I cried and cried. When he laid his hand on my head, I felt a flood of heat throughout my body and a total reassurance that was indescribable. The fear and uncertainty about my trip to the Rice Diet Program was gone. At that moment I truly understood forgiveness. I no longer wanted to live in yesterday or tomorrow, but could live for today. That day I knew I was on my way to recovering my physical health, as well as inner healing.

If the Greek adage is "Know Thyself," I was not even barely acquainted. I was out of touch with my feelings. When I felt something, regardless of what it was—sadness, happiness, anger, or joy—I ate. It had been a long, long time since I had felt anything. But, eating the simple foods on the Rice Diet three times a day, seven days a week, gave me no other choice but to feel my feelings again. I realized it was not food I was after. I was using food to fulfill other needs.

I really had not begun to come to terms with how much things in my past were affecting my response to the present. For example, as a child, there was always a lot of fighting in my family. Yet everything was slippery and never spoken about in an up-front kind of way. My father was an alcoholic and my mother took on raising us seven kids with very little money. Life was a constant battle. Supper time was a good time. A time when everybody instantaneously made up. The food seemed to make everything OK. Things in my family never got worked out, but I was finally starting to re-examine the comfort I was attempting to find in my food as an adult.

The groups offered at the Rice Diet Program really helped me gain a much deeper understanding of why I was doing what I was doing with food. And I believe that awareness of truth was the first big step out of the abyss. It is not over until it is over, but I am still losing weight at home, and have plans to follow up my investment in myself with a ten-day rejuvenation period at the Rice Diet Program this spring.

Kate is another patient who made a change in her life by trusting in a Higher Power. Here is her story:

I hope you don't think I'm crazy when I say that I heard God speak to me, but I did, and I might as well admit it. I was raised without a mother or a father, and God spoke to me and said that if I don't lose the weight I would not live to see my youngest son graduate from school. Around the same time I was hearing God say this, my family and I went to the beach for our summer vacation. I was unable to swim because I was too ashamed to be in a swimsuit or shorts with all my weight. Although I was at poolside, I feared I wouldn't be able to save my son even if he was drowning. At that point, I told God I was turning it over to Him because I could not do it by myself. I had been on every new weight loss program that had ever come out. I would lose the weight and then typically gain it back, and an extra 20 pounds. It was the following week that I found out about the Duke University Rice Diet Program. I have now lost 138 pound in the last fifteen months, with the medical staff's constant encouragement and my family's support. With my renewed energy and obvious progress, it has been easier than I would ever have imagined.

Despite that, I have had to learn some hard lessons and suffer some losses besides my weight. Being from a family with twelve children, I never liked to be alone. I first began walking in the mall with friends, but soon they deserted me, and God taught me that dieting is a lonely business. I also lost my best friend, who eventually admitted to me that she was jealous that I was getting so much smaller than she. But, my comfort is that God is my best friend, and He won't leave me. Although my husband never was particularly interested in my losing weight, he is now excited by the improvement in the quality of life I can now enjoy. My five-year-old is now enjoying a bike-riding partner, whereas my previous two children had a mother that was on the sidelines, an onlooker. I missed a lot of life with them. My family is just so happy to have me be all that I can be.

Robert is a nationally renowned psychologist who learned how to perceive and respond to life differently, after decades of trying to teach others. Years after he participated in the facilitation of the "Just Say No To Drugs" campaign championed by Nancy Reagan, he admitted that he had no idea how to "just say no" to his own addictions. In fact, he did not know he had an addiction—to thinking he could control his own life and the lives of others—until everything fell apart. Here is how he tells it:

> I came to the Rice Diet physically, emotionally, and spiritually bottomed out. I had hypertension, a recent history of successive congestive heart failures, and arrhythmias, and had ballooned up to 320 pounds. Between the excessive weight and the osteoarthritis in my left hip, I had lost almost all flexibility and ability to move. I was almost paralyzed with pain not only for these physical reasons, but also due to the emotional pain of my son committing suicide. I now know I was trying to eat myself to death to join my son. I was just so ashamed. I literally hobbled in with two canes. My referring doctors wanted me to lose some weight so that I could have hip surgery.
>
> But, you should see me dance the Lindy now, without the supposedly needed surgery! Six years later, at age sixty-seven, I am going strong. I'm the coordinator for narcotics and drug education for a school district, and the executive director for my own drug prevention agency. I have swum almost daily for the last six years, and I do weights and treadmill a couple of times per week. I am also still enjoying my vegetarian diet. And probably most important, I journalize daily. I am enjoying my own self-esteem and that ability to say no to myself, and yes to the Twelve Steps.
>
> Dr. Kempner showed me how to lose weight and Dr. Rosati taught me how to keep it off. Dr. Rosati and Kitty were just starting the Twelve Step-type groups at the Rice Diet Program when I arrived. Although I had just left three and a half decades of leading groups professionally, I knew that I was "hitting bottom" and had to at least show up. It was during that year of intense introspective journalizing and attending these groups that I finally learned the meaning of surrender.

I still periodically review the informational and spiritual components that I learned at the Rice Diet Program. They are like the cheeks of one behind; both are so important.

Let me share a recent journal entry: "Thank you Lord for my life and breath, clarity of mind, and freedom from pain. Thank you for your ongoing reality checks. Thank you, Lord, for all the people and things you have given me. Thank you for all that and those you have taken away. Thank you Lord for all that and those you have blessed me with. I am still insecure about certain thoughts and feelings. I surrender these and the upcoming concerns for today."

Finally getting to where I could thank God for giving and even taking away my son was the ultimate test of surrender. It took away all my self-pity. Until I got to this part of the healing process, I tended to get stuck in thinking about what I was missing, and then was truly missing the three kids I had left. But, that is over, thank God, and now I am really free to live my life.

4

LOWERING YOUR RISK OF HIGH BLOOD PRESSURE

High blood pressure strongly increases your risk of congestive heart failure and vascular disease and thus your risk of heart disease, stroke, and kidney disease. High blood pressure, also called hypertension, is considered one of the "big three" risk factors for heart disease, along with smoking and high cholesterol. But it's *the* biggest risk factor for strokes. Hypertension can be sneaky. Many people have it for years and don't know it until they have a heart attack, or stroke.

Fortunately, in the past two decades, many more people with high blood pressure have become aware of their condition before it did too much damage. Unfortunately, most of these patients are told to "reduce their sodium or salt-shaker use," but told in the next breath that they must now be on medications for life. Few are told the empowering fact that a dietary approach like the Heal Your Heart Program nutrition plan would likely enable them to control their symptoms quickly, for as long as they stayed on the plan, without ever needing medications.

Why am I against medications? After all, many people find it easier to pop a pill than to change their lifestyle habits. Well, in addition to frequent unpleasant side effects from these medications (sexual impotence in men is one of the most common side effects), only about half of those who take these medications succeed in lowering their blood pressure below 140/90. This blood pressure level is still considered high, and increased risk of heart disease occurs long before this level is reached. So, as with other heart disease risk factors, the Heal Your Heart Program will help you see how low you can go *naturally*.

"NORMAL" vs. "IDEAL" BLOOD PRESSURE

In our society, it is considered "normal" for a person's blood pressure to rise with age. But this gradual raising of blood pressure does not occur in societies that typically eat a low-fat and low-sodium diet, such as people in New Guinea, Venezuela, and Botswana, as well as unacculturated populations in the Pacific islands, Africa, Australia, and Central and South America.

What can we learn from these other cultures? The message is that we don't have to accept higher blood pressure as we age. A diet that is very low in sodium, and fat can bring existing blood pressure down or, even better, prevent it from going up in the first place.

While most doctors won't consider your blood pressure "high" until it reaches 140/90, I feel that the lower your blood pressure the better off you are. Is there a danger in going too low? It's true that if your blood pressure were too low you would not feel well; the first symptom is usually dizziness upon standing. But it is very rare that your blood pressure would ever get too low, even on a no-salt-added vegetarian diet.

So what do the blood pressure numbers mean and what should your blood pressure goal be? The *systolic* pressure (the top number) is the highest degree of pressure reached in the body's arteries when the heart pumps. The *diastolic* pressure (the bottom number) is the measurement of the pressure when the heart relaxes between beats. In 1992, the National High Blood Pressure Education Program (NHBPEP) released new classifications for blood pressures. This marked the first time a blood pressure classification system used the systolic as well as the diastolic pressure in assessing the severity of hypertension.

The new guidelines also emphasized the belief that there is no precise or distinct line between normal and abnormal, since the risk of death and disability from heart attack and stroke increase progressively with higher levels of pressure. They defined a systolic blood pressure between 130 and 139 and a diastolic between 85 and 89 as "high normal," followed by four stages with progressively higher blood pressures. They defined a systolic blood pressure between 120 and 129 and a diastolic blood pressure between 80 and 84 as "normal," and a systolic blood pressure less than 120 and a diastolic less than 80 as "optimal."

As usual, I take this even further, recommending that your best health goal should be a systolic pressure of less than 110 and a diastolic pressure of less than 70. While I agree with the NHBPEP that the line between normal and abnormal is not distinct, I think we need to go much farther in educating ourselves on the advantages of being well below "normal." In this case, "normal" does not mean healthy. Having a normal blood pressure means rather, that you share the normal blood pressure of an American, who is likely to suffer from premature heart disease and stroke. People in the "normal" and "high normal" ranges still suffer more than one-third of the preventable deaths caused by above-optimal blood pressures. If you add these with blood pressures in the "normal" and "high normal" ranges to those in the "high" blood pressure range (50 million), about 80 percent of Americans aged thirty-five or older have blood pressures that increase their risk of both heart disease and stroke! This is an epidemic that lifestyle changes can cure.

THE ORIGINAL RICE DIET AND BLOOD PRESSURE

Dr. Walter Kempner's Rice Diet was the first to treat hypertension with a low-sodium, low-protein, and high-potassium regimen. This was back before blood pressure-lowering medications were available, so patients were highly motivated to adhere to such a prudent diet plan. Their choice was to stick to what was then a monotonous and unimaginative diet or to die prematurely. Given these choices, the diet was an inspiring option!

Dr. Kempner's many studies, confirmed by others, showed that very low sodium and protein intakes could not only treat malignant hypertension (very high blood pressures), but could also help reduce the problems that result from these diseases, such as papilledema (swelling of the optic nerve often due to hypertension), hemorrhages (bleeding in the eyes), exudates (leaking of plasma from the blood vessels), and heart failure. Today, when so many are dependent upon pills to cure their ills, it may be difficult to imagine the response of thousands with malignant hypertension and kidney disease who realized that by following the Rice Diet they could reverse their disease and associated problems, rather than go untreated and likely die before the age of forty. Dr. Kempner's Rice Diet Program truly marked the birth of dietary therapy in the treatment of chronic diseases.

The most amazing part of this story is that the same diet could work today, but most patients are given medication instead. This may be the "easier" treatment, but medications often have side effects, such as raising uric acid, cholesterol, triglyceride, and blood sugar levels; lowering potassium levels; and creating problems with impotence. And choosing to treat their blood pressure with only medications rather than significant lifestyle changes usually leaves patients with many other problems.

As with all the modifiable heart disease risk factors, true and lasting healing of your blood pressure problem requires assessing the potential root causes, then embracing the numerous improvements needed in your lifestyle, including: nutrition, exercise, and spiritual renewal. I believe that you will be most successful only if you address all three of these areas. Simply eliminating added sodium in your diet may "fix" your hypertension for the moment, but with life's inevitable curve balls, continued success seems quite dependent upon some ongoing form of stress management and spiritual centering.

Again, I feel I should caution you that this program can produce profound results. I recommend that you consult with your doctor before embarking on these changes, and be sure not to change your medications without your doctor's advice.

YOUR BLOOD PRESSURE AND YOUR DIET

The Heal Your Heart Program nutrition plan will lower your blood pressure, lower and faster than you ever thought possible, by natural means. The plan works because it is very low in sodium, fat, and alcohol, and high in potassium, antioxidants, fiber, and phytochemicals. (Phytochemicals are non-nutritive substances in plants that provide health-protective effects.) Why low fat as well as low sodium? It's true that fat doesn't raise blood pressure directly, but limiting it will help you achieve or maintain a lean weight, which is very beneficial for your blood pressure. Let's examine the connection between blood pressure and salt, potassium, and other nutrients and food factors.

Hypertension and Salt

Although hypertension is, at least in part, inherited, it is most significantly influenced by sodium intake over a lifetime and particularly during the first few years of life. Studies have shown that blood pressure rises with age in societies where salt is traditionally added to food. In populations that do not add salt to food, blood pressure does not rise with age.

Many patients are told to reduce their salt usage by limiting sodium intake to 2,000 to 4,000 milligrams per day, but this amount is still far too high, as it produces very little improvement in blood pressure. I prefer to counsel people to reduce their sodium intake enough to produce impressive results, which will resolve the root of the problem rather than mask it. Experiencing significant results is also the biggest inspiration for continuing on the program.

The Rice Diet is the lowest-sodium nutrition plan that has ever been practiced in an out-patient setting, and its effectiveness has been proven for longer than any in the world. On Phase Two of the Rice Diet (the stage that inspired the Heal Your Heart Program nutrition plan), patients are served a diet that contains a variety of fruits, vegetables, whole grains, and beans, and provides less than 250 milligrams of sodium per day. Then, if and when their blood pressure and other symptoms reach optimal levels, they are allowed foods from the animal kingdom, such as fish and skinned chicken breast, but they still eat less than 500 milligrams of sodium a day. Since animal products contain significantly more sodium, are higher in calories and fats, and are more likely to be overeaten than vegetable products, I recommend you eat exclusively from the vegetable kingdom until your blood pressure and other risk factor goals have been reached.

How Much Sodium Do We Really Need?

Our bodies do need *some* sodium to function. The average American consumes 4,000 to 7,000 milligrams of sodium per day. The average cardiologist and dietition recommend 2,000 to 4,000 milligrams of sodium per day for people with high blood pressure. Both of these amounts are far more than is necessary for our bodies. In fact, the National Research Council's latest edition of the Recommended Dietary Allowances stated that 115 milligrams of sodium per day is a minimum average requirement for adults. Because of the wide variation of patterns of physical activity and climatic exposure, we at the Rice Diet Program counsel patients that they can go a bit higher than that, but should consume no more than 500 milligrams per day.

The bottom line is: the lower your sodium intake, the lower your blood pressure and the lower your risk of congestive heart failure, heart disease, stroke, and kidney disease.

It is difficult to justify adding salt to food once you realize salt's correlation not only to hypertension, but also to kidney and heart disease, diabetes, congestive heart failure, obesity, and osteoporosis. But, the good news is that salt is an *acquired* taste. Most of us were trained from infancy to like it, but we *can* retrain our taste buds to prefer foods without salt—it takes approximately two months—and teach the next generation about the preventive benefits of a salt-free lifestyle.

The Importance of Potassium

There is considerable evidence that a potassium-rich diet can keep your blood pressure low, or lower existing high blood pressure. Recommendations by the National Research Council for increased intake of fruits and vegetables would provide approximately 3,500 milligrams of potassium per day—a level that could significantly reduce the prevalence of hypertension and stroke. The Heal Your Heart Program nutrition plan provides plenty of potassium; if you follow this plan you will not have to worry about getting enough potassium. Most fresh fruits and vegetables and dried beans and peas are impressive sources of potassium. I stress *fresh* fruits and vegetables because the canning process destroys significant amounts of potassium, so fresh or frozen produce is much preferred to canned, even the no-salt-added canned varieties. The southeastern part of the United States has the highest incidence of hypertension in America, not only because of a high-fat and high-sodium diet (from favorite processed meats like fat back, bacon, and sausage) but also because of this region's high consumption of canned foods.

A word of warning: patients with kidney or liver ailments often need to limit their potassium, as well as their protein and sodium intake. So if you have one of these conditions, consult with your doctor and consulting nutritionist or Registered Dietitian for specifics on how to do this safely. Animal products are very high in potassium, as are some fruits, vegetables, and legumes. Chapter 7 provides more details.

Many people use salt substitutes when trying to control high blood pressure. It's worth noting that the ones that actually taste salty contain potassium chloride rather than sodium chloride. For most of us, their use would help us consume more needed potassium. But they can be very dangerous if you need to avoid potassium. Ask your doctor before using them. Note that a few of the Chinese recipes in this book contain a minimum amount of the potassium-chloride-rich very-low-sodium bouillons, so avoid these products if your doctor tells you to limit potassium.

Other Dietary Ways to Lower Blood Pressure

While it is most beneficial to your blood pressure for you to concentrate on a low-salt, low-fat (thus low-calorie), high-potassium diet, there are also other nutritional factors to keep in mind.

We are now fairly certain that antioxidants (Vitamins C, E, and beta carotene, a precursor of Vitamin A) help reduce our risk of heart disease by preventing plaque formation (see Chapter 2 for a full discussion), and they may also work to preserve the function of our blood vessel linings and help control our blood pressure. But, we are even more certain that eating foods rich in antioxidants is more beneficial than taking antioxidant supplements. This may be because these foods are also low in sodium and calories, and high in potassium, fiber, and substances called phytochemicals, such as those found in garlic and onions. These factors may actually provide more benefit than the antioxidants themselves.

Fiber also has the potential to control blood pressure. Although soluble fiber's most impressive contribution to preventing and reversing heart disease has been its ability to significantly lower cholesterol and blood sugar, it has also been shown to lower blood pressure. Here again, it may not be so much the fiber itself that is beneficial, but everything that comes with it. High fiber foods tend to be lower in fat, calories, and sodium than foods lower in fiber, and the reduction of these factors can help bring about weight loss, which in turn helps lower blood pressure. See Chapter 2 for a more detailed discussion of soluble fiber.

Fish is one of the few exceptions to the good advice to lower our caloric, fat, and sodium intake as much as possible to lower blood pressure. Although the cholesterol-lowering effect of fish has been rather inconsistent, its ability to lower triglycerides and blood pressure has been more impressive. If you have a history of heart disease, stroke, or elevated blood pressure, seafood can help—and is the only meat you can really justify.

Magnesium and calcium are other nutrients that have been researched extensively with respect to their blood pressure-lowering potential, the results have been less than convincing. Although heart attacks and strokes are less common in areas with hard water, which is high in magnesium, the research on its ability to lower blood pressure has been disappointing. In fact, the better the study, the clearer it is that magnesium supplementation does not effect blood pressure. The previous rumors that calcium would lower blood pressure have also proved less than newsworthy; only small effects have been noted with large doses.

However, there is strong and consistent scientific evidence that limiting alcohol intake will lower blood pressure. The research also shows that one alcoholic drink is not a problem, but two or more alcoholic drinks per day can substantially raise your blood pressure. So instead of turning to alcohol to wash the day's cares away, why not look into healthy alternatives, such as exercise and other stresss management techniques?

EXERCISE AND YOUR BLOOD PRESSURE

Regular exercise can be tremendously beneficial for preventing and treating high blood pressure. Sedentary and physically unfit people with "normal" blood pressures have a 20 percent to 50 percent increased risk of developing high blood pressure than their more active and fit peers. One of the most significant benefits of exercise is that it helps us achieve and maintain a healthier weight. In the Trials of Hypertension Prevention (*Journal of the American Medical Association,* 1992) the participants who lost an average of eight pounds through caloric restriction and modest exercise cut their risk of high blood pressure in half. Exercise can also prevent your blood pressure from increasing with age. More specifically, moderate-intensity aerobic exercise, like brisk walking, hiking, cycling, or swimming may actually be better than high-intensity workouts.

Regular aerobic exercise not only benefits your weight and blood pressure, the psychological advantages cannot be overestimated. The natural release of endorphins from aerobic activity is a healthy alternative to stimulants and depressants, such as caffeine and alcohol, which can raise blood pressures in addition to providing a psychological boost.

SPIRITUALITY AND YOUR BLOOD PRESSURE

You have probably heard of or even practiced stress management techniques to reduce blood pressure, but you may not have associated such practices with spirituality. Chronic stress can be managed fairly effectively through certain short-term relaxation techniques, such as biofeedback, deep breathing exercises, and other behavior modification practices, but long-term resolutions of stressful perceptions and responses more often come from a deeper inner exploration of self and a sense of purpose in life. I use the word "perceptions" because I think it is important to note that stress is not due to outside demands so much as it is a result of how we choose to respond to different challenges or stimuli. A certain crisis could be perceived by one person as the worst thing that could ever happen, while another person could receive a great deal of satisfaction in dealing with the challenge. How can you become the person who responds positively? There are a variety of answers. Here I'll discuss the connection between blood pressure and your psyche, and recommend some behavior modification strategies for immediate stress reduction, then offer some deeper inner healing paths which can help you examine why you respond in stressful ways and see how spiritual growth can inspire you to choose to respond differently.

The Mind-Body or Soul-Spirit-Body Connection

The "mind-body connection" is a popular catchphrase for the growing awareness that physical disease is not separate from our mental or thought processes. But I also firmly believe that we are more than mind and body. No doubt our mind effects our body, but so do the other components of our soul: emotions, will, and subconscious, as well as what I call our indwelling spirit. (See Fig. 2.1.) These inner components of self can all affect our physical responses and thus our health. Understanding this may inspire you to more seriously commit to stress management techniques and spiritual disciplines.

One of the main ways that our emotions produce direct physical responses in the body is through the *autonomic nervous system*. This incredible mechanism, which is actually two systems, enables our body to respond to many situations without conscious awareness. The *parasympathetic system* builds up the body and stores energy. Its functions include stimulating the organs that digest and assimilate food by dilating the blood vessels that supply these organs and at the same time slowing the heart and lowering the blood pressure. The *sympathetic system* prepares for quick release of energy, assisting the body to react to emergencies. Both of these parts of the nervous system originate in the *hypothalamus,* a part of the midbrain near the head of the spinal column.

The sympathetic system organizes the "fight or flight" response to danger or perceived danger. A complex chain reaction begins with a chemical discharge into your pituitary, which then alerts your adrenals and other glands to spread the command. Immediately the blood vessels to your stomach and intestinal areas are shut down, and blood is instead sent to the brain, lungs, and external muscles, where it will be needed for the escape or fight response. Your heart and lungs are stimulated to move fuel and oxygen faster; the bronchial tubes relax, admitting more oxygen. Your liver and other storage depots are directed to release carbohydrates as quickly utilizable blood sugar. And while your blood pressure and heart rate rise, the clotting time of your blood decreases as the body prepares itself for a possible wound or injury.

So this sympathetic system can prove invaluable if a bear is charging you, but can actually be disease-producing in modern industrialized societies where it is "falsely" activated all day long by pressures on Wall Street or the IRS, in traffic jams, or just from the frustrations of living. These obvious stresses stimulate the sympathetic nervous system, and so will your fears and resentments—even when you are not consciously aware of being afraid or angry.

Morton Kelsey, in his book *Psychology, Medicine and Christian Healing* (Harper & Row, 1988), shares not only the most well-researched account of this subject, but also rich practical wisdom from his personal counseling experience. He reports how aggressive emotions—resentment, hostility, or hatred—set the sympathetic nervous system in motion, as do more passive responses like concern, apprehension, anxiety, and an active emotional withdrawal. He states that: "Anger and fear are strangely similar; indeed they are opposite sides of the same coin. Both are reactions to a threatening situation. In anger we feel that we can meet the threat by attack, while in fear we feel that we are inadequate to deal with it and must run away or freeze, but the physiological response is almost identical."

So whether the stress is mental or emotional, conscious or unconscious, your body's response is the same. Meanwhile, the parasympathetic system is trying to return the body to "business as usual" but as long as you are consciously or unconsciously telling your body that you are not at peace, you can be contributing to your emotional, and thus physical, dis-ease.

Most of us have by now lived long enough to have experienced moments of awareness, when something we were thinking or feeling suddenly became conscious to us. But, you can be affected by the subconscious long before it is brought to your conscious awareness. In fact, research suggests that accidents are also highly correlated with emotional dis-ease, and likely the subconscious. When Flanders Dunbar and her associates were looking for a group of "normal," healthy people with whom to compare diabetic and heart patients, they chose as their control group some patients who had been admitted to the hospital because of accidents. They were amazed to find that the accident patients were on the whole more disturbed than other patients. Morton Kelsey comments, "What easier way to avoid meaninglessness than to let one's unconscious psyche produce an interesting or even fatal injury?" Carl Jung also observed that frequent physical injury often reflects inner conflict just as much as frequently hurt feelings. Unfortunately, some people have used these observations to blame afflicted people for their own ailments. My intention in sharing these ideas is not to blame anyone who is sick or suffering, but to help you bring your root issues to light, so that your connectedness of body, soul and spirit can be healthy and whole.

STRESS MANAGEMENT STRATEGIES TO TRY TO EXPLORE

1. Follow the Heal Your Heart Program nutrition plan as closely as you can. Give it your best try for at least a month to prove to yourself whether it is worth the effort to keep your diet this low in fat and sodium. You can handle stress more successfully if you are properly nourished and fueled!

2. Make a commitment to avoid any substances that are less than healthy, such as alcohol, tobacco, caffeine, and foods that trigger you into overeating. You may think these substances temporarily relieve your stress, but in the long run they promote disease. Keeping a food intake record (either Appendix C or D) can help you stay conscious of your success with this commitment.

3. Follow the Heal Your Heart exercise plan, which will prove to be a great stress reducer. The endorphins released during aerobic exercise really will make you feel better within minutes.

4. Do whatever it takes to insure yourself sufficient time for sleep. Your body needs sleep to process the day's stress. Insufficient sleep is a setup for emotional and physical dis-ease.

5. Periodically assess whether your life is balanced in a healthy way. Consider these factors:

   ❖ connection with your Higher Power or spiritual development
   ❖ care of the soul: reading, journalizing, meditating, and yoga
   ❖ relationships (quality time with family and friends)
   ❖ career and financial security
   ❖ physical health: nutrition, exercise, and rest
   ❖ social and cultural service

   Take the time to rank the amount of time you devote to these areas of your life, from 0 to 10, on the Wheel for Seeking Balance shown in Figure 4.1. You may want to photocopy this wheel so

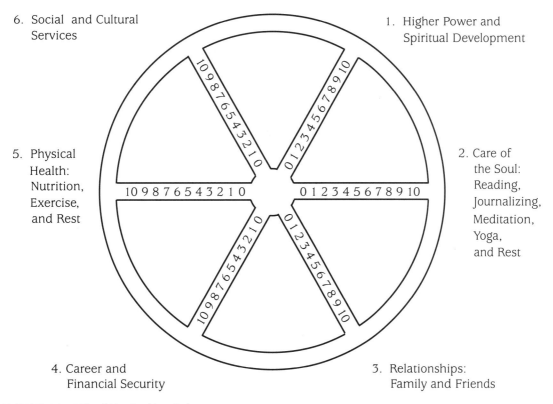

FIGURE 4.1 Wheel For Seeking Balance

that you can use it for periodic re-assessment of the balance in your life. Circle the numbers corresponding to the various areas in your life. A 0 would imply you neglect this area of your life, and 10 means you give it all the attention you think it needs. The lesson to be learned is that the wheel doesn't roll if any of these areas of your life are neglected or ill-attended. This wheel was inspired by a very successful Rice Diet participant, Morris Weisner, who appreciates how much planning and evaluation it can take to achieve balance in our lives. In addition to having fun with all of these everyday ventures, remember to regularly schedule vacations. Vacations are good for the body, soul, and spirit, and it is important to schedule them rather than waiting until you collapse, to slow down.

6. Seek healthy physical encounters, as touch can be healing. Dr. James Lynch, in his book *The Broken Heart* (Basic Books, 1977), reported on the power of human contact in healing not only the physical aspects of heart disease but also the emotional. And, of course, "the laying on of hands" has been a Christian healing tradition practiced since Jesus's example. Fortunately, this is now practiced in a growing number of churches, advertised as "healing services" weekly or monthly. As with other areas, there are many people gifted with healing power who do not hold an advanced psychology or divinity degree, or practice their gift within a center for organized religion. Personally, I have received physical, emotional, and spiritual healing via hands-on healing from priests and other believers, as well as from accomplished "body workers" or massage therapists. It is important to seek recommendations from friends whose spirituality you share or respect, and interview or get to know the healing practitioner first. Use your discernment.

7. Research available stress management courses or intensive workshops in your area. An ideal course would be similar to the one that Drs. Redford and Virginia Williams teach at the Rice Diet Program, where the behavioral characteristics that are correlated to heart disease are outlined and many behavior modification techniques to remedy them are taught, along with time to practice the techniques.

8. Seek a teacher, preacher, or rabbi to instruct you in a form of meditation that feels right for you. Although Chapters 2 and 10 describe the practice researched by Dr. Herbert Benson, which was found to lower blood pressures effectively, it is important to trust

your instincts on which method feels best to you. The "relaxation response" brought on by meditation, which is the opposite of the "fight or flight" response, can be evoked through many other techniques such as yoga, biofeedback and tai chi. Here, as with all of these introspective avenues, it is of utmost importance to feel that the teacher and the teaching strategy will honor your religious or spiritual orientation.

9. Develop a practice of prayer and faith. Read Dr. Larry Dossey's book *Healing Words* (Harper, 1993) to further convince your left brain (your analytical self) of the importance of prayer. Read Richard Foster's book *Prayer: Finding the Heart's True Home* (Harper, 1992) for inspiration for the spirit and soul. Also, commitment to a regular group practicing their faith may also prove to be emotionally, spiritually, and physically rewarding. In a large study in Evans County, Georgia, those who reported frequent attendance at church enjoyed lower blood pressures than did those who attended less often. You may also want to consider scheduling renewal retreats periodically (see Appendix B). Search your heart for which spiritual groups or associations are best for you, and once you find them, be dedicated in your commitment to them.

10. Join a community or group for support. This can not only increase your odds of surviving a heart attack, but it can also help you improve your quality of life considerably. Groups can offer you an invaluable environment in which to practice truly listening to others (without simultaneously practicing your brilliant response!) and learn to really feel and then articulate your feelings. This opportunity can be found in a cardiac rehabilitation support group, a Twelve Step group (such as Overeaters Anonymous, Codependents Anonymous, Adult Children of Alcoholics, to name a few) or any confidential group where you feel safe. If the group is already established, be sure to assess whether they are willing to share honestly from the heart and are not in the practice of "fixing" each other. Dr. Jerry Jampolsky's Attitudinal Healing groups, which are now found throughout the world, have been a profound inspiration for thousands ready to *perceive things differently* (see Appendix B). Finding the right group may, like many things in life, take a little shopping around; but take the time to seek and you will find what is right for you.

11. Keep a journal. There are many different approaches to this, but if you are interested in pursuing one of the best-known techniques,

try Progoff's Intensive Journal Process (see Appendix B). *The Power of Your Other Hand* (Newcastle Publishing Co., Inc., 1988) outlines a technique of journalizing with your nondominant hand to help access right brain function, or intuitive, introspective insights. It has also proven to be a pivotal tool for many who have tried it.

Although I believe that all of our answers lie within ourselves, and that in time, if we are open to them, they will be revealed to us, I think few of us slow down long enough to know ourselves. There are many other paths to get to know oneself and our higher power, but these techniques will provide a variety of ways for you to contemplate and explore. Note that the "Wheel for Seeking Balance" (Figure 4.1) prioritizes our spiritual development and care of the soul before all of our physical concerns. We need to seek our own inner healing before we can function at our best in our relationships with family and friends, in our careers, with our nutrition and exercise plan, and in serving others.

PART TWO

YOUR PERSONAL HEAL YOUR HEART PROGRAM

❖ ❖ ❖

5

ASSESSING YOUR HEART'S HEALTH

In this chapter and the next, I'll be showing you how to adapt the Heal Your Heart Program to your own specific needs. You'll learn how to assess your heart disease risk factors, and then, in Chapter 6, you'll discover how to turn that information into the best action plan for you.

YOUR HEART HEALTH PROFILE

There are modifiable and nonmodifiable risk factors for heart disease. You should be aware of both kinds and tailor your program to suit your own risk factors.

The modifiable risk factors include high total cholesterol, high LDL, low HDL, high blood pressure, high blood sugar, high triglyceride (if cholesterol is also high), excess weight, and tobacco use. If you don't do anything else recommended here, please stop smoking.

Of course, if you have already had a heart attack, that statistically increases your risk of another, unless you make significant lifestyle changes immediately. Other signs and symptoms of heart disease are also risk factors, such as angina (pain in the chest, shoulders, and arms), claudication (pain in the legs), congestive heart failure, an electrocardiogram that shows you have left ventricular hypertrophy (an enlarged heart muscle), and a history of atrial fibrillation (irregular heart beats). If you have any of these, you need to follow the strictest, lowest-in-fat version of the Heal Your Heart Program.

You can easily keep track of your modifiable risk factors by having a full lipid panel (meaning your blood is tested for cholesterol, LDL, HDL, and triglycerides), and your blood pressure and weight assessed. If you have not had this done in the past month, you should do so before starting this program. Not only do you need this information to tailor the Heal Your Heart Program to your own needs, but it is always more inspiring to continue on with your plan if you have a starting point from which you can compare your progress periodically.

The nonmodifiable risk factors are those that we have to accept: age and a family history of heart disease. Many people also include sex and race in this category but these are more tenuous. I'll explain why below. But if you are a man forty-five years old or older, or a woman fifty-five or older, or have experienced heart disease, or if a first-degree male relative less than fifty-five years of age or a first-degree female relative less than sixty-five years of age has died suddenly, you need to be extra careful.

AGE AND YOUR HEART

Many people think that heart disease is an old person's problem, and that the young do not need to worry about it. Neither is true. In fact, heart disease progresses throughout our lives if we live the traditional western lifestyle.

An estimated 36.5 percent of American youth age nineteen and under (26.7 million young people) have cholesterol levels of 170 or higher. Unfortunately, most people are not concerned with their cholesterol until they are middle-aged, or worse yet, until they have their first painful signs of heart disease. But simply not having symptoms of heart disease does not mean young people don't have to worry. An autopsy study of twenty-two-year-old soldiers killed in the Korean War, published in the *Journal of the American Medical Association* (1955) reported that 77 percent of the American men already had significant levels of atherosclerosis (plaque in their arteries). The researchers contrasted these sobering findings with the virtually nonexistent levels of atherosclerosis in the Asian males of the same age. Unfortunately, in developed nations we consider cholesterol to be "normal" for years until the arteries feeding the heart are approximately 70 percent blocked, and then more blatant physical signs of heart disease start to get our attention. Clearly it would be easier to prevent it in our youth than to try to change our lifestyle radically at middle-age.

That said, your advancing age should also not be an excuse to accept higher cholesterol levels or blood pressure. While it is "normal" for these to rise with age, "normal" is not healthy. You can maintain a low cholesterol level and low blood pressure no matter what your age, by making the appropriate adjustments in your lifestyle. Both young and old would benefit by maintaining a healthy nutrition plan, exercising moderately, and keeping their lives spiritually whole.

If You Have a Family History of Heart Disease

You may be thinking, "I have inherited some bad genes for heart disease, so it may not be worth all this effort." Let me assure you that having a genetic propensity gives you all the more reason to cut your fat and cholesterol intake dramatically and bring your cholesterol level to less than 150. Your family history need not be your fate if you do this.

This is not just my overly zealous opinion; it has been shown true for many different populations. In China, where people typically consume grains and vegetables and can't afford our higher-fat food, they enjoy cholesterol levels that are typically 100 to 150, with an average around 127, and heart disease is almost unheard of. Similar trends have been noted in many populations who typically eat very-low-fat diets, and have very low cholesterols, including the Bantus of Africa and the indigenous people of Brazil and New Guinea. The New Guinea natives enjoy cholesterols of about 100 that do not increase with age. And, studies of twenty-five other societies with similar diets have shown the same cholesterol results.

RACE, GENDER, AND OTHER FACTORS

Again, you may be thinking that the low instance of heart disease among Chinese has no meaning for you if you're not Chinese. But a major study has helped dispel the concern that race, vocation, climate, or nationality could exclude any of us from claiming these wonderfully low cholesterol and heart disease rates. This was the International Atherosclerosis Project, completed in 1965. In more than 22,000 autopsies in fourteen countries over a five-year period, pathologists found that the artery surface area damaged by plaque and overall plaque damage was directly proportional to both blood cholesterol levels and how much fat and cholesterol was eaten.

Other studies have shown that people who typically enjoy a low cholesterol level and thus low risk of heart disease will lose these advantages if and when their diets become higher in fat. A major study of Japanese who migrated to Hawaii and California found a threefold increase in heart disease rates within a generation in those who moved to California, and a twofold increase in those who moved to Hawaii. This unbiased effect of fat intake on cholesterol has also been seen on their home turf as well. In the past forty years Japanese fat consumption has increased from 10 to as much as

25 percent of calories (thanks to Western influences), and the heart disease rates have gone from almost nonexistent to about a third of the American rate. This certainly seems to indicate that lifestyle has a much stronger influence than race in your risk of heart disease.

Many people still falsely assume that women have a genetic blessing that protects them from heart disease. While it is true that women's higher levels of estrogen prior to menopause are associated with their relatively high levels of HDL, if a woman has undesirable cholesterol levels, her body will still develop plaque. It is just likely to cause symptoms later than it would in men. In fact, studies show that women's cholesterol levels are higher than men's from age twenty to thirty-four and from age fifty-five up. Another likely protective factor for females is that menstruation reduces the iron in their blood, and high iron levels have been associated with higher rates of heart disease. So lower iron levels likely slow the buildup of plaque as well.

But these protective factors are temporary, and shouldn't be relied on. Unfortunately, women catch up with men with respect to their incidence of heart disease soon after menopause, and many of their statistics quickly look worse. For instance, at older ages, women who have heart attacks are twice as likely as men to die from them within a few weeks; and 44 percent of women, compared with 27 percent of men, will die within one year after having a heart attack. Even more sobering, 63 percent of women who die suddenly of heart disease have had no previous evidence of disease, compared to 48 percent of men. Given this, it seems sensible to act preventively rather than bank on any sex-specific exemptions.

How to Tailor the Program to Your Risk Factors

Having reviewed your risk factors, you have a better sense of where you stand with heart disease, and the degree of change you need to achieve to enjoy the goals you seek. The most proactive approach to selecting your version of the program is to look at your risk factors and design your plan of action accordingly. Although each of the risk factors has been deemed a powerful enough predictor of heart disease to be considered and respected individually, they are certainly of greater concern when you have two or more of them. If you have heart disease or more than one risk factor for heart disease, go straight to the less-than-10-percent reversal guidelines outlined in Chapter 6. On the other hand, if excess weight is not your problem and a less than optimal blood pressure is your only risk factor, follow the guidelines for less than 500 milligrams of sodium—this will probably lower your blood pressure sufficiently within the first week.

In other words, read the chapter in Part I on your risk factors and see what is the main thing you need to do to produce results. Thus, for all risk factors except blood pressure, the lower your fat intake the faster and more assuredly you will reach your goals. If you have no risk factors, and want to stay that way, you may find that the 20 percent fat prevention guidelines will be the best plan for you.

Another strategy you might try is to follow the strictest approach for fat, sodium, and calories until you reach your goal, then try increasing these slightly if you think having a little more olive oil or fish will help your long-term compliance. The more years I work with heart patients and those struggling with overeating tendencies, the more convinced I am of the wisdom of this approach. Embracing the lower fat guidelines religiously for at least a month, then re-assessing your risk factors, will convince you more effectively of the power of this diet than anything I can say. It is actually much easier to stick with something that really works than to try to adhere to a less strict plan that would produce a fraction of the results.

Chapter 6 will give you the specifics on designing the Heal Your Heart Program that is perfect for you.

6

Designing Your Personal Heal Your Heart Program

While the general parameters of the Heal Your Heart Program are beneficial for everyone, you can tailor the program to your specific needs. This chapter will show you how to adapt each of the three areas, nutrition, exercise, and spirituality, to your own health goals and level of comfort.

Heal Your Heart Nutrition Guidelines

The following section will outline the nuts and bolts of the Heal Your Heart nutrition plan. You will gain a much clearer idea of how all of the nutritional specifics, such as fat, cholesterol, and calories translate into "allowances," or servings, of real food. You will also gain a firmer handle on just how much sodium, sugar, and fiber are desirable in general, and in particular for various special conditions. The summary of vitamin and mineral supplements will help you decide if these are right for you as well. This plan will show you how many allowances, or servings, you can eat per day of starch, vegetable, fruit, protein, dairy, and fat. At first, this allowance approach takes a little effort as you learn what foods go in what groups and the basic serving sizes. But it quickly becomes an easy way not only to be sure you limit your calories, fat, cholesterol, sodium, and sugar, but also to be sure you get enough of the good things, such as fiber and antioxidants. All this is built into the plan. Most people agree that learning this system is far easier than they imagined, and well worth the initial effort. Once you document your consumption for a week or two on your Food Intake Record with Allowances (Appendix C), you will start ''thinking in allowances.'' You'll begin to know automatically that your intake is appropriate on a given day and you will not feel a need to count calories, grams of cholesterol and fat, and milligrams of sodium.

How Much Fat You Can Eat

If you have heart disease, the Heal Your Heart nutrition plan allows you to eat no more than 10 percent of your calories from fat. This amount will likely get you the fastest and best results. If you are simply trying to prevent heart disease, you can go closer to 20 percent, although 10 percent certainly won't hurt! Needless to say, the more risk factors of heart disease you have, the more reasons you have for consuming less fat.

Following a vegetarian, 1,000 to 2,000-calorie nutrition plan is the easiest way for you to ensure that your fat intake is low enough. But, if you are interested in calculating your total fat intake, Table 6.1 will help you determine how many grams of fat you can have per day to attain your fat goal. It lists the amount of fat you can eat for different calorie amounts. (You'll be calculating your calories later in this chapter.) I have given a range of percentages, but if you have heart disease, stick to the 10 percent figure. Remember that this guideline for fat includes the grams naturally occurring in the whole foods you are eating, not just the grams of fat noted on the packages of processed foods. You can purchase an inexpensive pocket-size

❖ TABLE 6.1   TOTAL GRAMS OF FAT IN 10–20% FAT NUTRITION PLANS ❖

TOTAL CALORIES	FAT GRAMS FOR 10% FAT	FAT GRAMS FOR 15% FAT	FAT GRAMS FOR 18% FAT	FAT GRAMS FOR 20% FAT
1200	13	20	24	27
1300	14	22	26	29
1400	16	23	28	31
1500	17	25	30	33
1600	18	27	32	36
1700	19	28	34	38
1800	20	30	36	40
1900	21	32	38	42
2000	22	33	40	44

fat gram counter in most bookstores and at many grocery stores to help you figure out how much fat you are consuming.

Your body does need *some* fat to function. But the average person needs to consume less than 14 grams of fat per day to meet the daily requirements of essential fatty acids. This amount of fat can be found naturally in seven $\frac{1}{2}$-cup servings of starchy foods, without adding any oil. Don't worry that you won't be getting enough fat: essential fatty acid deficiencies are not a reported problem in anyone consuming a varied diet.

How Much Cholesterol You Can Eat

The American Heart Association recommends that you consume no more than 300 milligrams of cholesterol a day. But nine studies have shown that this amount produced a progression of atherosclerosis, meaning that 300 milligrams can still clog your arteries. Considering that the average American man and woman consume about 360 and 260 milligrams a day, respectively, and that one in two die prematurely of heart disease, I recommend that you eat less than 100 milligrams of cholesterol a day if you are truly serious about preventing or recovering from heart disease.

A cholesterol intake of less than 100 milligrams per day would bring about a significant drop in most people's blood cholesterol as well as reducing other risk factors. While ambitiously low enough for most healthy people, it is still generous enough to allow you to enjoy fish daily if you wish. Less than 5 milligrams of dietary cholesterol per day and less than 10 percent of calories from fat were two of the lifestyle changes that inspired a reversal of atherosclerosis in 82 percent of Dr. Dean Ornish's research participants. I allow slightly more dietary cholesterol than this because the foods that contribute the extra cholesterol have not been shown to aggravate risk factors of heart disease, and in fact are major components of the Mediterranean diet, which results in very little heart disease. To be more specific, I allow nonfat dairy and yolk-free egg products, as well as seafood (this is known as a lacto-ovo-pesce-vegetarian plan), because I have seen this plan produce dramatic results during my more than fourteen years of counseling heart patients. I have also personally practiced this nutritional lifestyle for more than twenty-five years. My professional and personal experience has been that more people are able to enjoy and stick to this type of vegetarian diet long term.

Does Dietary Cholesterol Affect You?

While the 100-milligram recommendation is generally a good idea for everyone, some people may be able to exceed the amount safely, while others would benefit from excluding all cholesterol from their diet. Research suggests that eating foods with cholesterol can elevate the blood cholesterol of one in four to five people, but does not raise cholesterol levels in most people. If you want to find out whether dietary cholesterol affects you, you can do a simple experiment, which only requires discipline. Begin by eating strictly vegetarian foods—in other words, grains, beans, fruits and vegetables—until you reach your ideal weight and your cholesterol level is less than 150. Then begin to eat 3 ounces of shellfish daily for approximately two weeks. I recommend shellfish for this test because they are one of the highest sources of cholesterol, while being one of the lowest animal sources of saturated fat. Eating saturated-fat-rich food during the testing period will make your results invalid. Also try to be sure that your stress level and weight remain fairly constant throughout the testing period.

After the two weeks, test your cholesterol again at the same lab. It is important to use the same lab, since cholesterol testing is not as accurate as most would think. You can only imagine how inaccurate it might be to compare values from different laboratories.

If your blood cholesterol levels go up significantly after this test, you are sensitive to dietary cholesterol. This means that you should continue to keep your cholesterol intake less than 100 milligrams per day, avoiding shellfish and other cholesterol-rich foods, while monitoring your cholesterol levels regularly. It would also be to your advantage to avoid all animal products except for nonfat dairy products, which have had most of their cholesterol and fat removed.

If your cholesterol does not go up after this test, you can enjoy cholesterol-rich foods as long as they are low in saturated fat. Shellfish is one of these foods. You need not concern yourself with staying under the 100-milligrams-a-day recommendation, because the Daily Food Allowances defined in Tables 6.2–6.7 will ensure that. As none of the nutrition plans outlined for you there allow for more than 3 ounces of meat per day, it would be difficult to exceed the 100-milligram cholesterol goal if you are limiting your meat intake to seafood. The only possible exception would be if you ate shrimp almost every other day, so try not to have shrimp more than once a week.

Finfish is a healthier seafood choice most of the time, not only because it is lower in cholesterol, but also because it tends to have fewer toxins than shrimp or other bottom feeders. And remember to continue to monitor your blood pressure and weight, as any animal product contains more sodium and fat than most vegetarian foods.

If you are not sensitive to dietary cholesterol, your blood cholesterol is less than 150, and your blood pressure and weight are ideal, you can enjoy fish as often as you like. If you follow one of the 10 to 20 percent nutrition plans, you will keep your total fat and sodium intake low enough to prevent other health problems. (The only exception to this may be people with liver and kidney disease, who may need to avoid all animal protein. If this applies to you, check with your doctor.) If you really want meat, you can add lean cuts of poultry and even the leaner red meats at least a month after your cholesterol sensitivity test. Be sure you test your cholesterol within a month of eating these foods so that you will know your body's response to the additional saturated fat intake. As long as your cholesterol level and other risk factors do not go up, you can eat what you want. If your blood cholesterol goes higher than 150, you should not consume any meat other than fish.

If you get one high cholesterol reading, try looking at a few readings over a six-month period and average them, observing a pattern rather than being worried about a 5-point difference that is statistically insignificant. Physical stresses, such as pregnancy and emotional stresses, such as those caused by shift work, or tax and exam time, can significantly elevate your cholesterol reading. I have also seen cholesterol readings rise when a person loses substantial weight. This is because fat we lose does not evaporate; part of it circulates through our bloodstream, often elevating significantly before a noticeable drop occurs. On the other hand, catabolic states, such as cancer, heart attacks, infections, and a variety of other diseases may be accompanied by lower lipid levels. These are only a few of the many factors that may affect your analysis, so be sure to ask your prevention-oriented cardiologist or dietitian to translate your individual lab findings.

I strongly recommend that you follow the order of this test, first cutting *all* foods with cholesterol and then adding them back in gradually, rather than trying to cut back on cholesterol-rich foods slowly. That approach will not tell you as easily if you are cholesterol sensitive. An Overeaters Anonymous participant once agreed with my strategy for other reasons. She said, "If you don't want to fall down, don't go to slippery places." I have yet to meet anyone who achieved significant reductions in saturated fat and cholesterol intake by trying to eat smaller portions of steak, fried foods, gravy, or cheesecake. Typically those who succeed in reversing heart disease do so by committing to vegetarianism first, then adding other foods when their risk factors are in the healthy range.

How Much Salt You Can Have

The low-sodium aspect of the Heal Your Heart nutrition plan sets it apart from many other cardiac diets. It follows the Rice Diet "going home" recommendation of less than 500 milligrams of sodium a day. In Phase

I of the Rice Diet, patients begin by eating less than 50 milligrams of sodium, then Phase II allows 250 milligrams of sodium. After that, if and when their risk factors reach optimal levels, foods from the animal kingdom, such as fish and skinned chicken breast are allowed, still keeping sodium intake to less than 400 milligrams a day. Because animal products have significantly more sodium, are higher in calories and fats, and are more likely to be overeaten than vegetable products, it is advantageous to eat exclusively from the vegetable kingdom until blood pressure, cholesterol, and weight goals are reached and kidney and liver tests are normalized.

Our bodies do need some sodium to function, it's true. But most Americans, even those on so-called low-sodium diets, consume far more than is necessary or healthy for our bodies. The National Research Council's latest edition of the Recommended Dietary Allowances states that only 115 milligrams of sodium per day is a minimum average requirement for adults. In consideration of wide variations in patterns of physical activity and climatic exposure, I feel a safe minimum intake is 500 milligrams per day.

How Much Sugar You Can Eat

It's important to your plan that you limit your refined sugar intake. Sugar has 16 calories per teaspoon, which is not a large amount. It's the sugar-loaded sweets that are really harmful. In addition to providing extra calories, leading to weight gain, refined sugars are harmful because they can elevate triglyceride and blood sugar levels, increase dental caries and inspire binge eating. Sugars are considered "empty" or "wasted" calories because all sweeteners basically offer *no* nutrition (except for molasses, which is very high in minerals). Syrups and ingredients ending in *-ose* mean sugar and should be avoided or strictly limited. Some new products, such as those made by Health Valley, are sweetened only with fruits and fruit juices. This is preferred since you would be getting a *little* nutrition from the fruit and some fiber from the fruit purees.

As 4 grams of sugar = 1 teaspoon = 16 calories, limit yourself to cereals with 6 grams or less per serving of sucrose and other sugars.

How Much Fiber You Should Eat

Eat primarily whole foods that are high in fiber to get at least 25 grams of total dietary fiber per day. Fiber is one area where more is better. If you can get up to 50 grams without exceeding your calorie limit, you may be even better off. But a good general recommendation is that you would be getting plenty if you eat dried beans or peas four to fourteen times per week, and eat whole grains rather than processed ones most of the time. That general rule of thumb will ensure sufficient fiber, especially when consumed in addition to the six or more allowances of fruits and vegetables built into every nutrition plan.

How Much Protein You Can Eat

In industrialized countries, consuming excessive protein is by far a greater problem than is protein deficiency. Grown adults do not really need more than 25 grams of protein per day, and there are at least 35 grams of protein available in the lowest-calorie, lowest-percentage-of-fat nutrition plans outlined in Tables 6.2 to 6.7. Protein from vegetable sources is really the only protein you need. So if you eat a variety of grains, beans, and vegetables, you will get more protein than you need. Animal protein, even with all fat removed, can raise cholesterol levels in your blood, which is one of the many reasons I consider vegetable protein of higher quality than animal protein.

How Many Calories You Can Eat

If counting calories helps you maintain a healthy weight, by all means do it. First complete the following worksheet: How Many Calories Do You Need?, then continue to find out how to convert your calorie and fat needs into servings of different food groups per day. This method is actually much simpler than dealing with the unending hassle of counting calories in every food consumed. Once you learn how to convert your calories into allowances, and do so for a week or two, you will have a valuable tool for life that will automatically help you eat in a balanced way while meeting all your prioritized goals.

Although many people like this kind of structure to help improve their nutrition, specifics are not for everyone. If the details overwhelm you, skip to the 1200 Calorie, 12% Fat, Sample Day and the Sample Week Menus 1 to 3, which follow Tables 6.2 to 6.7 to get a general idea of how tasty this nutrition plan can be. Or, if many of the recipes look too complicated for you now, be sure to try the 15-Minute Meals section in Chapter 14, Recipes with Results.

Losing one to two pounds per week is plenty if you are following the program at home. If you are getting frustrated with your inability to lose more than one pound per week, try reducing your calories further while increasing the calories you expend through exercise.

How Many Calories Do You Need?

Follow these steps to assess how many calories you should eat per day to meet or maintain your weight goal.

1. Find the best weight for your height and frame. The formulas below are for the midpoint of a healthy weight range, but your ideal weight may be plus 10 percent if you have a large frame, and minus 10 percent if you have a small frame. (To determine your frame size, wrap your thumb and middle finger around the narrowest part of your wrist: Large = fingers do not touch; medium = fingers touch or overlap; small = fingers overlap $\frac{1}{2}$ inch or more.)

    a. Women: 100 pounds for first 5 feet
                     +_____ (5 pounds for each additional inch)
    b. Men: 106 pounds for first 5 feet
                     +_____ (6 pounds for each additional inch)

2. Determine your activity factor. Pick the number that reflects your current exercise level and weight status most closely. If you are two or more pounds over or under the weight assessed as ideal in Step 1, use the "overweight" and "underweight" figures. If less than two pounds from your ideal weight, consider yourself at "ideal" weight.

	Sedentary	Moderate	Very Active
Overweight	10	11	12
Ideal	13	14	15
Underweight	16	18	20

3. Calculate your caloric energy needs. Multiply your healthy body weight from Step 1 by your activity factor from Step 2.

Healthy body weight × Activity factor = Energy Needs

_____ × _____ = _____

4. Adapt the number to fit your weight goals. If you want to maintain your weight as it is, enjoy the number of calories you calculated in Step 3. If you want to lose or gain weight, take the number you calculated in Step 3 and adjust for your weight goal as shown below. But also remember that it is easier and healthier to lose weight and keep it off by eating less and exercising more!

To Maintain Weight: Keep same caloric level calculated in Step 3, unless you want to change exercise habits. If you want to increase or decrease your exercise regimen, increase or decrease your caloric intake an equivalent amount.

To lose 1 pound per week:

| _____ | − | 500 Cals. | = | _____ |
| Caloric need (from Step 3) | | | | Calories allowed |

To lose 2 pounds per week:

| _____ | − | 1000 Cals. | = | _____ |
| Caloric need (from Step 3) | | | | Calories allowed |

To gain 1 pound per week:

| _____ | + | 500 Cal. | = | _____ |
| Caloric need (from Step 3) | | | | Calories allowed |

In addition to adding 500 calories per day, you should also increase muscle resistance exercise to gain weight.

Your final number is the approximate amount of calories you should eat per day to achieve your weight goal.

When you achieve your weight goal, you can stabilize your weight by eating a few extra allowances, or servings, preferably from food groups other than protein and fat. If you want to do this more scientifically, go back to the calorie worksheet and redo it with your new data. If you reached your ideal weight and now have to add some calories back in to maintain that weight, you may want to do this gradually by adding just a few hundred calories more per day. You could first see what an extra 280 calories per day would do by adding two more starches and two more fruit allowances. After a week, weigh yourself again. Equations are good general guides, but every individual's metabolism is different, so your body will teach you as much as any equation as you get more and more conscious of energy intake and energy expenditure.

Calories and Your Daily Food Allowances

Now that you know how many calories you should consume each day, let's go over *how* these should be distributed from different food groups

❖ TABLE 6.2   NUTRIENT CONTENT OF FOOD GROUPS ❖

FOOD GROUP	CALORIES	CARBOHYDRATE	PROTEIN	FAT
Starch	80	15	3	1–2
Vegetable	25	5	2	—
Fruit	60	15	—	—
Protein	55	—	7	3
Dairy	90	12	8	Trace
Fat	45	—	—	5

to provide the most well-balanced intake. Table 6.2 summarizes the caloric and macronutrient contents of the different food groups that are the basis of the Heal Your Heart Program nutrition plan. Chapter 7 will provide details on what specific foods are in each of these groups. Tables 6.3 to 6.7 then show you how many allowances of the various food groups would provide for 1,000-, 1,200-, 1,500-, 1,800-, and 2,000-calorie nutrition plans containing from 7 to 18 percent of their calories from fat. (Although my general recommendation for fat intake is less than 10 percent for heart disease reversal and less than 20 percent for prevention, I use 7 to 18 percent in these tables in order to give you whole allowances, rather than suggesting fractions, such as $1\frac{1}{2}$ teaspoons of oil and $2\frac{1}{2}$ ounces of meat.) Look up the amount of calories that your worksheet showed you can consume and then find the amount of fat you can have. Then

❖ TABLE 6.3   DAILY FOOD ALLOWANCES PER CALORIE LEVEL 1,000-CALORIE PLAN ❖

		NUMBER OF SERVINGS				
FOOD GROUP	% FAT	5	7	9	13	15
Starch ($\frac{1}{2}$ c.)		8	9	7	7	6
Vegetable ($\frac{1}{2}$ c.)		3	4	4	3	4
Fruit (1 pc.)		3	3	3	3	3
Protein (1 oz.)		0	0	1	1	2
Dairy (1 c.)		1	0	1	1	1
Fat (1 tsp.)		0	0	0	1	1

❖ TABLE 6.4   DAILY FOOD ALLOWANCES PER CALORIE
LEVEL 1,200-CALORIE PLAN ❖

FOOD GROUP	% FAT	NUMBER OF SERVINGS				
		7	9	11	12	17
Starch ($\frac{1}{2}$ c.)		11	9	9	7	8
Vegetable ($\frac{1}{2}$ c.)		5	3	4	5	3
Fruit (1 pc.)		3	4	3	4	3
Protein (1 oz.)		0	1	2	3	3
Dairy (1 c.)		0	1	1	1	1
Fat (1 tsp.)		0	0	0	0	1

follow down the appropriate percent fat column to learn how many "allowances" from each food group you can have per day.

Your Food Intake Record with Allowances (Appendix C) may help you choose the best plan to start with. For example, let us say you have calculated your caloric need to be 1,200 calories to reach your goal of one pound weight loss per week. And since you have high cholesterol and a family history of heart disease but no heart disease yourself, you choose a 12 percent-fat nutrition plan. As the guidelines in Table 6.4 show, this 1,200-calorie, 12 percent-fat nutrition plan would contain 7 starches, 5 vegetables, 4 fruits, 3 proteins, 1 dairy, and 0 fat allowances.

❖ TABLE 6.5   DAILY FOOD ALLOWANCES PER CALORIE
LEVEL 1,500-CALORIE PLAN ❖

FOOD GROUP	% FAT	NUMBER OF SERVINGS				
		10	11	12	15	17
Starch ($\frac{1}{2}$ c.)		13	14	12	11	9
Vegetable ($\frac{1}{2}$ c.)		3	3	4	5	5
Fruit (1 pc.)		4	4	4	3	5
Protein (1 oz.)		0	0	1	3	3
Dairy (1 c.)		1	0	1	1	1
Fat (1 tsp.)		1	1	1	1	2

❖ Table 6.6   Daily Food Allowances per Calorie
Level 1,800-Calorie Plan ❖

		NUMBER OF SERVINGS				
FOOD GROUP	% FAT	10	11	14	15	18
Starch ($\frac{1}{2}$ c.)		17	13	15	14	13
Vegetable ($\frac{1}{2}$ c.)		5	3	4	5	5
Fruit (1 pc.)		4	4	4	4	4
Protein (1 oz.)		0	0	1	2	3
Dairy (1 c.)		0	1	1	1	1
Fat (1 tsp.)		1	1	2	2	3

But, after a few days of recording your food intake, you see that when you ate 3 ounces of fish, you relapsed into the old habit of ordering it fried! Try to see this kind of thing as a learning opportunity rather than as a failure. In this case, you may instead decide to try the 1,200-calorie, 7 percent-fat nutrition plan to avoid the temptation of eating fish until your cholesterol level goes under 150. You can then add fish back later with more awareness when you reach your cholesterol goal. You might then make a pact with yourself to enjoy only broiled, grilled or poached fish until you lose that last ten pounds you had targeted.

Keeping a record of your food intake can also help you stay in touch with foods and patterns that may be getting monotonous for you. The Sample Day Menu on page 103 will help you understand how to translate the daily

❖ Table 6.7   Daily Food Allowances per Calorie
Level 2,000-Calorie Plan ❖

		NUMBER OF SERVINGS				
FOOD GROUP	% FAT	10	11	12	14	15
Starch ($\frac{1}{2}$ c.)		20	18	19	17	16
Vegetable ($\frac{1}{2}$ c.)		4	4	5	4	5
Fruit (1 pc.)		4	4	4	4	4
Protein (1 oz.)		0	1	0	2	3
Dairy (1 c.)		0	1	1	1	1
Fat (1 tsp.)		1	1	2	2	2

food allowances (given your desired calorie level) into a typical day's worth of food. And the Sample Weekly Menus can help you avoid the pitfalls that so often send people back into their old, unhealthy habits. It has been shown that people who plan their menus in advance, and even create a corresponding grocery list in advance, succeed more with their weight loss and maintenance than those who do not.

The Sample Weekly Menus provide approximately 1,200 calories, with 5 to 16 percent from fat, and 121 to 494 milligrams of sodium per day. The recipes printed in italics can be found in Part Four. Of course, these menus, as well as the recipes themselves, are not carved in stone; they are for you to use as an example of how delicious and fulfilling a nutrition plan this low in calories, fat, and sodium can be.

❖ 1,200-CALORIE, 12% FAT, SAMPLE DAY ❖

MEAL & TIME	FOODS EATEN/PORTIONS/PER CUP, TBS., OZ.	FOOD ALLOWANCES
10/5 Breakfast 7:15 am	¾ cup nonfat/no-salt cold cereal 1 cup skim milk 1 piece of fresh fruit 2 tablespoons of raisins	1 starch 1 dairy 1 fruit 1 fruit
Lunch 12:30 pm	1 cup of *Refried Beans* 10 no-fat/no-salt corn chips ⅔ cup of *Kitty's Sassy Salsa* ½ cup of spinach 1 piece of fresh fruit	2 starches + ½ vegetable 1 starch 1 vegetable 1 vegetable 1 fruit
Dinner 7:00 pm	3 ounces of *Blasting Blackened Red Snapper* 1 medium baked potato (1 cup) 2+ cups of *My Favorite Vegetable Salad* 2 tablespoons of *Dijon Vinaigrette* 1 slice of *Basic Whole Wheat Bread* 1 piece of fresh fruit	3 proteins 2 starches 2 vegetables ½ vegetable 1 starch 1 fruit

	STARCHES	PROTEIN	VEGGIE	FRUIT	DAIRY	FAT
Daily Food Allowances	7	3	5	4	1	0
Allowances Eaten	7	3	5	4	1	0
Difference	0	0	0	0	0	0

❖ Sample Menu: Week 1
1,200-Calorie Menu ❖

	Sunday	Monday	Tuesday
Breakfast	• 3 *Heart Healthy Hotcakes* • ½ C *Wonderful Pancake Topping*	• ¾ C oatmeal • banana	• 3 *Heart Healthy Hotcakes* • ½ C *Wonderful Pancake Topping*
Lunch	• 1½ C *Berry-Barley Fruited Salad*	• Tuna salad sandwich • ⅔ C raisins	• 1½ servings *Grilled Gourmet Vegetables* • 2 C pasta
Dinner	• 3 oz *Grilled Gourmet Vegetables* • 6 oz grilled tuna • ¾ C brown rice	• *Super Swift Spaghetti with Polenta* • *My Favorite Vegetable Salad* • 2 T *Dijon Yogurt Vinaigrette*	• *My Favorite Stir-fry w/ Almonds* • 2 oz Quinoa
Daily Values	1,177 calories 16% cals. from fat 175 mgs. sodium	1,205 calories 10% cals. from fat 121 mgs. sodium	1,206 calories 16% cals. from fat 195 mgs. sodium

Supplements and Your Plan

I recommend a basic multivitamin with the Heal Your Heart Program nutrition plan, especially if you are consuming less than 1,500 calories. Most affordable multivitamin/mineral pills seldom have 100 percent of the twelve vitamins and eight minerals for which there are United States Recommended Daily Allowances (U.S. RDAs). So you should buy a basic, inexpensive multivitamin-mineral pill and then buy individual supplements for any nutrient you are concerned about.

For example, a U.S. National Institutes of Health panel now states that calcium intake should be higher than the current RDA for selected age groups. For women at menopause, 1,000 milligrams with estrogen replacement, or

---

Average Daily Value: 1195 calories, 13% calories from fat, 215 mgs. sodium
C = cup; t = teaspoon; T = tablespoon; oz = ounce

Wednesday	Thursday	Friday	Saturday
• $1\frac{1}{2}$ C *Berry-Barley Fruited Salad*	• 1 oz no-fat/no-salt cold cereal • 8 oz skim milk • banana	• 1 C melon • 1 slice *Basic Whole Wheat Bread*	• $\frac{3}{4}$ C *Angelic Ambrosia* • $\frac{2}{3}$ C Health Valley granola
• *Veggie-stuffed Potato*	• *Refried Beans & Salsa w/ Chips* • *My Favorite Salad* • 2 T *Dijon Yogurt Vinaigrette*	• *My Favorite Stir-fry w/ Almonds* • $\frac{3}{4}$ C brown rice	• *Spontaneous Pizza* • *My Favorite Salad* • 2 T *Dijon Yogurt Vinaigrette*
• 2 C *Pasta w/ Escarole & Beans* • *An Italian Finalé Salad* • 2 T *Dijon Yogurt Vinaigrette*	• 2 C *Prudent Potato Latkes* • *My Standard Steamed Veggies* • 1 C applesauce	• *Salmon Black Bean Burrito w/ Cucumber Salsa* • 1 C *Mexican Bean Salad* • $\frac{1}{2}$ C *Banana Cream Kahlua*	• 2 servings *Vegetable Fried Rice* • *Bean Sheet Salad* • *Spicy String Beans*
1,182 calories 13% cals. from fat 243 mgs. sodium	1,182 calories 5% cals. from fat 318 mgs. sodium	1,208 calories 13% cals. from fat 292 mgs. sodium	1,203 calories 16% cals. from fat 159 mgs. sodium

1,500 milligrams without estrogen is recommended. Women and men over fifty years of age are advised to increase calcium intakes to 1,500 milligrams. The increased recommendations are to improve bone and tooth health, and possibly help prevent colon cancer and hypertension. If you are consuming a diet as low in sodium and protein as outlined in this book, you need only about half this amount of calcium because you won't lose as much through your urine.

If you are still worried about osteoporosis, because of your nonmodifiable risk factors, a supplement of 500 to 1,000 mgs. will likely not create a problem for you. But, there are a few dangers of supplementing with calcium that you should be aware of. Large calcium intakes may cause calcium-based urinary tract stones to develop in people who are susceptible. Vitamin D, which is often packaged with calcium to enhance absorption, can be toxic; more than 20 micrograms of vitamin D should not be taken without a doctor's recommendation to do so. Calcium carbonate, found in most antacids, may cause constipation, while calcium gluconate, or "chelated calcium," may

❖ Sample Menu: Week 2
1,200-Calorie Menu ❖

	Sunday	Monday	Tuesday
Breakfast	• *Fat-free Oatbran Muffin* • 8 oz skim or soy milk • $\frac{1}{2}$ C blueberries	• $\frac{3}{4}$ C oatmeal • 5 prunes • $\frac{1}{2}$ grapefruit	• 1 oz no-fat/no-salt cereal • 8 oz skim or soy milk • fresh fruit
Lunch	• 1 C *Refried Beans* • $\frac{1}{2}$ C *Guaca-Asparagus* • $\frac{1}{4}$ C *Green Chile Cream Sauce* • 2 oz *Kitty's Sassy Salsa* • 1 tortilla	• veggie sandwich (lettuce, tomato, cucumber, peppers, etc.) • apple • 8 oz nonfat yogurt	• 1 C *Vegetarian Chili Immediato!* • $\frac{1}{2}$ C spinach • pear
Dinner	• 1 C *Outta Banks Seafood Gumbo* • $\frac{3}{4}$ C brown rice • $\frac{1}{2}$ C spinach • $\frac{1}{2}$ C *Banana Cream Kahlua*	• 2 C *Indian Subzi* • $\frac{3}{4}$ C brown rice • banana	• *Blastin' Blackened Red Snapper* • baked potato • *My Favorite Vegetable Salad* • 2 T *Dijon Yogurt Vinaigrette*
Daily Values	1,200 calories 9% cals. from fat 430 mgs. sodium	1,184 calories 10% cals. from fat 493 mgs. sodium	1,202 calories 8% cals. from fat 374 mgs. sodium

produce diarrhea. Other calcium-rich sources, such as bone meal, oyster shells, and dolomite, often touted in health food stores as "natural," can be contaminated with heavy metals, such as lead and mercury. Winston Craig's excellent summary of this subject in *Nutrition for the Nineties* (Golden Harvest Books, 1992) shared reports that calcium supplementation has re-

---

Average Daily Value: 1195 calories, 13% calories from fat, 215 mgs. sodium
C = cup; t = teaspoon; T = tablespoon; oz = ounce

WEDNESDAY	THURSDAY	FRIDAY	SATURDAY
• 1½ C Kashi (7 grain hot cereal) topped w/ banana & 1 t cinnamon	• 1 oz no-fat/no-salt cold cereal • 8 oz skim milk • 1 C berries	• bagel • 1 T tahini • 1 T sugar-free jelly	• *Huevos Con Frijoles Y Chipotles* • 1 slice *Basic Whole Wheat Bread* • ½ cantaloupe
• 1 C *Outta Banks Seafood Gumbo* • ¾ C brown rice • apple	• *Fat-free Oatbran Muffin* • *Swift Summer Fruit Plate*	• baked potato w/ salad bar • 2 T *Dijon Yogurt Vinaigrette*	• *Bayou Baked Bourbon Beans* • *Fastest Slaw in the West* • 1 piece *D'Liteful Cornbread* • fresh fruit
• 1 C *Southern Succotash* • *Carolina Cukes* • *Twice Baked Garlic Sweet Potatoes* • 2 slices *Basic Whole Wheat Bread*	• ½ C *My Favorite Marinara* • 2 C pasta • *An Italian Finalé Salad* • 2 T *Dijon Yogurt Vinaigrette*	• *Fool Proof Fish* • *My Standard Steamed Veggies* • fresh fruit	• *Gnocchi "via Mangione"* • ½ C *My Favorite Marinara Sauce* • ¼ C *Marinated Roasted Peppers* • 1 slice *Basic Whole Wheat Bread* • *Poached Pears w/ Pomegranate Sauce*
1,205 calories 8% cals. from fat 131 mgs. sodium	1,190 calories 7% cals. from fat 235 mgs. sodium	1,195 calories 16% cals. from fat 494 mgs. sodium	1,188 calories 7% cals. from fat 280 mgs. sodium

duced iron absorption by 50 percent, and also has been shown to interfere with the blood clotting action of vitamin K. Clearly it makes more preventive sense to minimize all your modifiable risk factors of osteoporosis (as outlined in Chapter 2) rather than expect megadoses of one of the risk factors, inadequate calcium, to solve your problems.

Also make sure your multivitamin/mineral supplement contains 400 IUs of vitamin D, or 100 percent of the U.S. RDA, since this will help you absorb calcium. Many older people consume inadequate amounts of vitamin D and

❖ SAMPLE MENU: WEEK 3
1,200-CALORIE MENU ❖

	SUNDAY	MONDAY	TUESDAY
Breakfast	• $\frac{3}{4}$ C *Rancheros Frittata* • $\frac{1}{2}$ C *Guaca Asparagus* • $\frac{1}{3}$ C *Refried Beans* • 1 tortilla	• $\frac{3}{4}$ C oatmeal with cinnamon & 1 tsp maple syrup • 2 T raisins • grapefruit	• $\frac{3}{4}$ C Kashi (7-grain hot cereal) • banana • 4 prunes
Lunch	• 1 slice *Basic Whole Wheat Bread* • 1 *Best "Burger" Out* • tomato, sliced • $\frac{1}{2}$ C arugala • no-salt mustard • $\frac{3}{4}$ C *Fresh Fruit Soup*	• $\frac{2}{3}$ C *Refried Beans* • fresh tomato, sliced • 2 slices *Pane Paesano* • $\frac{3}{4}$ C *Carol's Fruit Salad*	• *Legal Lasagna* • 1 C *An "Italian Finalé" Salad* • 2 slices *Pane Paesano*
Dinner	• *Legal Lasagna* • 1 C *An "Italian Finalé" Salad* • 1 slice *Pane Paesano* • $\frac{3}{4}$ C *Carol's Fruit Salad*	• $\frac{3}{4}$ C jasmine rice • *Stir Fried Grouper & Asparagus* • $\frac{1}{4}$ C *Kim Chee*	• $\frac{2}{3}$ C *"Boss" Black Beans* • 1 C *Fastest Slaw in the West* • 1 piece *D'Liteful Cornbread* •1 C *Icy Melon Delight*
Daily Values	1,205 calories 8% cals. from fat 419 mgs. sodium	1,198 calories 9% cals. from fat 158 mgs. sodium	1,210 calories 7% cals. from fat 165 mgs. sodium

do not get enough through sunshine (approximately ten to fifteen minutes per day).

If you are avoiding animal products or are more than six years old, you also need to be sure that your multivitamin includes 100 percent of the U.S. RDA for vitamin B_{12}. In fact, vegans (people who do not eat any meat or dairy) should be sure to get 6 micrograms daily, as a B_{12} deficiency can cause irreversible nerve damage.

Average Daily Value: 1206 calories, 9% cals. from fat, 230 mgs. sodium.
C = cup; t = teaspoon; T = tablespoon

WEDNESDAY	THURSDAY	FRIDAY	SATURDAY
• 2 oz. no-fat/no-salt cold cereal • 1 C strawberries • 2 T raisins	• *Swift Summer Fruit Plate* • $\frac{1}{3}$ C Health Valley Granola	• 1 slice toasted *D'Liteful Cornbread* • *Swift Summer Fruit Plate*	• 2 *Heart Healthy Hotcakes* • $\frac{1}{2}$ C *Wonderful Pancake Topping* • 1 C fruit & $\frac{1}{2}$ C cottage cheese
• $\frac{2}{3}$ C *"Boss" Black Beans* (in burrito) • 2 tortillas • $\frac{1}{2}$ C *Kitty's Sassy Salsa*	• 1 *Salmon Cake* • $\frac{3}{4}$ C jasmine rice • 1 C *Fastest Slaw in the West*	• $\frac{3}{4}$ C *Pasta Bean Pronto!* (using *"Boss" Black Beans*) • $\frac{1}{2}$ C *Lorraine & Maria's Garlicy Greens*	• $\frac{3}{4}$ C *Barbequed Tempeh on Quinoa* • *Grilled Gourmet Vegetables* • 1 C pasta
• 2 *Salmon Cakes* • baked potato • $\frac{1}{2}$ C *Okra & Onions* • $\frac{1}{2}$ C *Lorraine & Maria's Garlicy Greens*	• 2 C *Broccoli Rabe & Artichoke Stir Fry* • pasta • $\frac{3}{4}$ C *Carol's Fruit Salad*	• 1 *Sushi Roll - Vegetarian Style* • 2 oz *Kung Pao Fish* • $\frac{1}{2}$ C basmati rice • $\frac{3}{4}$ C *Spicy String Beans*	• $\frac{3}{4}$ C *Tortilla Soup* • 1 *Potato Enchilada w/ Chili Sauce* • $\frac{1}{4}$ C *Green Tomatilla Glaze* • 1 C *Delicious Jicama-Chayote Salad*
1,173 calories 11% cals. from fat 242 mgs. sodium	1,202 calories 9% cals. from fat 185 mgs. sodium	1,225 calories 9% cals. from fat 155 mgs. sodium	1,227 calories 13% cals. from fat 288 mgs. sodium

If you have heart disease, you may also want to consider taking an antioxidant supplement, although it is difficult at this point to make a blanket recommendation on these. It would certainly be safe for you to take these supplements at their U.S. RDA levels: 60 milligrams of vitamin C, 30 IU of vitamin E, and 5,000 IU of beta-carotene (which meets the U.S. RDA for vitamin A). But the average antioxidant blend has more beta-carotene than I can confidently recommend. Most researchers agree that the evidence is strong that 200 IUs of vitamin E and 500 milligrams of vitamin C would prove helpful for a heart patient. But the evidence is strongest that eating foods with these antioxidants is better than using supplements.

HEAL YOUR HEART EXERCISE GUIDELINES

Men under age forty and women under age fifty who are apparently healthy do not generally need to be evaluated before starting an exericse program. If you're a man aged forty or more or a woman aged fifty or more, you should discuss with your doctor the most appropriate evaluation and exercise program for you. You should also discuss exercise with your doctor if you have two or more risk factors for heart disease or any signs or symptoms of heart disease such as fatigue, ankle swelling, intermittent leg pain, or known heart murmur.

Exercising for Your Fitness Level

When we use our muscles in a new way, they can become sore. This soreness is different from acute pain you may feel during exercise. You can avoid soreness by breaking into your exercise routine gradually. Your body did not become out of shape in one week, and you can't get back into shape in one week—so don't rush it! Try starting with short periods of activity a couple of times a day. For example, if you know you can walk 15 minutes two times a day, start with that (even if your goal is to walk 30 minutes in one bout), then gradually work your way up to 30 minutes. Also, start at an intensity that is easy for you. The following descriptions can help you decide which category suits you best, and how to safely design your ideal plan.

If You Are Sedentary

If you have been unable or unwilling to exercise, or your exercise has been extremely limited, you fall into the sedentary category. Establishing an exercise pattern is more important initially than duration or intensity. Try walking or another low-impact exercise for 5 to 10 minutes, two times per day. Do this everyday for two weeks. Over the next two months, very gradually increase your duration to 30 minutes, once a day, and five to six times per week.

If You Are of Average Fitness Level

The average fitness level can be best characterized by someone who is able to go to work and to perform daily activities but doesn't go for walks of more than 10 minutes at a time. If you are at this level of athletic practice, you should start to slowly but surely increase your activity. Start with a low-impact exercise, like walking, for 10 to 15 minutes, two times per day. Here again, establishing a habit is more important than trying to break any records. Over the next two months, continue increasing your duration until you are enjoying a brisk pace daily for 30 minutes, five to six times per week.

If You Are Moderately Active

If you exercise occasionally, you fall into the moderately active category. ("Occasionally" means you may exercise as little as once to twice every two weeks. An exercise session consists of moderate to heavy physical activity for at least 20 minutes.) If you are in this group, you could start with 15 to 20 minutes of low-impact exercise, twice a day, and within two months be exercising for 30 minutes or more daily, five to six times per week.

If You Are Already Healthy and Active

Healthy active people are those on a regular exercise program. This means exercise three or more times per week for 20 to 30 minutes. If you are in this category, continue your exercise. If you aren't already, try to exercise at least five times per week.

What Activities Are Right for You?

There are different types of exercise or activity. For most people, and especially those concerned about their heart health, aerobic exercise is the best. Aerobic exercise includes activities that require an increase in oxygen intake and produce beneficial changes in the respiratory and circulatory systems. To achieve this increase in oxygen uptake involves continuous, rhythmic activity of the large muscle groups that is sustained for at least twenty minutes. Aerobic exercise reduces high blood pressure, fat weight, and diabetes symptoms, and increases HDLs. Thus, for overall disease risk reduction, aerobic exercise is top dog.

Many people ask, "If I had to choose one aerobic activity what should it be? For most people the answer is walking, for a variety of reasons. It is easily accessible and inexpensive and requires no special equipment or instruction.

This does not mean that strength and flexibility training aren't important. Strength helps you do all your daily activities. Strength training helps build muscle, maintain posture, and strengthen bones. Flexibility helps you use your strength and endurance. If you were very strong but couldn't move your arm because your shoulder joint was inflexible, you wouldn't be able to produce any work or have as much fun.

As we age, we may see a decline in strength and flexibility. Because we need these two attributes to move through the world, we miss them greatly when they are diminished. Fortunately, this age-related decline in strength and flexibility is somewhat reversible. Strength exercises and flexibility stretches can help even octogenarians. Regular strength training, stretching, and aerobic exercises are essential components of a well-rounded health regime for people of all ages, enhancing bone density, balance, strength, and cardiovascular fitness.

If You Have Physical Limitations

Physical limitations are barriers to performing daily activities with ease. Such limitations include arthritis or other joint problems, fibromyalgia, blindness, deafness, and injuries. If you have any of these, or other physical limitations, it is important not to let them limit you more than is absolutely necessary. Doing what your body will allow is crucial to maintaining and restoring your abilities, as well as preventing or recovering from a cardiac event.

If you have a physical limitation, ask your doctor about exercising in a pool. People tend to be more flexible in the water due to buoyancy. The water helps support you and your limbs so you are able to do more in water than on land. Many people who can't walk on land find that they can swim just fine!

If swimming doesn't thrill you, try walking in the water. Water walking requires little skill, but can give you a great workout. Although the water is forgiving on your joints and legs, it also gives you resistance as you walk through it. Water exercise can really strengthen muscles as well as the heart. Running can also be adapted to the water. There are several water running vests that keep you afloat in deep water, thus allowing you to stride with no impact. If you are just starting out, begin with walking, as water running is an intense workout.

If you enjoy the company of others and the leadership of a fitness expert, find a water aerobics class. The freedom you find in water may surprise you. Many folks who liked playing in the water as children rediscover their love of water as adults.

On dry land, you may find that stationary biking is tolerable when land walking isn't. Or you may need to do activities with just your arms. The main thing is to be creative, think of ways that you can be active, and then try them. If you have great discomfort during an activity, then it is not the best choice for you—at least not the way you were doing it. Try modifying the activity or try a different activity.

Cross-Training Is Not Just for Triathletes

Cross-training has been touted as the best way to prepare athletes for their competitions. The secret to the success of cross-training is injury prevention and well-rounded conditioning. These assets will work for you just as they do for more experienced athletes.

When you cross-train, you do different activities every workout. For true cross-training, you need to choose at least two activities, but there is no advantage to choosing more than four cross-training activities. For example, on Monday you might cycle. Tuesday, you might swim. Wednesday, you might stair-climb. Then, Thursday, you might go back to cycling. Generally, choosing only one high-impact activity, like running, is recommended. For your other activities, you should choose low-impact ones like walking, cycling, stair-climbing, and cross-country skiing. Other high- and low-impact activities are listed on page 114. You could also choose all low-impact activities. If you prefer, you don't *ever* have to participate in high-impact aerobic activities to make your heart healthy. All the benefits of exercise can be achieved through low-impact aerobic exercises with a decreased risk of injury.

You can also cross-train during one exercise session. You could exercise on the stationary cycle for 10 minutes. Then, move to the treadmill for 10 minutes, and finish with 10 minutes on the stair-climber. However, if you choose this type of workout, you need to move quickly to the next activity. If you have to wait in line for a piece of equipment, you will lose aerobic benefits.

When you cross-train, you are using muscle groups in different ways during the different activities. You tone different muscles and you reduce the repetitive stress on your muscles, joints, and bones. Using the same muscle group over and over again in the same manner is called repetitive stress. This can lead to over-use injuries such as shin splints, tendonitis, stress fractures, plantar fasciitis, and some back discomfort. Cross-training helps you avoid repetitive stress and eliminate injuries. Cross-training can also reduce boredom. Instead of doing the same old routine day in and day out, the varied challenges of cross-training can give you an increased sense of well-being.

How to Get Started

If you have already been exercising on a regular basis, great! Before starting your exercise regime, read over the following as a guide to your program and review the Quick Health and Safety Tips in Chapter 9. If you haven't been exercising, that's okay, too. Now you have an excellent opportunity to start, using the following exercise recommendations.

Choosing a Specific Activity or Activities

As discussed above, regular aerobic exercise is the best type of exercise for a healthy heart. To ensure you are getting a good healthy dose of aerobic exercise, gradually work up to 30 minutes of exercise five to six times a week.

When choosing activities that you would like to do for your exercise, consider whether the activities are low impact or high impact. High-impact activities are those most likely to cause injury. They require both feet to be off the ground or floor at one time. This increases the forces on your foot when you land on it. Increasing the forces absorbed through your feet increases the shock felt up your leg. Increasing shock can lead to injuries.

If you decide to choose a high-impact activity, also choose a low-impact activity and cross-train. Try not to do two high-impact workouts consecutively. Here are some examples of low- and high-impact exercises:

Low-impact	**High-impact**
Walking	Running
Low-impact aerobic dance	High-impact aerobic dance
Swimming	Jumping rope
Cycling	
Cross-country skiing	
Stair-climbing (machine)	
Water aerobics/walking	
Rowing	

You may have noticed that I didn't mention step aerobics. Although step aerobics falls in the low- to moderate-impact category, technique is crucial to avoid injuries. Many knee injuries have been caused by improper step height and the repetitive deep knee bending. If you are going to choose step aerobics, please cross-train with another low-impact activity. Try not to do two step aerobics classes on consecutive days.

Popular sports, like tennis, racquetball, and basketball are not considered to be aerobic because they involve so much stop-and-go activity. Thus, they are better for strengthening bones and muscles than for improving cardiovascular conditioning.

How Often to Exercise

You will get better cardiovascular results if you exercise at least five times per week. Studies show that the average person will receive minimal aerobic benefits if he or she exercises three times per week for 20 minutes. Unfortunately, minimal benefits do not include the best possible improvements in HDL levels, blood pressure, or blood sugar control. Also, most people find minimal exercise doesn't reduce fat weight as much as they desire. Thus, to get good aerobic benefits, you need to do consistent, long-duration aerobic exercise like walking.

Exercise does increase your metabolic rate, meaning that you burn more calories after exercising. However, the amount per person varies tremendously, so don't depend on this elevated metabolic rate to eliminate your need to exercise the next day. Go ahead and stick to your routine. You will see better weight loss results and physiological changes. Remember, *consistency* is the key to seeing the benefits of exercise.

The Duration of Your Exercise

The number of minutes you spend exercising each session is the duration. Try doing a manageable number of minutes per session for you. If 10 minutes is manageable, start with that. Listen to your body. Think about what you are able to do comfortably now, then gradually work up to more as your body becomes adjusted to the activity. Your goal is at least 30 minutes of exercise at a time.

The Intensity of Your Exercise

The intensity is how hard the activity is to you. Your body knows how hard an activity is for you. It tells you something is too hard by making you out of breath or greatly fatigued. Here are some ways you can tell if you are exercising too intensely:

❖ *The talk test.* You should be able to carry on a conversation while exercising. You may be breathing more frequently, but you should be able to string phrases together without gasping for breath. If you are gasping for breath, slow down—you are exercising too fast and hard. If you cannot talk naturally while exercising, you are burning carbohydrate, not fat.

❖ *Borg Perceived Exertion Scale.* Speaking of too hard, there is an easy scale you can use to determine if you are doing the right amount of work for you. The Borg Perceived Exertion Scale, shown on page 116, consists of phrases and numbers that correlate to your exertion level.

❖ The number 6 corresponds with "rest," for example, sitting in a chair doing nothing at all. Number 20 is absolutely all that you can do. When you are exercising, you want to be in the 10 to 13 range—ideally around "somewhat hard." Although you will have an increase in your breathing, you will be able to string together phrases in conversation before taking another breath. If you are working at the 15 level, slow down. At 15 you would be "huffing and puffing," or taking a breath after almost every word spoken. If you are at 9, pick up your pace. Learn to trust your body. Ask yourself, "on a scale of 6 to 20, where am I now?"

Borg Perceived Exertion Scale

6	rest
7	
	very, very light
8	
9	
	very light
10	
11	
	light
12	
13	
	somewhat hard
14	
15	
	hard
16	
17	
	very hard
18	
19	very, very hard
20	maximal exertion

(Borg, G. A. Medicine and Science in Sports and Exercise, 14, 1982, pp. 377–378.)

❖ *Find your target heart rate.* Another way to determine if you are getting the right amount of exercise is to take your heart rate during exercise. Your heart rate goes up in response to increased activity. When your heart rate gets to a certain number you know you are getting aerobic benefits. If you exceed a certain number, you are working too hard and not receiving optimal aerobic benefits.

This range of heart rate numbers at which you receive optimal aerobic benefits is called your *target heart rate zone.* It gives you the high and low number of heart beats per minute that it will take to get aerobic benefits. (See Table 6.8 for age-related heart rate ranges.) Although many assume your target heart rate is a more technical means of assessing your exercise intensity, the former two means of assessment (the talk test and the Borg Perceived Exertion Scale) are just as effective and usually easier. Learn to listen to, and trust, your body.

❖ TABLE 6.8   AGE-RELATED HEART RATE CHANGES ❖

AGE	HEART RATE IN BEATS/MINUTE
20	100–150
25	98–146
30	95–142
35	93–138
40	90–135
45	88–127
50	85–127
55	83–123
60	80–120
65	78–116
70	75–113

The most accurate target heart rate zone can be derived from a maximal exercise treadmill test or a stress test. If you have had a maximal exercise treadmill test in the recent past, your doctor can calculate your target heart rate range.

❖   *Taking your pulse.* Check your pulse during the middle and at the end of your workout. (If you are just starting and exercising less than 15 minutes, checking your heart rate at the end of your workout is sufficient.)

To get your pulse:

1. Stop exercising. Place the tips of your first two fingers of one hand on the thumb side of your opposing wrist. Your pulse will be between the tendons that run down the center of the inside of your wrist and outside of your wrist. Apply a light pressure to your pulse.

2. Count the number of pulses/heart beats that you feel during 10 seconds. Multiply that number by six to find out how many times your heart beats per minute.

3. Compare that number to the target heart rate range for your age (given in Table 6.8) or your personal target heart rate range.

Please note: If you are taking medications that keep your heart rate down, the table will be inaccurate for you. Consult your doctor.

If you are below your range, you can speed up; by speeding up, you increase your intensity. If you are above your range, slow down; by slowing down, you decrease your intensity. Most important, remember that *you* are in charge of your intensity. No piece of equipment controls you.

How to Work Up to Your Exercise Goal

You need to progress gradually in order to reach your exercise goal safely. The exercise progressions recommended here are based on starting a walking program. If you are interested in doing other activities, you may substitute that activity for walking, but use the same time frames. Beside walking, the activities that work best in these progressions are stationary cycling, stair-climbing on a machine, rowing on a machine, and stationary cross-country skiing. Swimming and water exercises work better when you are only exercising once a day.

When your workouts reach 20 minutes or more, a warm-up and cool-down can help your cardiovascular system adjust.

The standing exercises given in Chapter 9 are easier to do than the floor exercises. So if you haven't been exercising, choose the standing exercises. First, try doing ten repetitions. If you can't do ten, that's okay. Try for ten the next time. If ten doesn't seem very difficult, try fifteen. If you haven't been exercising, stick with fifteen or fewer for the first three sessions even if you feel that you can do more. Gradually increase your repetitions from ten (or fifteen if you feel able) the first week, three times per week, to thirty repetitions by the fifth week. When you are able to do thirty repetitions of those exercises consistently, move to the floor exercises. When you achieve your goals for these exercises, definitely consider moving into weight training.

You'll find guidelines on specific exercises in Chapter 13.

YOUR INNER HEALING PLAN

Your spiritual growth and development, or inner healing plan, is similar to the nutrition and exercise aspects of the program in that it also needs to be personalized. We need to take some time to know ourselves, or reflect on what is our preference or orientation, before we go blazing down someone else's trail rather than our own. The importance of this truth with respect to spiritual formation first became clear to me when I was auditing a personal transformation course at Duke University's Divinity School.

One night Professor Westerhoff discussed the four ways of approaching God, or our spiritual selves. (I'll cover these in more detail in Chapter 10.)

Professor Westerhoff was wise to encourage most of the soon-to-be preachers that it was their responsibility to become familiar with the varied paths or routes to God, as their different parishioners would relate to different ways of being spiritual. He shared how he tried to go to four retreats each year, one aligned with each of the different paths, to become more understanding of the many paths to God. He felt that this better equipped him to help those who sought his guidance. So if you know any spiritual persons—priest, rabbi, preacher, or anyone whose spirituality you respect—ask them if they know of spiritual retreats that you might be comfortable with.

I first speak of retreats because I found retreat centers to be one of my most rewarding paths (see Appendix B for specific recommendations). If you are not comfortable with groups and prefer to be alone in your spiritual endeavors, you may want to read books, listen to tapes, and watch videos on meditation before signing up with a group endeavor. There are many different paths, and the joy of life is in finding your own.

As you begin to think about the inner healing methods that may work best for you, consider these options:

❖ Consulting a therapist, minister, or caring physician

❖ Meditation

❖ Prayer

❖ Keeping a journal

❖ Interpreting your dreams

❖ Confession

❖ Twelve Step programs

Chapter 10 will provide further details on each of these methods.

COMBINING THE THREE COMPONENTS TO HEAL YOUR HEART

The following worksheet will help you create your own version of the Heal Your Heart Program. The first one is a sample based on a hypothetical heart patient so that you can see how it's done. The blank one is for you to copy and fill in for yourself. Yours will of course be personalized to your needs. Once you have filled out the worksheet, post it where you can see it often, or keep it in a place where you can frequently refer to it.

MY PERSONALIZED HEAL YOUR HEART PLAN (Sample)

My current health status: *Had a heart attack on 3/20/97: have high cholesterol and blood pressure*

My goals (with projected date for accomplishing them): *Want to lower cholesterol to less than 150: also want BP less than 110/70 by 5/20/97*

My Nutrition Plan

My nutrition plan will include:

__2000__ calories per day

__10__ % of my calories from fat

__50__ mgs. of cholesterol

__500__ mgs. of sodium

My general strategy on nutrition: *Eat only vegetarian foods, then add fish when I get to my goal: will keep a food record.*

If I do not meet my nutrition goals by my projected date, I will: *Seek weekly counsel from a consulting nutritionist who can support my initial goals; re-commit to my food record.*

My Exercise Plan

My exercise goals include:

__60__ minutes per day of aerobic exercise __5__ times a week

__10__ minutes per day of stretching __6__ times a week

__45__ minutes per day of strength training __3__ times a week

My general strategy on exercise: *Continue participating in cardiac rehab (CR) program 3×/week, and working out at spa with friends*

If I do not meet my exercise goals within my projected date, I will: *Hire a trainer to give me an extra push, and organize some fellow heart patients from CR group to walk more with me*

My Inner Healing Plan

My plans for spiritual renewal and inner healing include: *I will strive for 15—30 minutes of meditation/day, and explore church options with my wife*

My general strategy for accomplishing this emotional and spiritual growth: *I will meditate early in the day and document my spiritual pursuits with my food and exercise record*

If I do not honor my spiritual goals by my projected date, I will: *Join a meditation class and attend it weekly; keep a journal of my thoughts and feelings; join an Anonymous group*

MY PERSONALIZED HEAL YOUR HEART PLAN

My current health status: _____

My goals (with projected date for accomplishing them): _____

_____

My Nutrition Plan

My nutrition plan will include:

_____ calories per day

_____ % of my calories from fat

_____ mgs. of cholesterol

_____ mgs. of sodium

My general strategy on nutrition: _____

_____

If I do not meet my nutrition goals by my projected date, I will: ____

_____

My Exercise Plan

My exercise goals include:

_____ minutes per day of aerobic exercise _____ times a week

_____ minutes per day of stretching _____ times a week

_____ minutes per day of strength training _____ times a week

My general strategy on exercise: _____

_____

If I do not meet my exercise goals within my projected date, I will:

_____

My Inner Healing Plan

My plans for spiritual renewal and inner healing include: _____

_____

My general strategy for accomplishing this emotional and spiritual growth: _____

If I do not honor my spiritual goals by my projected date, I will:

_____

The important thing to remember as you put together your own personal Heal Your Heart Program is that your healing must involve the emotional or spiritual components, as well as the physical ones of diet and exercise. Diets alone are not effective in the long run. After experiencing this in my own healing, as well as those of many Rice Diet participants, I am convinced we need to honor the *whole* person. If we have not contemplated the true purpose of our lives, and our connectedness with self, others, and our Creator, how could we possibly be emotionally content and truly healthy?

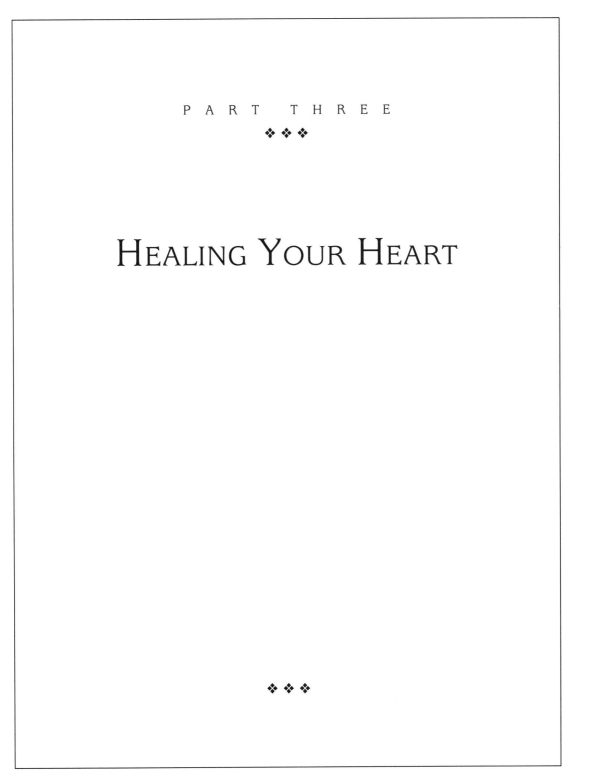

PART THREE

❖ ❖ ❖

HEALING YOUR HEART

❖ ❖ ❖

7

Healing Your Heart
Through Nutrition

My most important advice for a healthy diet is to eat only foods that grow out of the ground, in their whole, unprocessed form. It is truly that simple. If we all would eat only foods that look like they were just picked, no more than a cup of nonfat dairy products daily, and 3 to 6 ounces of fish a couple of times per week, I would need to find another profession! Research has shown that when people eat only unprocessed vegetarian foods (without nuts, seeds, or added oils) they lose weight without having to count calorie portions or allowances.

Despite the simplicity of this advice, I find that many people want a more specific strategy. The Heal Your Heart nutrition plan provides you with more detailed direction. Now that I have translated nutritional recommendations into allowances and menus (see Chapter 6), I will now define the allowances more specifically, and share tips on maintaining appropriate vitamin and mineral levels. It is important to consult your physician before reducing your fat, salt, and calories to this extent. **Remember, do not make any changes to your diet or medication regimen without your physician's advice.**

Your Food Group Allowances

Let's get started with the food group part of the plan. People often find this plan easier to follow than simply trying to cut fat and salt and eat healthy. Foods are divided into these categories: Starches, Vegetables, Fruits, Protein, Dairy Products, and Fats and Oils, as well as condiments, conditionally acceptable foods, and foods you should eat only rarely. I'll explain how big an allowance is, and give you tips on preparing each in the healthiest way.

Starch

The foods in the starch group contain an average of 80 calories, 15 grams of carbohydrate, 3 grams of protein, 1 gram of fat, trace amounts of saturated fat, no cholesterol, and 5 milligrams of sodium per allowance, or small serving size. Choose a minimum of six servings from this group per day, with the majority coming from the higher-fiber items. This group includes whole grains; slightly processed cereals, breads, and crackers; and starchy vegetables, such as potatoes, corn, peas, and winter squash. All whole grains—such as brown rice, oat groats (or steel-cut oats and oatmeal), barley (preferrably hulless type), buckwheat groats, quinoa, millet, whole wheat berries (or cracked wheat), and rye kernels—are the ultimate base for your nutrition plan. Whole grains have more fiber and nutrients than do their processed counterparts, despite efforts to enrich these processed foods. Although all whole grains are good for you, rice is especially beneficial, offering some of the highest quality protein of any grain. If these whole grains constitute the majority of your grain intake, then you can occasionally eat slightly processed grains, such as whole-grained crackers, breads, fat-free cookies, and pasta. Generally speaking, you would be getting plenty of fiber and nutrients as long as three quarters of your grain intake is whole grain. If you can do that much, then you would not need to be concerned if one quarter of your grains are slightly processed.

Dried beans and peas can be counted as a starch or as a protein allowance. These are the highest protein members of the starch group, and among the richest in cholesterol-lowering soluble fiber. Other nutrient and fiber rich starches are the starchy vegetables, such as yams, sweet and white potatoes, corn, peas, and winter squash. To increase your fiber and nutrient intake, consume the peelings of vegetables whenever possible.

Try to eat a nice variety of starches. Your body would prefer a cup of rice and $\frac{1}{3}$ cup of black beans to 2 cups of potatoes. This is much more of a concern if you have unstable blood sugars, since refined, processed grains and potatoes become blood sugar faster than do these other carbohydrates. (See Chapter 3 for more details on fibers' ability to slow blood sugar absorption.)

Tips on Making the Most of Your Starches

Whether you are preventing or reversing heart disease, the following tips will prove useful in healthfully lowering your fat and sodium intake and increasing your fiber:

❖ As most commercially prepared starches—such as biscuits, muffins, cookies, pancakes, and croissants—are not made with the recommended fats, it is smartest to enjoy such baked goods primarily at home, where you can modify the recipes to use preferred oils, and less fat and sodium. Homemade versions could be prepared with egg whites or egg substitutes instead of whole eggs and you can substitute fat-free moist ingredients like skim milk, yogurt, pureed fruit, fruit juices, or Wonderslim for the fat.

❖ Bread can have more cholesterol-lowering potential if you use oats, oat bran, or barley flour for some, if not all, of the wheat flour called for in a recipe. Cholesterol-lowering beans, such as limas, can be cooked and mashed and substituted for a third of the flour in many recipes without imparting a beany taste! Try the *Pumpkin Bean Bread* and see what you think.

❖ Since most low-sodium canned soups still contain more than our 500 milligram sodium recommendation per day in just a single cup, it is smartest to enjoy only homemade soups in which you can control the sodium and fat (or no-salt-added soups). Although soups vary widely in ingredients, most 1-cup servings of soup contain at least 1 starch allowance, or approximately ½ cup of cooked grain or starchy vegetable. You can guestimate how many (starch) allowances are in a serving by comparing the nutritional analysis on the label to the nutritional information given in the first sentence defining each food group.

❖ If you add significant amounts of any kind of bran to your diet you should also drink more water to prevent constipation. You can add bran to cooked cereal and casseroles, or to moist items, such as applesauce.

❖ Drink 4 to 8 cups of water or beverages daily to assure proper fluid intake with your high-fiber, complex carbohydrate-rich, starch-based diet. Respect your thirst mechanism, as fluid needs vary with sodium intake and perspiration losses (influenced by exercise, temperature, and humidity). For example, someone who is eating a salt-free vegetarian diet and exercising moderately will likely desire only 32 ounces of water, while someone eating an additional 500 milligrams of sodium and running a summer marathon may need twice this fluid intake. When you are eating a no-salt-added vegetarian diet it is important not to force fluids, as is often recommended with higher-salt diets. Drinking a lot of water for "dieting" reasons can cause electrolyte imbalances if you are truly eating a no-salt-added vegetarian diet.

Unless you are taking medication that alters your thirst mechanism, or are running marathon distances, then relax, tune into your body, and trust your thirst mechanism.

❖ Try eating breads and starchy foods with no salt added. You may want to request your favorite salt-free bread at the nearest bakery. If they do not want to stock a salt-free bread, they will often make you a batch upon request. You may have to buy a large batch at once, but bread freezes beautifully. Also become friendly with the grocery store managers who will often stock your favorite no-fat/no-salt snacks if you let your desires be known. Diplomacy and tenacity with these requests usually produces healthful results.

Portion Size for 1 Starch Allowance

The allowances, or serving sizes, for starches, as for most groups in this nutrition plan, may be smaller than you would find typical. But, the different calorie diet plans include *between six and twenty starch allowances per day*. So even on a 1,000-calorie plan, you can have two starches per meal. Here are the amounts that equal one allowance of starch. An asterisk (*) indicates a high-fiber item.

Breads:

Bagel: $\frac{1}{2}$

Bread stick, 4″ long by $\frac{1}{2}$″ diameter: 2

Bread (whole wheat,* rye,* oatmeal,* pumpernickel*): 1 slice

Croutons: 1 cup

English muffin (whole wheat,* oatmeal*): $\frac{1}{2}$

Hamburger or hot dog bun (whole wheat*): $\frac{1}{2}$

Pita bread, 6″ diameter (whole wheat*): $\frac{1}{2}$

Roll, plain (whole wheat*): 1

Tortilla, corn* or flour, 6″ diameter (without lard): 1

Crackers, chips, and snacks:

Frito-Lay Baked Tostitos, no fat or salt added: $\frac{3}{4}$ ounce

Harry's Whole Wheat Honeys Pretzels: $\frac{3}{4}$ ounce

Health Valley Oat Bran Graham Crackers: $6\frac{1}{2}$

Matzo crackers: $\frac{3}{4}$ ounce

Popcorn, popped with no fat: 3 cups

Rice cakes: 2

Ryvita Sesame Rye: $2\frac{2}{3}$

Smart Temptation's no-fat/no-salt corn chips: $\frac{4}{5}$ ounce

Guiltless Gourmet no-fat/no-salt corn chips: $\frac{4}{5}$ ounce

Grains (cooked):

Barley (hulled*): $\frac{1}{2}$ cup

Buckwheat groats*: $\frac{1}{2}$ cup

Flake-type cereals (oat* and whole grain*): $\frac{3}{4}$ cup

Grits: $\frac{1}{2}$ cup

Oat bran*: $3\frac{1}{2}$ Tbs.

Oatmeal (oat groats*): $\frac{1}{2}$ cup

Polenta: $\frac{1}{2}$ cup

Quinoa: $\frac{1}{2}$ cup

Rice (brown*): $\frac{1}{3}$ cup

Wheat bran: $3\frac{4}{5}$ Tbs.

Starchy vegetables (cooked):

Acorn* or Butternut squash*: $\frac{3}{4}$ cup

Corn*: $\frac{1}{2}$ cup

Corn on the cob*: 1 ear, 6″ long

Dried beans*, peas, lentils*: $\frac{1}{3}$ cup

Green peas*: $\frac{1}{2}$ cup

Lima beans*: $\frac{1}{2}$ cup

Plantain, or yam*: $\frac{1}{2}$ cup

Potato, baked with skin*: 1 small ($\frac{1}{2}$ c.)

Sweet potato*: $\frac{1}{4}$ cup

Vegetables

An allowance of vegetables has about 25 calories, 5 grams of carbohydrate, 2 grams of protein, trace amounts of fat, no saturated fat or cholesterol, and 10 milligrams of sodium. Note the large differences in calories and carbohydrate between the starchy vegetables, with 80 calories and 15 grams of carbohydrate, and these nonstarchy vegetables, with only 25 calories and 5 grams of carbohydrate. The sodium content of vegetables can vary widely, with an allowance of cooked celery and spinach offering 48 and 63 milligrams of sodium, respectively. But you don't need to worry about naturally occurring sodium unless you have kidney or liver disease.

Choose a minimum of three servings per day, but you should try to have more. Again, it would be advantageous to enjoy plenty of the higher-fiber items. Since vegetables are the lowest calorie food group and are packed with nutrition, it would be difficult to eat too many—if, of course, they contain no added fat or salt.

Tips on Making the Most of Your Vegetables
The following tips can enhance your ability to retain the highest nutrient, antioxidant, and fiber content of your vegetables, as well as to minimize their contribution of fat and sodium:

❖   Fresh and frozen vegetables are the most nutritious. Canned vegetables are the least preferred, not only since most canned products have very high sodium contents, but also because they have approximately half the potassium of the fresh or frozen versions. Since low potassium intakes have been associated with high blood pressure, the more fresh or frozen fruits and vegetables the better.

❖   Eat the skin on vegetables whenever possible for more fiber and vitamins. (Of course scrub the skin before eating.)

❖   Avoid fried vegetables as well as those prepared with butter, cream, or cheese, as these are high in saturated fat. Instead, eat vegetables raw, steamed, or microwaved. Vegetables can be stir-fried with a teaspoon of olive oil, plenty of fresh herbs and spices, and a little vegetable stock or wine to preventing scorching. If you like some kind of topping on your vegetables, try squeezing a fresh lemon on them.

❖   Eat as much of the following raw vegetables as you want, without counting each as an allowance. They are considered "free" because they have less than 20 calories per cup, raw. Those high in fiber are marked with an asterisk (*).

Celery	Chinese cabbage
Cucumbers	Green onion*
Peppers	Mushrooms
Radishes	Zucchini

Endive	Escarole
Lettuce	Romaine
Spinach*	Hot peppers

Portion Size for 1 Vegetable Allowance

The allowances, or serving sizes, for vegetables is fairly typical for those of us from industrialized nations, where meat has typically been the meal's centerpiece. The main difference is that more allowances than usual are recommended for you. Three or more allowances per day, plus as many vegetables as you want from the free group, are not only packed with nutrients and antioxidants, but will give you lots of chew and fiber with few calories. One cup raw or ½ cup cooked of the following vegetables equals one allowance or serving. High fiber items are marked with an asterisk (*).

Artichoke (½ medium)*	Asparagus
Beans (green, wax, Italian)*	Bean sprouts
Beets*	Broccoli*
Brussels sprouts*	Cabbage*
Carrots*	Cauliflower
Eggplant*	Greens (collard, mustard, turnip)*
Kohlrabi	Leeks
Mushrooms	Okra*
Onions	Pea pods
Peppers	Rutabaga
Spinach	Squash (crookneck, zucchini)
Tomato (1 large)*	Tomato/vegetable juice, no salt
Turnips*	Water chestnuts

Fruits

Fruit allowances contain about 60 calories, 15 grams of carbohydrate, 0 protein, trace amounts of fat, 0 saturated fat and cholesterol, and 1 milligram of sodium. As you may notice, the fruit group has the lowest content of fat, protein, and sodium per serving, which is why fruit is great for people with many chronic diseases. It is also one of the highest sources of cholesterol-lowering soluble fiber.

Choose a minimum of three servings per day, and frequently from the higher-fiber items. Remember, the darker the orange color in fruit, the higher the betacarotene content, so enjoy plenty of oranges, peaches, apricots, cantaloupes, and mangoes.

Tips on Making the Most of Your Fruits

The following tips will prove helpful in your efforts to maximize the nutrient, antioxidant, and fiber content in fruits.

❖ Choose fresh, frozen, or dried fruit more often than canned fruit or juice, because canned fruits lose significant potassium during the canning process. And canned fruits and juices often have syrup or sugar added, which offers calories without nutrition. If you drink juice, make sure it is one hundred percent fruit juice with no sugar added, and do not drink more than 4 ounces per day. Whole fruit is preferrable to juice because the whole fruit offers more cholesterol-lowering soluble fiber and makes you feel more full per serving.

❖ Eat the skin on fresh fruit whenever possible for more fiber and vitamins. As with vegetables, scrub fruits carefully before eating.

❖ For a great frozen dessert, try freezing bananas, seedless grapes, or any fruit. To prevent their browning from oxidation, pour a little pineapple or lemon juice over them before freezing. They are great straight or whizzed in a blender with nonfat yogurt, skim milk, or juice, and a little vanilla and cinnamon to make a "fruit smoothie." You can also freeze this blend in an ice-pop maker or in ice cube trays.

Portion Size for 1 Fruit Allowance

The allowances for many fruits are just what you would expect them to be—one piece if it is raw, or $\frac{1}{2}$ cup if it is cooked or juiced. Dried fruit may be the only surprise; $\frac{1}{8}$ to $\frac{1}{4}$ cup of dried fruit is all you get because it is so calorically dense. Three or more allowances are recommended per day. In fact, if you ever want more food than your plan suggests, vegetables, then fruits, would be your two best options. Higher-fiber fruits are marked with an asterisk(*).

Fresh, frozen, or canned fruit:
Apple (raw, 2" across)*: 1
Applesauce (unsweetened): $\frac{1}{2}$ cup
Apricots (medium, raw): 4
Apricots (canned): $\frac{1}{2}$ cup or 4 halves
Banana (9" long): $\frac{1}{2}$
Blackberries (raw)*: $\frac{3}{4}$ cup
Blueberries (raw)*: $\frac{3}{4}$ cup
Cantaloupe (5" across): $\frac{1}{3}$
Cantaloupe (cubes): 1 cup
Cherries (large, raw): 12
Cherries (canned): $\frac{1}{2}$ cup
Figs (raw, 2" across): 2
Fruit cocktail (canned): $\frac{1}{2}$ cup
Grapefruit (medium): $\frac{1}{2}$

Grapefruit (segments): $\frac{3}{4}$ cup
Grapes (small): 15
Honeydew melon (medium): $\frac{1}{8}$
Kiwi (large): 1
Mandarin oranges: $\frac{3}{4}$ cup
Mango (small)*: $\frac{1}{2}$
Nectarine (2$\frac{1}{2}$" across)*: 1
Orange (2$\frac{1}{2}$" across)*: 1
Papaya*: 1 cup
Peach (2$\frac{3}{4}$" across): 1
Peaches (canned): $\frac{1}{2}$ cup or 2 halves
Pear: $\frac{1}{2}$ large or 1 small
Pear (canned): $\frac{1}{2}$ cup or 2 halves
Persimmon (medium, native): 2
Pineapple (raw): $\frac{3}{4}$ cup

Pineapple (canned): $\frac{1}{3}$ cup
Plum (raw, 2″ across): 2
Pomegranate*: $\frac{1}{2}$
Raspberries (raw)*: 1 cup

Strawberries (raw, whole)*: $1\frac{1}{4}$ cup
Tangerine ($2\frac{1}{2}$″ across)*: 2
Watermelon (cubes): $1\frac{1}{4}$ cup

Dried fruit:

Apples*: 4 rings

Apricots*: 7 halves

Dates*: $2\frac{1}{2}$ medium

Figs*: $1\frac{1}{2}$

Prunes: 3 medium

Raisins: 2 tablespoons

Fruit juice:

Apple juice/cider: $\frac{1}{2}$ cup

Cranberry juice cocktail: $\frac{1}{3}$ cup

Grapefruit juice: $\frac{1}{2}$ cup

Grape juice: $\frac{1}{3}$ cup

Orange juice: $\frac{1}{2}$ cup

Pineapple juice: $\frac{1}{2}$ cup

Prune juice: $\frac{1}{3}$ cup

Protein

One protein allowance averages 55 calories, 0 carbohydrate, 7 grams of protein, 3 grams of fat, $\frac{4}{5}$ gram saturated fat, 25 milligrams of cholesterol (varies widely), and 51 milligrams of sodium. This group includes high protein foods such as legumes, seafood, and, if you are preventing rather than reversing heart disease, poultry and lean meats. If you have heart disease or cholesterols over 150, it is important to remember that red meat (beef, pork, lamb, and veal) is highest in saturated fats; it is best to cut it entirely or limit it to very special occasions. Depending on your need to lose weight and your motivation to reverse atherosclerosis (and its risk factors such as high blood pressure and cholesterol), choose between 0 and 3 servings from this group every day.

I would recommend that you eat animal products and dairy foods only if your health indicators suggest that you can. For instance, you should avoid animal products if you have heart disease or a cholesterol that is greater than 150. You should limit them if your fasting blood sugar is more than 100, blood pressure is greater than 110/70, or weight is more than ideal. See Table 7.1 for animal products that you should avoid if you have heart disease or high cholesterol. Your best nutrition plan is one that respects your body's red flags!

Although I call this food group "Protein," there is also plenty of protein in the starch and vegetable groups. But the highest protein foods are in this group, with only the leanest choices allowed. Legumes (beans and peas) are the preferred source of high protein, and can be counted in this group or the starch group. They are preferrable to meats in that they offer similarly high protein and iron, without the accompanying sodium, saturated fat, and cholesterol, and with lots of cholesterol-lowering, blood sugar-stabilizing soluble fiber.

Tips on Making the Most of Your Protein Sources

Whether you are preventing or reversing heart disease, here are some tips to keep in mind:

❖ Legumes such as dried beans, peas, lentils, tempeh, and soybean curd (tofu) are good sources of protein and iron, so you should use them in place of meat as often as possible. If you have heart disease and are seeking to reverse it, legumes should be your only Protein selection, with the possible exception of fish.

❖ Regular ground beef (even extra lean) has more fat than a heart patient should consume, and people with preventive goals should certainly limit it. Try texturized vegetable protein (TVP) as a substitute. TVP is sold in health food stores, or can be ordered (see Harvest Direct, in Appendix A). If your

❖ TABLE 7.1   ANIMAL PRODUCTS TO AVOID IF YOU HAVE HEART DISEASE ❖

MEATS	DAIRY	SEAFOOD
Beef	Butter	Clams
Lamb	Cheese	Crab
Organ meats	Egg yolks	Crayfish
Pork	Ice cream	Lobster
Poultry	Whole milk	Oysters
Veal	Whole milk products	Shrimp

risk factors are ideal and you want an occasional hamburger, select a lean cut such as round steak and have it trimmed and ground, or try ground skinless turkey breast.

❖   Avoid liver and other organ meats completely. They are very high in cholesterol.

❖   Although crustaceans, such as shrimp and crayfish, have about twice as much cholesterol as beef and chicken, they are so low in saturated fats you can enjoy them in moderation if your cholesterol is less than 150.

❖   When eating poultry, have white meat rather than dark because it has only one third the saturated fat per ounce. Trim all visible fat and remove skin from poultry *before* cooking. Even with these precautions, eat poultry sparingly. Remember that although the skin contains approximately half of the fat found in half of a chicken breast (3.5 ounces), the remaining fat within the lean tissue is still 31 percent saturated.

❖   Trim all visible fat from meats. After cooking meat in a stew or soup, allow it to cool, and refrigerate. After the fat rises to the top, remove it before adding vegetables.

❖   Rarely prepare meat, poultry, or seafood by frying, basting, or sautéing, as this adds extra fat. Remember to count this added fat in your daily fat allowance if these cooking methods are used.

Portion Size for 1 Protein Allowance
Protein is the only food group where an allowance is much smaller than the average serving. Of course if you only have one meat allowance per day you could accumulate that 7 ounces for a week, and divide it into two meals. Then you could enjoy a 3-ounce piece of cooked fish one night, and a 4-ounce piece of cooked fish a few days later. All meats are cooked portions. (4 ounces raw meat = 3 ounces cooked meat.) Here are the amounts that equal one allowance of each of the following protein sources:

Beef: 1 ounce (Round is the leanest, use ground round instead of hamburger.)

Dried beans, peas, lentils, cooked: $\frac{1}{4}$ cup

Eggs: 1 whole, 3 egg whites, or $\frac{1}{4}$ cup egg substitute

Fish: 1 ounce, or $\frac{1}{4}$ cup flaked

Lamb: 1 ounce

Meat, any type, lean, diced: $\frac{1}{4}$ cup

Pork: 1 ounce (Tenderloin is the lowest in saturated fat.)

Poultry: 1 ounce (skinned)

Veal: 1 ounce

Wild game, except duck: 1 ounce

Four ounces of raw meat becomes 3 ounces once it is cooked, which is typically considered a small serving. A 3-ounce serving of cooked meat is about the size of a deck of cards. For those of you whose risk factors allow this much meat, the following examples of 3 allowances are given to help you get a visual image of more typical portions:

Beef, round: 3 ounces

Fish, canned, flaked: $\frac{3}{4}$ cup

Fish patty: 3 ounces

Hamburger patty: 3 ounces

Pork tenderloin: 3 ounces

Poultry, skinned: $\frac{1}{2}$ breast = 3 ounces

The Best Meat Choices, for Protein
Remember that meat, other than fish, is not included in your plan if you are trying to reverse heart disease. However, if your goal is prevention, here are your best bets:

❖ *Seafood:* any finfish, such as tuna or salmon (fresh, or canned in water, preferably no-salt-added "dietetic" type) or some types of shellfish such as crab, lobster, scallops, clams, and oysters (no deviled crab or mixed seafood dishes with butter or cream). Other seafood choices vary greatly in their calorie, fat, protein, cholesterol, and sodium content. See Table 7.2 for your favorite seafood choices compared to popular meat choices.

❖ *Poultry:* Chicken (white meat without skin); turkey (white meat without skin).

❖ *Pork:* Lean pork, such as pork tenderloin. Avoid higher-fat pork chops and processed meats, such as sausage and bacon.

❖ *Beef:* USDA Select or Choice grades of lean beef, including round steak, sirloin tip, tenderloin. To assure the leanest ground meat, buy round steak and have it ground (ground round has one sixth the

❖ TABLE 7.2   SURPRISING SEAFOOD COMPARISONS ❖

SEAFOOD (3 OZ. COOKED)	CALS.	PROTEIN (GMS.)	FAT (GMS.)	SATURATED FAT (GMS.)	CARBO-HYDRATE (GMS.)	CHOLES-TEROL (MGS.)	SODIUM (MGS.)
Catfish	120	19	5	1	0	60	65
Clam (12 sm.)	130	22	2	0	4	60	95
Cod	90	19	1	0	0	50	60
Crab, blue	90	19	1	0	0	80	310
Crayfish	96	20	1.2	.3	0	149	57
Flounder	100	20	1	0	0	50	85
Halibut	120	22	2	0	0	30	60
Haddock	90	20	1	0	0	60	70
Lobster	100	20	1	0	1	100	320
Mackerel	190	21	12	3	0	30	95
Mussel	93	13	2.4	.6	4	31	305
Orange roughy	70	16	1	0	0	20	70
Oyster (12 med.)	120	12	4	1	7	90	190
Salmon, Atlantic coho	150	22	7	1	0	50	50
Scallop (6 lg. or 14 sm.)	150	29	1	0	2	60	275
Shrimp	115	23	2	.4	1	164	159
Tuna (yellow fin)	118	25	1	0	0	48	39
Tuna, light, chunk, Star-Kist	90	20	1.5	.3	0	30	465
Tuna, white chunk, Star-Kist dietetic	105	23	1.5	.3	0	30	45
Chicken, light	186	34	5	1.3	0	90	76
Turkey, light	184	35	6	1.9	0	89	82
Pork tenderloin	194	34	5.7	2	0	110	79
Beef round	164	27	5.3	2	0	72	53

The above data was obtained from Food Values of Portions Commonly Used, *Jean A.T. Pennington and* Journal of the American Dietetic Assoc., *Oct. 1992, p. 1254.*

saturated fat of most lean ground hamburger!). On all cuts, trim visible fat.

❖ *Lamb:* Roast, chop, and leg are leanest cuts.

❖ *Veal:* Remember to trim visible fat on all cuts. All cuts are fairly lean except for veal cutlets, so avoid them.

❖ *Wild Game:* Venison, rabbit, squirrel, pheasant, buffalo, ostrich; except for duck, wild game is typically very low in fat.

What About Luncheon Meats, Processed Meats, and Eggs?
Luncheon meats are highly processed, usually made from leftovers from other cuts or meat products. *Avoid them.* The lowest-fat ones are still loaded with sodium and chemical preservatives, such as nitrates, a proven carcinogen (cancer-causing agent). Processed meats get the same recommendations—*never.* When a fellow dietitian once called a producer of ground turkey to find out how their product could possibly contain more than 50 percent fat, the ground turkey producer told her that they used "parts" of meat, grinding the dark meat and skin and the less expensive remnants. She asked him to be more specific about "parts" and he said "Use your imagination, darling!" After this frank admission that his product was garbage, I have a difficult time viewing this product as human food. If you want to eat ground turkey, I recommend you go to a butcher where you can request and watch the grinding of skinned turkey breast, with 29 percent of calories coming from fat.

To stick to the cholesterol recommendation of less than 100 milligrams per day, it is necessary to avoid egg yolks as much as possible. One large whole egg contains 6 grams of fat, 2 grams of saturated fatty acids, and 274 milligrams of cholesterol, so it doesn't fit into our game plan often. Instead, try one fourth cup of cholesterol-free egg substitute or 2 egg whites for one egg in recipes, such as muffins or cornbread. Prepare your scrambled eggs, or omelets by scrambling egg whites with a little skim milk and turmeric to create a yellow egglike appearance, then top with sauteed herbed vegetables. As many prepared foods contain eggs, it is probably wiser for you to cook with your own egg whites or substitutes. As you will agree after trying the recipe in Chapter 14 for *Huevos con Frijoles y Chipotles,* if you have enough other flavors, you will never know it is not made with whole eggs.

Dairy Products

This group includes only those dairy products that are fat-free with no salt added, and an average allowance contains 90 calories, 12 grams of carbohydrate, 8 grams of protein, 0 fat, 0 saturated fat, trace amounts of cholesterol, and 150 milligrams of sodium. Select a maximum of two servings per day.

Tips on Making the Most of Your Dairy Choices

The following are helpful tips in preventing and reversing heart disease and its risk factors:

❖   Skim milk has had the fat removed to less than .4 grams per cup, whereas $\frac{1}{2}$% and 1% milk still have the equivalents of $\frac{1}{4}$ and $\frac{1}{2}$ pat of butter remaining in each cup, respectively. So, skim milk is the best choice. If you need to ease into the lower-fat options, many feel that the 1% Sweet Acidophilus milk is the best tasting of the low-fat varieties. (Acidophilus, like yogurt cultures, is often recommended after an antibiotic series to restore helpful organisms to your gut.)

❖   Nonfat yogurt has had the fat removed to less than .4 grams of fat per cup. Low-fat yogurt has the equivalent of $\frac{3}{4}$ pat of butter remaining in each cup and usually 4 to 6 teaspoons of sugar added in each cup of the flavored types. Nonfat yogurt is a good substitute for sour cream on baked potatoes or bean burritos and for mayonnaise in pasta or tuna fish salads. The *Yogurt Cheese* recipe in Chapter 14 is a good cream cheese substitute. (Try adding some sugar-free jelly to it for a delicious bagel topping.)

❖   Experiment with homemade frozen yogurts: blending and freezing non-fat yogurt with fruit, vanilla, and cinnamon. See the *Banana Cream Kahlua* recipe for the basic technique, then your imagination is the only limit. (I like this frozen in ice-pop makers or blended soft before serving.)

Portion Size for 1 Dairy Allowance

Most of the following dairy product allowances are similar to portions that you would typically consume, except for the frozen desserts. Here are the amounts of popular dairy choices that equal one allowance, or serving:

Cottage cheese, $\frac{1}{2}$% dry-curd type with less than 65 mgs. sodium: $\frac{1}{2}$ cup

Dry powdered nonfat milk: $3\frac{1}{2}$ tablespoons

Frozen dessert, no added fat or sodium: $\frac{1}{2}$ cup (limit to once a week if weight or triglycerides are a problem, as these can be high in sugar)

Milk, skimmed: 1 cup (1% milk still gets 22% of its calories from fat)

Plain yogurt, nonfat: 1 cup

Sour cream, nonfat: 7 tablespoons

Sugar-free fruited yogurt, nonfat: 1 cup

Fats and Oils

An average allowance from this group contains 45 calories, 0 carbohydrate and protein, 4½ grams of fat, ¾ gram of saturated fat (although this varies widely), 0 cholesterol and 0 sodium. Depending on your need to lose weight and motivation to reverse atherosclerosis, choose from 0 to 3 servings per day from this group.

All fats and oils contain *some* saturated fat, so use all sparingly and choose those with the least saturated fat. As Table 7.3 shows, the fat sources highest in saturated fat are typically animal in origin, such as butter and meat fats. The most highly saturated vegetable oils are coconut, palm kernel, and palm oil.

❖ TABLE 7.3   COMPARISON OF DIETARY FATS ❖

Dietary Fat	Cholesterol MG/TBSP	Fatty Acid Content Normalized to 100%
Almond Oil	0	8% / 18% / 74%
Beef Tallow	14	52% / 4% / 44%
Butterfat	33	66% / 4% / 30%
Canola Oil	0	6% / 36% / 58%
Chicken Fat	11	30% / 21% / 43%
Coconut Oil	0	92% / 2% / 6%
Corn Oil	0	13% / 62% / 25%
Cottonseed Oil	0	27% / 54% / 19%
Lard	12	39% / 11% / 50%
Olive Oil	0	14% / 9% / 77%
Palm Oil	0	51% / 10% / 39%
Palm Kernel Oil	0	82% / 1% / 17%
Peanut Oil	0	18% / 34% / 48%
Safflower Oil	0	9% / 78% / 13%
Sesame Seed Oil	0	14% / 42% / 44%
Shortening	0	26% / 30% / 44%
Soybean Oil	0	15% / 61% / 24%
Sunflower Oil	0	11% / 69% / 20%
Walnut Oil	0	9% / 63% / 28%

■ Saturated Fat   ▨ Polyunsaturated   □ Monounsaturated

Tips on Making the Most of Your Fats and Oils (While Lowering Your Bad Cholesterol)

The following tips will help you further prevent and reverse heart disease:

❖   Research now suggests that cholesterol lowers best when our fat intake is primarily from monounsaturated fats, with slightly less from polyunsaturated fat, and even less (4 percent) from saturated fats. The oils highest in monounsaturated fats are olive and rapeseed oil. Rapeseed oil, better known by the name canola, appears to be lowest in saturated fat, but it has not been researched as extensively as has olive oil. So, I recommend using primarily olive oil.

❖   Not all monounsaturated fats can be recommended. Peanut oil is one of these—and peanut butter contains plenty of peanut oil. Although peanut oil does not appear to be very high in saturated fat, it has been shown to raise cholesterol and produce atherosclerosis in rat studies. If you crave a spreadable nut or seed butter, try using small amounts of walnut, or almond butter, or tahini, which is ground sesame. Although these nut and seed butters are primarily polyunsaturated, they can be used sparingly.

❖   Oils rich in polyunsaturated fats have been shown to lower both the bad LDLs and the good HDLs. The oils highest in polyunsaturated fats include safflower, sunflower, and corn oil.

❖   Dairy (butter) and animal fats, cocoa butter (chocolate), coconut, coconut oil, palm kernel oil, and palm oil contain high amounts of saturated fatty acids. Because saturated fats raise cholesterol more than any other factor in food, they should be limited as much as possible. Look for the listing of these fats on food labels, so that you can avoid them. Select products that contain as few saturated fatty acids as possible.

❖   Margarines and shortenings contain partially hydrogenated fats that can destroy the helpful omega-3-fatty acids (found in tofu and seafood) and raise your cholesterol level. To help you kick the margarine habit, try using olive oil instead of margarine, or try *Roasted Garlic, Skordalia, Chahine's Eggplant Spread,* or *"High Five" Hummus* on your bread instead of high-fat spreads. When consuming these healthier and tastier alternatives you will find yourself feeling sorry for people who still eat margarine! Generally, recipes are fine if a reduced volume of olive or canola oil is substituted for the hydrogenated fats such as margarine or shortening. Baked goods will be less flaky, but you can produce nice desserts if Wonderslim, or applesauce, or other pureed fruits are substituted for most (if not all) of the oil in a recipe.

❖   Most nuts and seeds are an excellent source of heart-friendly fats because they tend to be low in saturated fat and high in vitamin E. The exceptions to this are coconuts and peanuts, and to a lesser extent brazil, macadamia, and cashew nuts. These are higher in saturated fat than others. Avocado should also be limited because of its high saturated fat content. The other potential danger of these foods is that because they taste so good, many people are "triggered" into eating compulsively large amounts.

Portion Size for 1 Fat Allowance
An allowance of fat is 1 teaspoon, though few people actually consume this little when they use it. Although you do not really need any added fat or oil to realize your optimal potential for health, it is included for your enjoyment and to enhance the odds that you can maintain this low a saturated fat intake long term. The following food portions are equal to one allowance of fat or oil:

Oils:

Canola oil, or rapeseed oil: 1 teaspoon

Corn oil: 1 teaspoon

Olive oil: 1 teaspoon

Safflower oil: 1 teaspoon

Sesame seed oil: 1 teaspoon

Soybean oil: 1 teaspoon

Walnut oil: 1 teaspoon

Nuts, seeds and other high-fat foods:

Almonds: 6 nuts

Avocado: $\frac{1}{8}$ medium

Filberts: 1 tablespoon

Hazelnuts: 1 tablespoon

Pumpkin seeds: 1 tablespoon

Sesame seeds: 1 tablespoon

Sunflower seeds: 1 tablespoon

Tahini (sesame seed butter): $1\frac{1}{2}$ teaspoons

Walnuts: 1 tablespoon

Condiments

The following foods can be enjoyed as flavor enhancers or condiments if you use their no-fat and no-salt-added forms. They contain fewer than 20 calories per portion and are great anywhere you previously would have used salt. You can use as much as you like of any except catsup.

Catsup, no-salt-added type: 1 tablespoon

Herbs and spices

Horseradish

Lemon

Lime

Mustard, no-salt-added type

Salad dressing, no-fat/no-salt type

Vinegar, no-salt-added type

Wines, except for "cooking wines" or others with salt

Conditionally Acceptable Foods

There are some foods that are allowed on occasion under this plan, but discouraged. They include salt substitutes, sugar substitutes, cocoa as a chocolate substitute, and certain beverages. In general, you are much better off without these foods, as they are not whole and unprocessed.

Salt substitutes and low-sodium bouillons can cause problems if you already have high potassium levels or liver or kidney disease (so check with your doctor before using them). Sugar substitutes, though fat- and calorie-free, can "feed" your addiction to sweet flavors and have been associated with visual problems and migraines. Although cocoa contains caffeine, it is defatted, and thus a healthier substitute for most chocolate desserts; the challenge is to honestly assess if you can enjoy just one *Oat Bran Brownie*! Decaffeinated beverages (coffee, tea, or soda) still contain hundreds of other substances that are less than helpful, such as polyphenols that can bind the majority of iron consumed with that meal.

With the exception of cocoa, these manufactured food substitutes are just unnatural; they consist of a slew of artificial ingredients, and no one really knows what they do to you. So, if you can make the radical shift to a no-fat, no-salt vegetarian, whole food diet that is free of salt and sugar substitutes and dairy products, more power to you. And it may be easier than you think. See Table 7.4 to see just how much salt your favorite foods have, and how you can substitute less salty varieties. However, if you have trouble going cold turkey on sugary and salty flavors and you find that substitutes help, you can use them occasionally. Just don't allow them to become a habit.

Recommended Maximums for Conditionally Acceptable Foods

The following are recommended *maximums* per day, not recommended servings, since these foods are less than desirable. I allow these in the plan because many of the people I counsel ask not to have every "dietary crutch" taken away at one time. And although the sugar and salt substitutes and cocoa are not the best foods, they do not harm your health in the way that saturated fat, salt, and refined sugar do. It is healthiest to admit that you use these foods as crutches and, as with real crutches, plan for a not-too-distant day when you will not need them.

Drinks:

Bouillon or broth without fat or sodium: 1 cup

Carbonated drinks, sugar and caffeine-free: 1 cup

Cocoa powder, unsweetened: 1 tablespoon

Coffee or tea, decaffeinated: 2 cups

Sweet Substitutes:

Candy, hard, sugar-free: 2 pieces

Gelatin, sugar-free: 1 cup

Gum, sugar-free: 2 pieces

Jam or jelly, sugar-free: 2 teaspoons

Pancake syrup, sugar-free: 2 tablespoons

Sugar substitutes (saccharin or aspartame): 2 packages

Sodium Replacements

Remember that lowering your sodium intake is important not only if you have hypertension and kidney disease, but also to prevent you from getting these diseases, as well as stomach cancer, osteoporosis, and obesity. It is not easy to train yourself to prefer no-salt foods, but you can do it within a few months. Table 7.4 can help you make this transition. It compares the sodium content of typical foods to that of some lower-sodium alternatives. You can also make these assessments on your own with a little label-reading practice. Most of the low-sodium foods listed in the table must be found in a good health food store, but a growing number of better chain grocery stores are starting to carry them, too. This has come to pass because many customers, for many years, have been requesting these foods. So please help by asking your grocery store manager to stock these items—supply and demand is fueled by the consumer's voice.

❖ TABLE 7.4   SODIUM COMPARISONS OF POPULAR FOODS ❖

FOOD	SODIUM (IN MILLIGRAMS)
Cereals:	
Kelloggs Rice Krispies (1 ounce)	340
Grainfield Crispy Rice, No Salt, Fat, or Sugar (1 ounce)	35
Post Fortified Oat Flakes (1 ounce)	247
Health Valley Oat Bran Flakes (1 ounce)	10
Instant Quaker Oatmeal, plain (1 package, cooked)	160
Quaker Oats Quick Oatmeal, plain ($\frac{2}{3}$ cup, cooked)	0
Dairy Products and Substitutes:	
Cottage Cheese, 1% and 2%, creamed (1 cup)	918
Cottage Cheese, $\frac{1}{2}$% dry curd, no salt added (1 cup)	20
Skim Milk (8 ounces)	126
Buttermilk (8 ounces)	257
Yogurt (8 ounces)	174
Health Valley Fat-Free Soy Moo	60
Main Meals and Basic Staples:	
Prego Spaghetti Sauce (4 ounces)	623
Prego Spaghetti Sauce, No Salt Added	21
Canned Tomato Sauce ($\frac{1}{2}$ cup)	738
Heinz Tomato Sauce, No Salt Added	20
Chili with Beans (1 cup)	1,330
Health Valley Mild Vegetarian Chili (1 cup)	54
Canned black beans (1 cup)	922
Eden Organic Black Beans (1 cup)	30
Rice-A-Roni, Chicken Flavor ($\frac{1}{2}$ cup cooked)	500
Brown or enriched white rice ($\frac{1}{2}$ cup cooked)	3
Potatoes, au gratin ($\frac{1}{6}$ of 5.5 ounce package)	601
Baked potato	16
Del Monte Whole Kernel Corn, canned ($\frac{1}{2}$ cup)	360
Corn kernels, fresh or frozen ($\frac{1}{2}$ cup)	14
Calumet Baking Powder (1 teaspoon)	426
Featherweight Baking Powder, Sodium-Free	0

❖ TABLE 7.4 *(Continued)*

FOOD	SODIUM (IN MILLIGRAMS)
Whole Wheat Bread (1 slice)	159
Kroger Low Sodium Whole Wheat Bread	8
Heinz Mustard (1 teaspoon)	71
Westbrae Stoneground Mustard, no salt added (1 teaspoon)	2
Fish sandwich (average fast food value)	621
Star-Kist tuna, light, chunk (2 ounces)	310
Star-Kist tuna, dietetic (2 ounces)	30
Campbell's V-8 Vegetable Cocktail (6 ounces)	593
Campbell's V-8, No Salt Added (6 ounces)	41
Snacks:	
Bachman Stix pretzels (28 grams)	1,460
Harry's Honeys (1 pretzel = 24 grams)	20
Canned refried beans (1 cup)	1,068
Bearitos Vegetarian Refried Beans, No Salt Added (1 cup)	32
Corn chips (1 ounce)	218
Smart Temptations, No Fat, No Salt	0
Dill pickle, 1 medium ($3\frac{3}{4}'' \times 1\frac{1}{4}''$)	928
Featherweight Low Sodium Dill Pickle	5
Pace Thick and Chunky Salsa (2 tablespoons)	359
Enrico Chunky Style Salsa (2 tablespoons)	75
Soups:	
Campbell's Vegetarian Vegetable Soup (8 ounces)	790
Health Valley Organic Vegetable Soup, No Salt Added	65
Progresso Chicken Minestrone (9.5 ounces)	1,220
Health Valley Minestrone Soup (7.5 ounces)	110

Foods You Can Eat Only Rarely

Sugar and alcohol-rich foods lead this category. They should be used rarely if at all and only in very small portions. They are "empty calorie" foods, meaning they have significant calories but very little nutritional value. In some cases they may contain fat but little saturated fat or cholesterol. If you eat them frequently they can cause weight problems and may cause a rise in triglycerides. Some of those you may have on very rare occasions include:

> Desserts (cakes, pies, cookies, pudding), but only those made at home with allowed oil, skim milk, egg substitute, or egg whites. Angel food cake, Gingersnaps, Newton cookies, Entenmann's fat-free desserts/cookies and other brands of no-fat cookies are among the least harmful choices of store-bought desserts.

> Regular (nondiet) carbonated beverages

> Regular (nondiet) lemonade

> Sugar candy (candy corn, gum drops, mints, hard candy)

> Fruit ice or sherbet

> Regular (nondiet) fruit-flavored gelatin

> Sugar, syrup, and jam or jelly with added sugar

> Beer and liquor

The Dangers of Olestra—and Other "Magic Bullets" for Weight Loss

You may wonder why I have not included such new items as foods with Procter and Gamble's new fat substitute, olestra. This is only one of the most recent substitutes that promises something for nothing. In this case, we are promised the taste of fat without the calories. However, there is always a down side to this kind of substitute. Olestra, for example, has several potential adverse side effects. The label itself admits that "olestra may cause abdominal cramping, loose stools, and inhibit the absorption of some vitamins and other nutrients." But it fails to elaborate on some of the other more profound risks of those olestra-laced chips and crackers.

Olestra can deplete the body of fat-soluble vitamins, including A,D,E, and K, as well as carotenoids, such as beta carotene. Since Vitamin E and beta carotene have been shown to offer protection against heart disease and certain cancers, why would anyone willingly eat something that would reduce these benefits? One of the manufacturer's own studies found that eating sixteen olestra potato chips a day for 8 weeks reduced blood carotenoids levels by 50 percent. A Dutch study showed that even a small amount of olestra, 3 grams over 4 weeks, lowered the carotenoid called lycopene by 40 percent. This is of special concern as lycopene, found in high amounts in tomatoes, is a popular source of carotenoids for Americans. Other studies show similar problems with other carotenoids.

The effects on Vitamin K are also worrisome. Any effect olestra has on blood levels of K could be dangerous for people with bleeding disorders. Dr. Myra Karstadt, of the Center for Science in the Public Interest, reports that all studies done so far have intentionally excluded people taking a blood thinner called Coumadin. Since 1.5 million Americans are presently taking this drug, the potential dangers are staggering.

The other less-than-attractive side effect of olestra is the high risk it offers of diarrhea, bloating, flatulence, cramping, and a condition called fecal urgency—the need to go *right now*. One study showed that half the subjects developed diarrhea after eating 3 ounces of olestra-laced potato chips. And, even one ounce of chips has caused diarrhea and cramps in other studies. And if that is not enough to dissuade your "free fat" desires, olestra can cause anal leakage in some people, which is visible as yellow/orange stains on your underwear!

There is also concern about a potential cancer risk with olestra use, since some animal studies have found questionable liver-cell changes. Procter and Gamble argues that such liver changes in lab studies do not indicate cancer, and that long-term evidence in mice has not found cancer to be a problem. But what happens when olestra makes the leap from small lab studies to more than 200 million potential consumers who may eat it obsessively for years? We will never fully know. It is frightening when you realize that one of the longest-duration studies Procter and Gamble submitted—using pigs—lasted only 39 weeks. And the longest human study done on olestra thus far has been only 8 weeks!

I recommend you avoid this product because of what we do know and what we don't yet know about it.

Many of us are intent on finding an answer to our problems that is outside of ourselves, and outside of the simple whole food answer. We are actually much better off giving up the search for that "magic bullet" and embracing the natural goodness of grains, beans, fruits, and vegetables.

Nutritional Balance on the Plan

Although the Heal Your Heart Program nutrition plan is likely the most health-providing food plan you could enjoy, you'll want to ensure that you're getting enough of certain nutrients through both dietary means and supplements.

Multivitamin and Mineral Supplements

I recommend you take a basic multivitamin supplement, especially if you plan to consume less than 1,500 calories per day. Which one should you take?

The September 1994 issue of *Consumer Reports,* as well as most professional nutrition journals, encouraged the vitamin consumer to go for the bargain price. The following supplements are just as good as, if not better than, many of the more expensive brands:

Nature Made Mature Balance

Your Life Natural Multi-Vitamin and Mineral, iron free

Your Life Central-Vite Plus for postmenopausal women and men

Eckerd Central-Vite

Kmart Sentral-Vite

Kroger Complete for premenopausal women

Longs Central-Vite

Nature Made Century-Vite

Safeway Central-Vite

Although most multivitamin/mineral and single-supplement products generally contain the amounts stated on their labels and dissolve within an acceptable time period, it is still a good idea to buy one with a "dissolution test" guarantee on the label.

Most affordable multivitamin/mineral pills seldom have 100 percent of the twelve vitamins and eight minerals for which there are U.S. RDAs, so you may want to take an additional supplement of any nutrient you find lacking, such as antioxidants or calcium.

Antioxidants

It is best to get most of your antioxidants from your food, which provides not only fiber but many other known and unknown beneficial substances. But supplementing with antioxidants at levels higher than would be typically attainable through foods—for example, vitamin E at 200 I.U. and vitamin C at 500 milligrams—has produced very beneficial findings with respect to preventing and reversing heart disease. So you may want to supplement in those amounts. But also be sure to maximize the naturally occurring antioxidants by following these tips:

❖   Eat six or more fruits and vegetables daily, especially the root and dark orange and green vegetables and fruits that are especially high in vitamins E and C and beta-carotene.

❖   Use freshly cut fruits and vegetables when possible, as air and light can destroy many nutrients and antioxidants.

❖   Strictly limit or avoid meats rich in saturated fats and other fats. As you eat less and less meat and dairy products, you will likely increase your fruit and vegetable intake.

Also realize that your choice, method of use (temperature), and storage of oils can dramatically influence how many antioxidants you need to combat oxidized fats. The following fat tips reduce your intake and potential to create oxidized fats, which in turn will reduce your need for antioxidants:

❖   Limit your fat intake (to less than 20 percent or 10 percent, dependent upon heart disease risk factors) and use primarily monounsaturated oils, such as olive and canola oils. These oils cause LDL to be less susceptible to oxidation than diets high in polyunsaturated fatty acids.

❖   Avoid fried foods, especially in restaurants where the fat in fryers can go unchanged for weeks. Fats that have been heated to high temperatures are very volatile and very saturated with oxygen. As oxidized fats and cholesterol are the primary culprits in the plaque process, fried foods are not good dietary choices!

❖   Keep your oils, and fatty foods such as nuts and seeds, covered and less exposed to oxygen.

Calcium

Do you need a calcium supplement? Assess your individual risk factors for osteoporosis, discuss these with your doctor, and decide whether calcium supplementation is necessary for you. If you are following the Heal Your Heart Program—are eating a diet very low in sodium, alcohol, caffeine, and soda, and relatively low in animal protein, sufficient in calcium and vitamin D; are not smoking; are practicing stress management techniques; and are exercising regularly—you probably don't need to supplement with calcium. The low-fat, calcium-rich foods listed in Table 7.5 could provide you with sufficient amounts of calcium. You may be surprised at how much calcium you can get from food even without eating a lot of dairy products. Table 7.5 will give you an idea of how quickly naturally occurring calcium can add up without lots of fat and calories.

On the other hand, if you are still struggling to embrace all these positive lifestyle choices, you may choose to supplement to be on the safe side. Before you commit to a daily calcium supplement, be sure that you have educated yourself on the possible dangers; see Chapter 6 for a summary of concerns on calcium supplementation.

Vitamin B₆, Vitamin B₁₂, and Folic Acid

A growing amount of research has revealed many benefits of sufficient intake of folic acid, ranging from a reduction of homocysteine—and thus heart

❖ TABLE 7.5   HEALTHY CALCIUM-RICH FOODS ❖

FOOD AND QUANTITY	CALORIES	FAT (GMS.)	CALCIUM (MGS.)
1 cup acorn squash	114	.2	90
½ cup amaranth	14	.1	138
1 artichoke	53	.2	47
1 cup black turtle beans	241	.6	206
1 cup chickpeas	269	4.3	80
1 cup kidney beans	219	.2	116
1 cup navy beans	259	1	128
1 cup broccoli	46	.4	178
1 tablespoon blackstrap molasses	43	0	137
1 cup butternut squash	82	.2	84
1 cup carrots	70	.2	48
1 cup collards	54	.6	296
1 cup dandelion greens	34	.6	146
1 cup kale, scotch	36	.6	172
1 cup skim milk*	86	.4	302
½ cup rhubarb, sweetened	139	.1	174
2 sardines, canned in soybean oil (with bones)	50	2.8	92
1 tablespoon sesame butter (tahini)	89	8.1	64
1 cup spinach	42	.4	244
½ cup tofu, raw, firm*	183	11	258
1 cup turnip greens, frozen	48	8	250

disease—to prevention of birth defects and protection against cervical cancer and possibly colorectal and lung cancers. So, many were pleased when the Food and Drug Administration (FDA) announced in February 1996 that most grain products (those already enriched with several other B vitamins and iron) will be fortified with folic acid. Although many companies have already begun to fortify their grain products, manufacturers have until January 1998 to do so. But even then, fortified foods will probably supply only a portion of your daily folic acid needs.

Despite the fact that the 1989 Recommended Dietary Allowances reduced the recommendations from 400 micrograms for all adults to 200 for men

The above data was obtained with permission from Food Values of Portions Commonly Used, *15th Ed., by Jean A.T. Pennington, Harper & Row Publishers, New York, 1989. Foods are cooked unless followed by an asterisk (*).*

and 180 for women, the U.S. Public Health Service still recommends that all women capable of becoming pregnant should consume 400 micrograms of folic acid daily. Because folic acid stores must be sufficiently high at least a month before becoming pregnant to prevent birth defects, and an estimated 50 percent of all pregnancies are unplanned, women of child-bearing age should keep intakes this high at all times.

Any time we start trying to short-cut our nutritional needs with a pill or artificially created solution, complications inevitably arise. The main concern with folic acid supplementation or fortification is the fact that it can cover up or mask a vitamin B_{12} deficiency. It fixes the anemia (too few red blood cells) caused by too little B_{12}, but another symptom, nerve damage, can

❖ TABLE 7.6   HEALTHY SOURCES OF FOLIC ACID ❖

FOOD (1 CUP COOKED, UNLESS SPECIFIED OTHERWISE)	FOLIC ACID (MCG.)
1 artichoke	54
Asparagus	176
Baby lima beans	273
1 medium banana	22
Beets	90
Black beans	256
1 cup frozen blackberries	51
1 tablespoon brewer's yeast	313
Broccoli	108
Brussels sprouts	94
Cauliflower	64
Chickpeas	282
Cowpeas	356
Kidney	229
Lentils	358
Navy beans	255
Okra, frozen and boiled	268
1 cup orange juice, from frozen concentrate	109
1 cup pineapple juice	58
Pinto beans	294
1 cup romaine lettuce, shredded	76
Spinach	131
Split peas	127
2 tablespoons wheat germ	50

❖ TABLE 7.7   HEALTHY SOURCES OF VITAMIN B$_6$ ❖

FOOD (1 CUP COOKED, UNLESS SPECIFIED OTHERWISE)	VITAMIN B$_6$ (MGS.)
4 ounces cooked Atlantic salmon	1.4
1 banana	.7
Brown rice	.9
Brussels sprouts	.5
Carrots	.4
Chick peas, canned	1.1
1 piece of corn on the cob	.4
Green peas	.3
4 ounces cooked halibut	.5
Lentils	.4
Lima beans	.3
4 ounces cooked mackerel	.4
1 medium mango	.3
Mixed vegetables, frozen	.3
Navy beans	.3
$\frac{1}{4}$ cup rice bran	.6
Soybeans	.4
$1\frac{3}{4}$ cup watermelon	.5

worsen. The challenge is educating physicians and the public to recognize the early signs of neurological damage due to vitamin B$_{12}$ deficiency, because about a third of people with it never get anemia. Instead they will experience an unpleasant feeling, a tingling or burning pain, in their hands or feet, then up their legs. Once they lose muscle strength the damage is rarely reversible. In younger people these symptoms are easier to diagnose, but, unfortunately, many elderly people suffer from numerous diseases that share similar symptoms, such as diabetes, and Alzheimer's (which produces a similar dementia to that seen in vitamin B$_{12}$-deficient seniors). If these symptoms are familiar to you and if your vitamin B$_{12}$ blood test produces results at or below the normal range, further blood tests for methylmalonic acid and homocysteine would be needed to conclusively diagnose a vitamin B$_{12}$ deficiency.

As with all nutrients, it is safer and smarter to get your nutrients from whole foods which also come with many other healthful factors that are yet to be discovered. But if you find that you are not always able to ensure 400 mcg. of folic acid through the natural sources listed in Table 7.6, taking a multivitamin/mineral with this amount may help reduce your risk of heart disease, certain cancers, and birth defects. And if you are sixty-five years or older and you take a multivitamin/mineral pill that contains folic acid, it may be prudent to also take 500 mcg. of vitamin B_{12}. Although this amount is far higher than most of us need, there is apparently no known risk, and it is sufficiently high to treat people with pernicious anemia who lack the intrinsic factor that ordinarily ferries vitamin B_{12} into the bloodstream.

Because a high prevalence of vitamin B_6, B_{12}, and folic acid deficiencies have been observed in men with high homocysteine, and supplementing with these nutrients has been shown to reduce homocysteine levels dramatically, if you have heart disease or high homocysteine levels (or a family history of either) a multivitamin/mineral supplement ensuring 100 percent of the RDA would be prudent. If you would prefer to ensure adequate vitamin B_6 intake by natural food means, Table 7.7 may also prove helpful. To put these foods into perspective, the adult RDA for vitamin B_6 is 1.6 mgs. for women and 2 mgs. for men.

Foods fortified with vitamin B_{12}, such as specific brands of nutritional yeasts, some breakfast cereals, soy milks, and meat analogs, or a vitamin B_{12} supplement (which is generally included in multivitamin/mineral pills) are recommended if you choose a strict vegetarian plan. Look for 6 micrograms if you are following a vegan diet. If you are not on a strict vegetarian diet, the best food choices for B_{12} (those lowest in saturated fat content) are seafood, nonfat dairy products, and egg whites.

Iron

Remember that too much iron has been correlated with an increased incidence of heart disease. Remember, too, that iron deficiency is one of the most likely nutritional deficiencies, especially among menstruating women. You will probably never have a problem with iron inadequacy if you follow the Heal Your Heart nutrition plan (especially if you eat the highly recommended legumes). But if you are female, still menstruating, a vegetarian, and an athlete, it will help if you practice these iron tips:

❖ Frequently eat foods rich in iron along with vitamin C-rich foods to greatly enhance iron absorption. Foods rich in iron include dried beans and peas, dark green leafy vegetables, dried fruits, blackstrap molasses, and fortified breads and cereals. Vitamin C is found in many fresh fruits and vegetables, especially citrus, tomatoes, green leafy vegetables, and green peppers.

❖ Cook often in an iron skillet. Significant amounts of iron can leach from the skillet into your food, especially when you cook acidic foods such as tomato sauce. Food cooked in an iron skillet may have an iron content up to 10 times greater than if it had been cooked in a glass or stainless steel pan or pot.

❖ TABLE 7.8   HIGH- AND LOW-POTASSIUM FOODS ❖

HIGH POTASSIUM/LOW SODIUM (MORE THAN 250 MGS. POTASSIUM)	LOW POTASSIUM/LOW SODIUM (LESS THAN 200 MGS. POTASSIUM)
Fruits:	**Fruits:**
Apricots, 3 (313)	Apple, 1 (159)
Banana, 1 (451)	Applesauce, ½ cup (91)
Cantaloupe, 1 cup (494)	Blueberries, 1 cup (183)
Dates, 10 (541)	Cherries, 10 (152)
Honeydew, ½ cup (502)	Fruit cocktail, ½ cup (115)
Kiwi, 1 (252)	Grapefruit, ½ (158)
Mango, 1 (322)	Grapes, 1 cup (132)
Nectarine, 1 (288)	Mandarin oranges, ½ cup (165)
Orange, 1 (250)	Peach, 1 (171)
Papaya, 1 (780)	Persimmon, 1 (78)
Pomegranate, 1 (399)	Pineapple, 1 cup (175)
Prune juice, 1 cup (602)	Plum, 1 (113)
Raisins, ⅓ cup (373)	Tangerine, 1 (132)
	Prunes, 5 (194)
	Raspberries, 1 cup (187)
Vegetables:	Watermelon, 1 cup (186)
Artichoke, 1 cooked (316)	
Asparagus, ½ cup cooked (279)	**Vegetables:**
Lima beans, ½ cup cooked (477)	Onions, ½ cup (159)
Navy beans, 1 cup cooked (669)	Cauliflower, ½ cup cooked (129)
Okra, ½ cup cooked (257)	Mushrooms, ½ cup raw (145)
Parsnips, ½ cup cooked (287)	Eggplant, ½ cup cooked (119)
Potato, ½ cup cooked (556)	Green peas, ½ cup frozen (134)
Pinto beans, ½ cup cooked (400)	Mixed frozen vegetables, ½ cup (154)
Sweet potato, 1 cooked (397)	Peppers, ½ cup cooked (88)
Tomato juice, no-salt, 1 cup (549)	Cabbage, ½ cup cooked (105)
Winter squash, ½ cup cooked (473)	

❖   Avoid coffee and tea with meals. Coffee and tea can decrease iron absorption by as much as 39 percent and 87 percent, respectively. The culprit does not appear to be caffeine but substances called polyphenols. So, decaffeinated coffee and tea (except for herbal teas) are also a problem.

Other Nutrients

Although you don't need much Vitamin D or zinc, the small amounts needed by your body are very important. Vegetarians and older people, especially, tend to be deficient in these nutrients. Among many other things, vitamin D is important in absorbing calcium, and zinc is necessary if the immune system is to function properly.

You can get enough Vitamin D if you are in the sun for 10 to 15 minutes per day. But if you cannot ensure that, it is a good idea to take a supplement that provides 400 IUs, which is 100 percent of the U.S. RDA. As for zinc, it is also found in high levels in seafood, but substantial amounts are also available in whole grains and legumes.

Potassium

A high potassium intake can prevent hypertension and lower existing high blood pressure, but if you have kidney disease, you may need to limit the amount of potassium (as well as protein and sodium) in your diet. Check with your doctor. Table 7.8 shows the potassium content of many fruits and vegetables. The foods in the left column are good sources of potassium as they contain more than 250 milligrams, while those in the right column are good if you need to limit potassium, because they contain less than 200 milligrams. The foods in both columns are low in sodium, and so fit the Heal Your Heart nutrition plan perfectly. The potassium value in milligrams follows each food item.

8

Deciphering the New Food Labels

New food labeling rules, passed by Congress as the Nutrition Labeling and Education Act of 1990, went into effect in May 1994. While an improvement over the old ones, they still do not provide clear nutritional information to people trying to promote health and prevent or reverse chronic diseases. The guidelines on these labels are based upon a diet that has 30 percent of calories from fat and 10 percent of calories from saturated fat. As we discussed earlier, these dietary guidelines have repeatedly been shown to promote atherosclerosis rather than prevent or reverse it. So, until more ambitious guidelines are implemented, you will still face the challenge of translating food label information as you pursue a healthy diet.

The Positive Side of the New Label Laws

The most significant advantage of the new labels seems to be the inclusion of information on saturated fat and calories from fat. Because saturated fat intake is the most respected predictor of who gets heart disease, the lower the saturated fat content in a food, the better. I recommend that you get less than 4 percent of your daily calories from saturated fat rather than the 10 percent suggested on the food label.

Another advantage of the new labeling law is that servings are set by the FDA rather than by manufacturers. It will be easier to compare like products because they will *usually* be stating the same serving size. Previously, one butter company could give values for a tablespoon serving and another company give values for a teaspoon serving. But as you read the labels be sure to note the serving size, as there are a few exceptions to this new rule.

The rules for claiming a food is "low-cholesterol" have also improved. In order to make that claim, a food must now have less than 20 milligrams of cholesterol and less than 2 grams of saturated fat per typical serving. Previously, package labels could proclaim "low-cholesterol" even if the food was high in saturated fat. This was very deceptive because saturated fat intake causes high blood cholesterol levels even more than does dietary cholesterol itself.

Generally speaking, most of the thousand or so pages of new labeling rules are an improvement. It is easier for you to find out what nutrients are in a food and there are tighter restrictions on deceptive claims. But keep reminding yourself that the recommendations on the labels are based on fat and sodium guidelines that are too high if you are interested in prevention or reversal of heart disease. I'll explain a few of the loopholes and give you tips on how to make your own judgments.

The Factual Part of the "Nutrition Facts"

"Nutrition Facts" is the title of the column that now summarizes the nutritional information provided on most packaged foods in the United States. Although far from ideal, it does provide more information than we previously received to assess our food purchases and their relationship to current health concerns. These labels must provide the following information: total calories, calories from fat, total fat, saturated fat, cholesterol, sodium, total carbohydrate, dietary fiber, sugars, protein, vitamin A, vitamin C, calcium, and iron. Other vitamins and minerals as well as the further breakdown of monounsaturated and polyunsaturated fat or soluble and insoluble fiber may be listed but are not required.

Foods served in restaurants and cafeterias or on airplanes, food purchased from vending machines or mall cookie and candy counters, and ready-to-eat food prepared and sold primarily on site (such as bakery and deli items) do not have to have the food labels. But, the "Nutrition Facts" will be required on most packaged foods sold in grocery stores except raw fruits, vegetables, and fish. A 1990 amendment requires the Food and Drug Administration (FDA) to implement the nutritional labeling of the twenty most frequently consumed raw fruits, vegetables, and fish, so we will likely begin to see nutrition labels on these foods soon as well.

THE MANY LOOPHOLES TO LOOK OUT FOR

Of course, there are numerous loopholes to the labeling laws. Some serving sizes have been set too large or too small, dependent upon the strength of each food's lobbyists. For instance, the serving size for fresh meat, poultry, and seafood is 3 ounces, cooked. This is an admirably small serving size, but it doesn't fit the definition of a serving size, which is "the amount of food customarily consumed" in developed nations. I found it especially curious that protein was the only macronutrient that was not required in the "% daily value" column. Companies can voluntarily include a percentage based on a daily value for protein of 50 grams, or 10 percent of a 2,000 calorie diet, but I wouldn't hold your breath while looking for a meat product to admit this! Most Americans now consume far more than 50 grams, and they can easily obtain that much from vegetable sources that are free of cholesterol and saturated fat.

The carbohydrate versus sugar area on the label is also misleading. Complex carbohydrates are not listed because they cannot be distinguished from some sugars in food analyses. Where you see "other carbohydrates" listed, this includes complex carbohydrates plus sugars. I am not sure why sugars could not have been defined as "sugars added to a product that have no nutritionally redeeming qualities." But instead, "sugars" include those occurring naturally from nutrient-dense ingredients, as well as added sugars (like corn syrup) that offer only calories. So, foods like yogurt, milk, and fruit juices will appear high in sugar despite the fact that these are naturally occurring sugars found amidst an abundance of nutrients and beneficial factors, such as fiber, antioxidants and phytochemicals. Also of concern is the fact that "sugar" can be a gross underestimate because it does not include sugars that comprise up to two-thirds of some corn syrups.

Note the contrasting food labels in Fig. 8.1, which reflect how deceiving the sugar analyses can be. The Health Valley Fat-Free Apricot Delight Cookies label states that a serving (3 cookies) contains 11 grams of "sugars," but the uneducated reader may not realize that these naturally occurring sugars found in honey and fruits will not adversely affect the blood sugars or lipids nearly as much as the refined sugars in Nabisco Snackwell's Cookie Cakes (Devil's Food). Not only does fructose (which is high in honey and fruits) elevate a blood sugar less than do the refined sugars, which are primarily sucrose, but the fruits, soy flour, and organic oats also provide soluble fiber, which lowers cholesterol and helps stabilize blood sugars, whereas, the Snackwell's cookies made from refined wheat and sugars would inspire more dramatic blood sugar swings, likely raise your triglycerides more, and not offer the cholesterol-lowering effect of the soluble fiber-rich fruits, soy flour, and oats. But the sugar analyses would confuse the consumer to think otherwise; they would likely assume that the Snackwell's cookies were lower in "sugar" since they claim 9 grams of sugar per serving, while Health Valley cookies have 11 grams of sugar per serving. Few would note that the Snackwell's analysis refers to a 50-calorie cookie, while the Health Valley analysis refers to a more realistic 3-cookie serving totaling 100 calories.

Health Valley Fat-Free Apricot Delight Cookies

Nutrition Facts	Amount/Serving	%DV*	Amount/Serving	%DV*	*Percent Daily Values are based on a 2,000 calorie diet. Your daily values may be higher or lower depending on your calorie needs:
Serving Size 3 cookies (33g)	Total Fat 0g	0%	Total Carb. 24g	8%	
	Sat. Fat 0g	0%	Fiber 3g	12%	
Servings about 5	Cholest. 0mg	0%	Sugars 11g		
Calories 100	Sodium 50mg	2%	Protein 2g		
Fat Cal. 0	Vitamin A 2% • Vitamin C 4% Calcium 2% • Iron 4%				

	Calories	2,000	2,500
Total Fat	Less Than	65g	80g
Sat Fat	Less Than	20g	25g
Cholesterol	Less Than	300mg	300mg
Sodium	Less Than	2,400mg	2,400mg
Total Carbohydrate		300g	375g
Dietary Fiber		25g	30g

Calories Per Gram:
Fat 9 • Carbohydrate 4 • Protein 4

Ingredients: Organic 100% Whole Wheat Flour, Organic Cane Juice, Organic Oats, Dates, Honey, Dried Apricots, Dried Pineapple, Soy Flour, Natural Apricot Flavor, Baking Soda, Glycerin (Vegetable Source), Natural Vanilla, Cream of Tartar, Soy Lecithin, Concentrated Lemon Juice, Carob Beans, Carrageenan, Tri-Calcium Phosphate, Vitamin C (Calcium Ascorbate), Natural Beta Carotene. Organically grown and processed in accordance with the California Organic Food Act of 1990.

Nabisco Snackwell's Cookie Cakes (Devil's Food)

Nutrition Facts

Serving Size 1 Cookie (16g)
Servings Per Container 12

Amount Per Serving

Calories 50   Calories from Fat 0

	% Daily Value*
Total Fat 0g	0%
Saturated Fat 0g	0%
Cholesterol 0mg	0%
Sodium 25mg	1%
Total Carbohydrate 13g	4%
Dietary Fiber Less than 1g	1%
Sugars 9g	
Protein 1g	

Vitamin A 0%	•	Vitamin C 0%
Calcium 0%	•	Iron 0%

* Percent Daily Values are based on a 2,000 calorie diet. Your daily values may be higher or lower depending on your calorie needs:

	Calories:	2,000	2,500
Total Fat	Less than	65g	80g
Sat Fat	Less than	20g	25g
Cholesterol	Less than	300mg	300mg
Sodium	Less than	2400mg	2400mg
Total Carbohydrate		300g	375g
Dietary Fiber		25g	30g

INGREDIENTS: SUGAR, ENRICHED WHEAT FLOUR (CONTAINS NIACIN, REDUCED IRON, THIAMINE MONONITRATE [VITAMIN B_1], RIBOFLAVIN [VITAMIN B_2]), HIGH FRUCTOSE CORN SYRUP, CORN SYRUP, WATER, COCOA* (PROCESSED WITH ALKALI), SKIM MILK, GELATIN, BAKING SODA, CORNSTARCH, CHOCOLATE*, SALT, SOY LECITHIN* (EMULSIFIER), POTASSIUM SORBATE (TO PRESERVE FRESHNESS), ARTIFICIAL FLAVOR.

*ADDS A TRIVIAL AMOUNT OF FAT

FIGURE 8.1 The Sugar Seduction

Why the "% Daily Value" Is Misleading

In an attempt to help consumers assess how a particular food fits into their overall daily intake, the nutrition labels are now required to compare the amount of fat, saturated fat, carbohydrate, fiber, cholesterol, and sodium in the food to what a person should supposedly eat in a day. This "% daily value" reference is based on the assumption of a daily intake of 2,000 calories, and on these traditional dietary goals:

❖   60% calories from carbohydrate

❖   10% calories from protein

❖   30% calories from fat

❖   no more than 10% calories from saturated fat

❖   at least 11.5 grams of fiber per 1,000 calories.

But remember, since research has repeatedly shown that a diet with 30 percent of calories from fat promotes atherosclerosis, these values are not the best yardstick from which to measure your optimal dietary intake.

Because this "% daily value" data is based on guidelines that have been shown to promote heart disease, the column can be more confusing than helpful. If you did not understand that you need to eat less than 20 percent of your calories from fat to prevent heart disease and less than 10 percent to reverse heart disease, you might assume that the given "% daily value" for fat was an accurate way for you to achieve a healthy diet. The other confusing variable is that many people interested enough in their health to even read this nutritional information are trying to eat less than 2,000 calories a day, to lose weight. Thus, the "% daily value" numbers are based on too many guidelines that are irrelevant for people seeking to prevent or reverse diseases to justify the effort needed to convert them. It is far simpler for you to assess the product directly, as you will be instructed to later in this chapter.

The same concerns hold true for the sodium recommendations. The 2,000-calorie daily value for sodium is 2,400 milligrams, which is certainly far more than someone with high blood pressure (hypertension) should ingest and is also much more than anyone needs. The tables do not explain that heart patients and those with heart disease risk factors (hypertension, high cholesterol, diabetes, and obesity) would benefit from far lower fat and sodium intakes. Nowhere on the label are you told that the daily values are based on data that supposedly represent the *uppermost* limit that is thought desirable when considering public health concerns, rather than what is best for half of the American population that will die prematurely from heart disease.

Deceptions on the Front of the Label

Not only is the information on the back of the label enough to confuse dietitians and food scientists, but the hype on the front of the label can be misleading as well. One of the most important deceptions in the labeling law is in the standard for claiming that a food is "low-fat." A food can make this claim as long as it has no more than 3 grams of fat per typical serving. (In my opinion, a food is not truly low-fat unless it has no more than 2 grams of fat for every 100 calories, or less than 20 percent of calories from fat). Thanks to pressure from the dairy lobby, milk is exempted from this rule, so 2 percent fat milk will be called "low-fat" even though 35 percent of its calories are from fat. Given the atherogenic effect of butterfat and the naturally high sodium content of milk, the only dairy products truly low enough in fat and sodium to be considered healthy choices are: skim milk; ½ percent dry curd cottage cheese; and nonfat yogurt, sour cream, and ricotta (the low-sodium types).

Memorizing the new definitions for "low," "lean," "extra lean," "reduced," and "less" versus "light" would be far more troublesome than reading the "Nutrition Facts" for the most relevant information: calories, cholesterol, fat, and percentage of calories coming from fat and saturated fat. Since the claim that a food is "light" or "lite" can mean that it has one-third fewer calories than the regular version, *or* half the fat and half the sodium, *or* light in such properties as texture and color, it quickly becomes apparent that you need to learn how to translate the "Nutrition Facts" on the label to ensure that you make health-promoting food choices.

HOW TO READ FOOD LABELS

As you read through this section on how to read a food label, pick a favorite food and complete the "Food/Nutrition Label Worksheet" that follows. Make several photocopies of the worksheet and later complete them for all of your most frequently eaten foods, then keep them in a notebook for future reference. I have also included two filled-in worksheets to give you the idea of how this is done.

The most important pieces of information to note on a food label are the ingredients, serving size, calories, fat grams (gms.), saturated fat grams, percentage of calories coming from fat, milligrams (mgs.) of cholesterol and sodium, grams of fiber, and kind and amount of any additives such as refined sugar, artificial sweeteners, preservatives, or colorings.

The Ingredients

First, check the ingredients. They are listed in the order in which they are found in a product, by weight. For example, if sugar is the first ingredient listed, that means there is more sugar in the product than any other ingredient. It is important to choose foods that list only whole, unadulterated ingredients and that are naturally low in fat, sodium, and refined sugar.

Serving Size

Next, look at the serving size. The nutritional information provided on the label is given for the stated serving size. It is crucial to first note the serving size, as many packaged foods state unrealistically small servings. For instance, some low-calorie cereals state ¾ cup as a serving size, whereas many higher-calorie types (such as granolas) may state a serving size as small as ¼ cup. While it is true that your portion would likely be smaller for a dense, granola-type cereal, a ¼-cup serving is very unlikely. It also may surprise you that a 15-ounce can of soup is considered to be three servings by some companies. So be aware that many products may contain more than one serving per container.

Total Calories and Fat Calories

Next, check out the total calories and calories from fat. In assessing these, it will be helpful to remember the typical amounts naturally available in the various food groups as I defined them in Table 6.2. Table 8.1 shows the amount of calories and fat each group's food contains on average (cooked).

This information helps you "guestimate" what food groups (allowances) you have eaten within a mixed food. For instance, if you read that two nonfat cookies contain only grains and fruits and have 140 calories, it is a safe guess that the two cookies could be calculated as a starch (80 calories) and a fruit (60 calories). (See Chapter 6 for details on how many of each food group you can eat each day to achieve or maintain your weight goal.) Knowing the amount of fat naturally occurring in the food groups also helps

❖ TABLE 8.1   CALORIE AND FAT CONTENT OF FOOD GROUPS ❖

FOOD GROUPS	CALORIES	GRAMS OF FAT
Starches/breads (½ cup)	80	1–2
Vegetables (½ cup)	25	0
Fruits (1 piece)	60	0
Milk (1 cup skim)	86	0.4
Fat (1 teaspoon)	45	4.5
Meat (1 ounce lean)	55	3
Sugar (1 teaspoon)	16	0

you assess how much fat the manufacturer has added to the product. For example, some oat bran packages state a ½-cup cooked serving contains 2 grams of fat, while some state 3 grams. But, with no other ingredients listed but oat bran, and the knowledge that there is naturally occurring fat in all grains (1 to 2 grams on average), you would be equipped to "guestimate" that the 3-gram package of oat bran simply has a little more fat inherent in the oats than did the 2-gram-per-serving package. The naturally occurring fat is not a problem; it is needed for our health.

If you have chosen to just count calories rather than use the food group method (or in addition to it), simply multiply the total calories per serving by the number of servings you are eating. Of course, you would also need to purchase a pocket-sized reference for calories (and preferrably fat and sodium contents) in foods to also keep up with the calories coming from "whole foods." I hope that "whole foods"—such as whole grains, beans, and fresh fruits and vegetables—that are not surrounded by packages complete with labels and nutritional analysis will be the largest part of your diet.

To assess the amount of fat in a food, a good visual is

1 teaspoon of fat = 1 pat of butter = 4.5 grams of fat = 45 calories

Food labels now often tell you how many of the calories are "calories from fat," but two more steps are necessary before you know "percentage of calories coming from fat." Fat is listed in grams (28 grams = 1 ounce), and 1 gram of fat equals 9 calories. In case your label does not provide "calories from fat," simply multiply the number of fat grams by 9 to find out how many calories per serving come from fat. Then as the equation below shows, divide this "calories from fat" number by the total calories per serving; that number multiplied by 100 is "percentage of calories coming from fat."

$$\frac{\text{grams of fat per serving} \times 9}{\text{total calories per serving}} \times 100 = \% \text{ calories from fat}$$

Remember that if you have heart disease, less than 10 percent of your calories from fat per day will likely promote a more rapid and significant reversal of atherosclerosis. All vegetarian foods except nuts, seeds, avocados, and soy products naturally contain well under 10 percent of their calories from fat. So, if you eat only from the low-fat vegetarian foods and from processed labeled foods calculated to be less than 10 percent fat, you will be safely within your goals.

Now check saturated fats. If your cholesterol is high, less than 4 percent of your calories should come from saturated fats. In fact, limiting your saturated

fat to less than 4 perc
total fat intake. Your sa
diet has no more than
meat and dairy intake
the percentage of calo
"fat" in the percentag

$$\frac{\text{grams of saturated fa}}{\text{total calories}}$$

The oils that are
cholesterol *if* substit
relative. If you have
your added oil to no
This includes those
fine print in the ingr
for olive oil and car

Now look at the sugar
grams of sugar state
or quality. As th
"empty calori
must be ed
mean su
have
justi

Cholesterol Content

Next, look at the amount of cholesterol the food has. Limiting your cholesterol intake to less than 100 milligrams per day is a good goal. If the label does not reveal this information (as you may find with vending machine or deli foods), beware of foods that contain rich sources of cholesterol such as eggs, liver or other organ meats, dairy products that are not made from skim milk, high-fat meats, and shellfish.

Sleuthing for Added Sodium

Next, note the milligrams of sodium listed in a product. This is of utmost importance because a product can be advertised as "no salt added" yet still contain other sodium-rich ingredients. So it is necessary to avoid any products containing salt and anything with added sodium in it—that includes mono*sodium* glutamate (a flavor enhancer), *sodium* benzoate (a preservative), baking soda, and previously salt-cured items like olives.

Remember that the naturally occurring sodium found in grains, beans, fruits, and vegetables is not a problem. The goal is to avoid consuming *added* sodium whenever possible. For instance, the no-salt added Enrico's Salsa has 60 milligrams of sodium per 2-tablespoon serving, but the ingredients list includes only vegetables. This naturally occurring sodium should not be a concern unless you have severe liver or kidney disease.

content. As explained previously in this chapter, the
d on the label are not a very clear description of content
e sugar grams value includes justifiable sugars as well as
e" sugars, such as syrups and refined sugars, the consumer
cated and discerning. Syrups, and ingredients ending in "-ose,"
ar and should be avoided or limited. As fruits, honey, and molasses
eneficial factors accompanying their calories, these foods can be
able sugars even for people who are diabetic, hypoglycemic, and/or
verweight. Obviously, an accurately kept food record will let you know if any
of these justifiable sugars are triggering binging or excessive consumption.
Remember: 1 teaspoon (of most sugars or sweeteners) = 16 calories, and
1 to 2 teaspoons per day is not a problem. Limit yourself to cereals with 6
grams or less of sucrose and other sugars.

Fiber

Next, look at fiber. All labels list total fiber, and some break this down into
soluble and insoluble fiber. You can also read the ingredients list to look for
good sources of fiber. The highest sources of insoluble fiber include wheat
bran and most whole grains and vegetables. Soluble fiber-rich foods include
oat bran, oatmeal, dried beans and peas, barley, cornmeal, and fruits.

Again be cautioned about comparing the product's contribution of fiber
to your day based on the "% daily value," which is also less than ambitious.
Their 11.5 grams of fiber per 1,000-calorie intake guideline is less than half
the fiber consumed by most vegetarian populations that do not typically
suffer from our chronic diseases.

Additives

Last, but not least, check for artificial additives. Although some of the commercially used preservatives, starches, artificial flavors, colors, and sweeteners are safe, there is insufficient space here to list those that have been
shown to increase the risk of cancer. The safest bet is to eat foods that have
ingredients you can recognize and pronounce, like whole foods that have
grown from the ground. Why should we willingly treat our bodies to a poorly
designed biology experiment, where we subject ourselves to innumerable
unnatural fuels that have never been ingested by humans until this generation? A growing number of us choose not to. With the largest variety and
selection of fresh and organically grown whole foods, and processed foods
which by and large must list their ingredients, why not make the best choices?

Food/Nutrition Label Worksheet

Product: _____

Ingredients: _____

_____

Serving size: _____ Calories/serving: _____ Fat: _____ gms. Fat Calories: _____

$$\% \text{ of calories from fat} = \frac{_____ \text{ gms. fat} \times 9 \text{ calories/gm.}}{_____ \text{ total calories}} \times 100$$

% of calories from fat = _____%

List the fat-rich ingredients: _____

Does the product contain more than 4% saturated fat? _____

Does the product contain cholesterol? _____

Sodium content: _____ mgs. Naturally occurring or added salt? _____

Does it contain justifiable (nutritionally redeeming) sugars? _____

_____ Sugars: _____ gms.

Is it a significant source of fiber? _____

Product evaluation/comments: _____

_____

Highly recommend: _____

Conditionally recommend; alternatives: _____

_____

Avoid; list reasons: _____

_____

Food/Nutrition Label Worksheet

Product: *Armour Chili with Beans (New and Improved—Thick 'N Zesty)*

Ingredients: *water, beef, beans, wheat flour, spices, natural flavorings, sugar, paprika, caramel coloring, salt, monosodium glutamate, lecithin*

Serving size: *1 cup* Calories/serving: *370* Fat: *21* gms. Fat Calories: *189*

$$\% \text{ of calories from fat} = \frac{\underline{\quad 21 \quad} \text{ gms. fat} \times 9 \text{ calories/gm.}}{\underline{\quad 370 \quad} \text{ total calories}} \times 100$$

% of calories from fat = _____*51*_____ %

List the fat-rich ingredients: *beef*

Does the product contain more than 4% saturated fat?

$$\frac{9 \text{ gms. saturated fat} \times 9 \text{ cals/gm.}}{370 \text{ total cals}} \times 100 = 22\%$$

yes

Does the product contain cholesterol? *yes; 50 mgs.*

Sodium content: *1220* mgs. Naturally occurring or added salt? *added salt and MSG*

Does it contain justifiable (nutritionally redeeming) sugars? *no, refined sugar*   Sugars: *2* gms.

Is it a significant source of fiber? *yes; 10 gms. is high, primarily due to beans*

Product evaluation/comments: *this product typifies the fat and sodium-packed foods typically eaten by those with chronic diseases*

Highly recommend: *no*

Conditionally recommend; alternatives: *this product could not be recommended to anyone seeking to reverse or prevent disease*

Avoid; list reasons: *this product should be avoided because of its high fat (especially saturated fat), cholesterol, and sodium content*

Food/Nutrition Label Worksheet

Product: *Health Valley Mild Vegetarian Chili, no salt added*

Ingredients: *water, organic tomatoes, organic pinto beans, onions, tomato paste, organic carrots, soy granules, green bell pepper, chili pepper, honey, unsulfured molasses, garlic powder, cumin, organic potato flakes, paprika, ground bay leaves, organic sage, organic basil, oregano.*

Serving size: *1/2 cup* Calories/serving: *80* Fat: *0* gms. Fat Calories: *0*

$$\% \text{ of calories from fat} = \frac{0 \text{ gms. fat} \times 9 \text{ calories/gm.}}{80 \text{ total calories}} \times 100$$

% of calories from fat = *0* %

List the fat-rich ingredients: *none*

Does the product contain more than 4% saturated fat? *no*

Does the product contain cholesterol? *no*

Sodium content: *35* mgs. Naturally occurring or added salt? *naturally occurring*

Does it contain justifiable (nutritionally redeeming) sugars? *yes, honey and unsulfured molasses*   Sugars: *4* gms.

Is it a significant source of fiber? *yes; 7 gms. of fiber is high—beans are very high*

Product evaluation/comments: *this chili is the best I've tried on the market; the "soy grannules" are heavy and meatlike; my favorite ready-made, no-added-fat-and-salt meal*

Highly recommend: *this product epitomizes how delicious no-added-fat-and-sodium processed foods can be*

Conditionally recommend; alternatives: *undoubtedly my favorite chili; no other product comes close to being this "clean" and this good!*

Avoid; list reasons: *no problem; just precede it with a salad so that 1/2 can will satisfy, rather than a whole can, which previously made me uncomfortably "full"*

The Food/Nutrition Label Worksheet can not only assist you in assessing the healthfulness of a food product, it can be taken a step further to help you assess how that product would fit into a day's intake. A One-Day Intake Analysis form for calories, fat, and sodium would obviously be easy to complete if your favorite and most commonly eaten foods had already had their label's nutritional information summarized on the Food/Nutrition Label Worksheet. The One-Day Intake Analysis form can really help put the nutritional analysis for each food choice into a daily perspective. For example, although no-salt-added Bearitos Refried Beans offers 22.5 percent of calories coming from fat, when served with the no-fat/no-salt corn chips and salsa, they average far less than the 20 percent fat goal for the day. Our ultimate nutritional goals are outlined at the bottom of the form: to average less than 20 percent of calories coming from fat if your goal is to prevent heart disease, or 10 percent fat to reverse heart disease, and to average less than 500 milligrams of sodium per day.

One Day Intake Analysis

Complete this form by writing down each food and drink you have in one day, along with the approximate portion size of each, in the first column. Calculate the calories, grams (gms.) of fat, and milligrams (mgs.) of sodium for each food or drink. You can find these on the food label or by consulting a book of nutrient values, such as the pocket-sized T-factor books available in most supermarkets. At the end of the day, calculate your daily total for calories, the percentage of those calories from fat, and your total amount of sodium. Compare these totals to your dietary goals to see if you need to make changes.

Portion and Food	Cals.	Fat (gms.)	Sodium (mgs.)
Breakfast: _____	_____	_____	_____
_____	_____	_____	_____
_____	_____	_____	_____
_____	_____	_____	_____
Lunch: _____	_____	_____	_____
_____	_____	_____	_____
_____	_____	_____	_____
_____	_____	_____	_____
_____	_____	_____	_____
Supper: _____	_____	_____	_____
_____	_____	_____	_____
_____	_____	_____	_____
_____	_____	_____	_____
_____	_____		_____

$\times$ 9 cals./gm.
_____
/total cals.
$\times$ 100 =

_____   __% cals.   __mgs. sodium
from fat   (<500 mgs.)
(10–20%)

9

HEALING YOUR HEART THROUGH EXERCISE

Our bodies are incredibly resilient; their ability to come back after years of inactivity and abuse is nothing short of miraculous. But successful physical conditioning is best done with patience and consistency. Follow the guidelines in this chapter to ease into an exercise program without injury, and with plans for consistency and long-term commitment.

The first rule of exercise is: Listen to your body. Your body has been talking to you all your life. You may not have understood those terms in the past, but now you have an opportunity to get reacquainted with your body. The only way your body can tell you that something is very wrong for you is to give you pain. If you experience pain during exercise, *stop.* The activity you have chosen may not be well suited for you or you may not be doing the activity correctly. Ask for advice from your doctor, nurse, exercise physiologist, or cardiac rehabilitation professional.

The following are all signals that your body wants to stop exercising immediately:

❖ Discomfort: pressure, tightness, squeezing, burning, numbness in the chest, back, jaw, neck, or arms

❖ Undue shortness of breath

❖ Numbness or tingling in your arms

❖ Rapid or irregular heartbeats

❖ Dizziness, confusion, or fainting

❖ Cold sweating or nausea

If you experience any of these symptoms, stop exercising and sit down. If the symptoms are persistent and last several minutes, call your emergency services number. If your symptoms subside on their own, call your doctor. He or she can evaluate your ability to exercise.

Other signs that you need to stop exercising are headache or anxiety. These symptoms may not need emergency medical attention, but you should tell your doctor if you experience them during exercise.

When we use our muscles in a new way, they can become sore. This soreness is different from acute pain with exercise. You can avoid this soreness by breaking into exercise gradually.

Quick Health and Safety Tips

Use the following health and safety tips to enhance the odds that your reentry into a more active lifestyle is a positive one. And continue to keep these tips in mind as you commit to exercise regularly:

1. Listen to your body. If you hurt, stop.

2. If you have any warning signs of heart problems, stop.

3. Do what you are able to and increase the intensity and duration of your exercise gradually.

4. Avoid doing two high impact workouts in a row.

5. Drink plenty of water unless you are instructed by your physician otherwise. But, if you are truly following a no-salt-added diet, your fluid needs will rarely be much more than six cups a day. Drink more if you are thirsty, but not just out of habit. Drinking unnecessarily large volumes of water for preconceived "dieting" reasons can create electrolyte imbalances in those consuming no-salt added vegetarian diets.

6. The Heal Your Heart nutrition plan, a diet rich in complex carbohydrates, is the preferred fuel for your body. Carbohydrate fuels you for peak performance. Unfortunately, many athletes, especially weight trainers, have been misled to believe that they need more protein than they actually do. For reasons described in Chapter 2, this nutrition plan offers more than enough protein for any athletic endeavor. Another popular sports-nutrition myth is that we need

to replenish lost electrolytes with sodium-packed "sports drinks." The amount of sodium and fluid lost in exercise lasting less than a marathon can be found in a nutrient- and fiber-rich tossed vegetable salad and an extra two or three glasses of water. Only people who run more than 20 miles without stopping could justify ingesting the excessive sodium found in the commonly advertised "sports drinks."

7. Be consistent with your exercise. If you fall off your program, get right back on track.

8. Whatever you do, be active. Be active in your daily life. Take the stairs instead of the elevator. Walk instead of driving short distances. Garden. Do your own yardwork. Plan activities that require movement.

9. Avoid exercising in extreme temperatures. If you live in an extreme climate or are sensitive to heat or cold, you may find exercising indoors more to your liking. If you experience angina (chest discomfort due to lack of blood flow to your heart), exercising in the cold can be especially troublesome. The cold temperatures can precipitate anginal symptoms.

10. If you exercise vigorously every day, take a rest day every fourteen days to prevent overtraining.

11. If you lift weights, avoid lifting two days in a row with the same muscle groups. You can alternate body areas by lifting for your upper body one day and lower body the next.

When you begin your exercise session, prepare your heart and other muscles with a warm-up by exercising at a slower pace for 3 to 5 minutes, then gradually increase to your exercise pace. The warm-up helps bring warm blood to the working muscles and increases your heart rate and blood pressure.

A cool-down, which means walking or exercising at a slower pace at the end of your workout, will help bring your heart rate and blood pressure down gradually. If you don't cool down, you may feel light-headed. When your heart is pumping fast and hard and you suddenly stop moving, blood pools in your legs. When blood pools in your legs, it isn't circulating in your system very well. Blood isn't getting back to the brain and heart the way it was when you were moving; thus you feel light-headed.

If you want to start lifting weights at a gym or health spa, look into personal training sessions. Weight lifting can be very beneficial, but it can also hurt you if done improperly. Seek advice before trying unfamiliar weight lifting machines.

Not being able to get to a spa or gym is no excuse for obesity and poor health. There are many strength training exercises you can do at home. The following section will explain some of these to you.

EXERCISES FOR SPECIFIC MUSCLE GROUPS

Exercising specific muscles strengthens them. When you exercise a muscle (or muscle group), it contracts and contributes to a primary movement. This primary movement is the action you need to make that muscle work. Whenever you complicate movements, you increase your chances for injury and decrease the effectiveness of the exercise.

While doing strength exercises, exhale on exertion and inhale on relaxation. Breathing this way can prevent your blood pressure from increasing too much due to increased chest pressure.

You may feel a discomfort associated with fatigue in the muscle group you are working. Many people describe this discomfort as a burning sensation. This is caused by a build up of lactic acid. It does not strengthen the muscle to work through the burn, so stop, rest, and maybe massage the area before completing your total repetitions.

Toning Your Abdominals

There are three abdominal muscles that you'll want to exercise: the rectus abdominus, and your internal and external obliques.

The Rectus Abdominus

Your rectus abdominus is the longest muscle in your body. It attaches at the lower ribs and at the pubic bone—the prominent bone in the groin area. When the rectus abdominus contracts, it flexes the trunk slightly. It does not bring the trunk all the way to the knees nor does it have any connection to the legs or feet. Thus, the movement caused by the rectus abdominus is only a slight movement of the trunk. While doing an abdominal crunch, if you need to lift your feet or pull with your legs, you are not working the rectus abdominus.

If you have ever done a full range sit-up where you bring your chest or elbows to meet your knees, you may have noticed that at a certain place you felt a "sticking" point. This sticking point is where you changed muscle groups from your rectus abdominus to the hip flexor (iliopsoas and rectus femoris) muscles. Because you are trying to work the rectus abdominus, stop when you reach the sticking point. Many people have been taught to do sit-ups improperly. Doing full-range sit-ups (the type where you bring your chest or elbows to your knees) may actually do more harm than good. Full-range sit-ups past the sticking point strengthen the hip flexors, not the abdominals; this can cause undesirable tension in the lower back.

The proper way to work the rectus abdominus is to begin on your back with your knees bent and feet on the floor near your buttocks. Cross your hands over your chest or place them in front of you. If you need support for your head and neck, place only your finger tips at the sides of your neck, slightly toward the back. Placing your hands around the back of your head can lead to neck and upper back injuries due to hyperflexion of the neck. If you feel neck fatigue because your neck is not supported, take a rest. You don't have to complete all of your abdominal crunches in a row. Lift the upper portion of your trunk off the floor until you reach the sticking point (about 30 degrees off the floor). As you inhale, return to the resting position, then repeat.

Internal and External Obliques

To work the internal and external obliques (your side abdominal muscles), start in the same position as the abdominal crunch. Lie on your back, with knees bent and feet close to buttocks. Place your hands across your chest. As you exhale, pretend you are drawing a line from your right shoulder to your left knee while you are lifting your upper trunk off the floor. When you reach the sticking point, inhale as you return to the resting position. Repeat this exercise, making a line from your left shoulder to your right knee.

Strengthening Your Outer Thighs

The outer thigh muscles (abductors of the leg), only move the leg from the midline of the body to beside the body. To isolate this primary movement, you need to prevent rotation of your leg while moving it. If you rotate the leg, other, stronger, muscles will take over. You may do this exercise lying on the floor or standing up.

While standing, you may want to use a chair to steady yourself. Stand behind the chair with your hands on the chair back, with knees slightly bent. Lift one of your legs to the side keeping the toes pointed forward or slightly turned inward. Use slow and controlled movements. Return to resting position and repeat until slightly tired, then do the other leg.

If you prefer to exercise on the floor; lie on your side. Keeping your body straight, bend your bottom leg at the knee and pull it slightly forward. This will give you more support. Relax your head on your out-stretched (bottom) arm to keep your spine in alignment. You may use your other arm to touch the floor in front of you for support. Lift your top leg up. Try not to bend at the hip, because you will change muscle groups if you do. Try to keep your toes pointing forward or slightly down, to isolate the abductor muscles. When you have lifted the leg as far as you can without bending at the hip or rotating the leg, return to the resting position. Do this exercise in a slow and controlled manner. Remember to have a distinct stopping and starting point for this exercise to help you proceed slowly with focus, which helps the muscle do more work. Repeat until slightly tired, then repeat with other leg.

Toning Your Buttocks

The buttocks (gluteus maximus muscles), are the large muscles that we sit on. They extend our legs. Moving your leg in one plane (forward and backward) helps isolate this muscle group.

While standing behind a chair, lift one leg directly behind you. Keep your knees slightly bent and toes pointing forward. Try not to move your back. Return to the resting position, then repeat.

While lying on the floor, lie on one side. Keeping your body straight, bend your bottom leg at the knee and pull it slightly forward. This will give you more support. Relax your head on your out-stretched (bottom) arm to keep your spine in alignment. You may use your other arm for support. Pull your top leg forward close to the floor, bending it at the knee. This is the resting position. Then, extend your top leg, pressing it behind you. Return to the resting position. Repeat with the same leg. Do this exercise in a concentrated and controlled manner. Remember to have a distinct stopping and starting point for this exercise to help you stay focused and slow with your movements. Then do on the other side.

Strengthening Your Inner Thigh Muscles

Your inner thigh muscles (adductors) bring your leg inward toward the midline of your body. Take care to keep your body in alignment while trying to work this muscle group to help prevent back injuries.

Lie on your side on the floor and bend your top leg, allowing it to rest on the floor in front of the bottom leg. The foot of your top leg will rest on its side on the floor. You can also rest your top leg on a cushion or pillow to help keep your body in alignment. Relax your head on your out-stretched (bottom) arm so that your spine stays in alignment. With your bottom leg straight, lift it slightly off the floor. Try to make sure that your body is not leaning forward or backward. Repeat until slightly tired, then repeat on the other side.

Toning Your Chest Muscles

Your chest muscles (pectoralis muscle group) help move your shoulder joint. They also help you breathe and maintain posture. Unfortunately, to isolate this muscle group, you need to use many joints—your wrists, elbows, hips, knees, perhaps ankles, and of course, the shoulder. You need to take special care to protect these joints.

Basically, you will be performing a regular old push-up, but you will be standing. Stand about $2\frac{1}{2}$ to 3 feet away from a wall with your feet shoulder-width apart. Place your hands on the wall at chest height, about shoulder-width apart. Keeping your knees slightly bent, bend your elbows. Your trunk will move closer to the wall, creating resistance in your chest muscles. When your face is close to the wall, exhale as you push against the wall. Your trunk will move away from the wall. Even at the end of your push-up, keep your elbows slightly bent. Repeat.

To do this exercise on the floor, lie face down. Bend your knees and pull your feet up toward the backs of your thighs. Place your hands under your shoulders. As you exhale, push against the floor, straightening your arms. Your trunk will move away from the floor. Try to keep your back in the same position it was in while lying on the floor. Try to move your body as one unit; do not allow yourself to bend at the middle. (If you cannot do this, stick with the wall push-up.) At the end of this movement, remember to keep your elbows slightly bent. Return to the resting position on the inhale. Repeat. These bent-knee push-ups are better than the old traditional push-ups done with straight legs because the latter can create extra tension on the lower back. Since the goal of this exercise is to strengthen the chest muscles, why put your back at risk?

STRETCHING

Stretching increases your flexibility. Flexibility is the amount of movement tolerable in a joint. Thus, your shoulder joint may be very flexible while your hip joint is not. Listening to your body and obeying its signals guides you in determining how far you need to stretch. When you feel discomfort, you have gone too far. You should feel as if you are challenging your joints to be more flexible, but not forcing them.

Muscles, tendons, and ligaments are more flexible when they are warm, so the best time to stretch is immediately after your workout. You may also want to stretch before your exercise session, but it is best to stretch immediately *after* your warm-up. When stretching, avoid bouncing. Instead, hold your stretches from 15 to 30 seconds to take full advantage of the muscle relaxation response.

Stretching the Calf

The calf muscle (gastrocnemius), is located on the back of the lower leg. This muscle can become very tight, especially if you walk long distances, wear high heeled shoes, or do aerobic dance. Any activity that requires you to point your toes uses the calf muscle.

To stretch this muscle while standing, place one foot flat on the ground behind you and bend your front knee. Your feet should be widely spaced from front to back. Your front knee should be right over your front heel. This supports your knee. You should not feel pressure in your front leg, but you will feel your back calf stretch. Hold for 30 seconds, then repeat with your other leg.

Stretching the Upper Thigh

Your quadriceps are the large muscles of your front thigh. These muscles can get very tight after performing aerobic exercise. To stretch this muscle group, hold onto a wall or chair while standing. Bend one of your knees, bringing your foot close to your buttocks. Reach for your ankle to hold your leg in this position. Keep the leg you are standing on slightly bent, so that you do not lock that knee. Hold this stretch for 30 seconds, then repeat with the other leg.

If you have trouble with this stretch, try this: Instead of holding your ankle, prop your leg in a chair behind you. This allows your leg to be supported at a lower level (below the buttocks).

Stretching the Back of the Thigh Muscles

The hamstrings are the muscles in the upper back of the thigh. They can become very tight and cause problems with your lower back. To stretch these muscles, lie on the floor on your back. Bend your knees, bringing your feet toward your buttocks. Extend one leg above you. Place your hands behind the knee of your extended leg to support it. Try to keep this leg straight. Hold this stretch for 30 seconds, then repeat with the other leg.

Stretching the Lower Back Muscles

Your lower back can become tired and tight from overuse. To stretch the muscles in your lower back, lie on the floor on your back. Bend your knees and bring them halfway toward your torso. Place your hands around the back of your knees, then hug your knees. Avoid holding onto the front of your knees. Hold this stretch for 30 seconds.

Stretching the Upper Back

Often we carry stress in our upper backs, which stretching can relieve. Place your right hand on your left shoulder and your left hand on your right shoulder and give yourself a big hug. Hold this stretch for 15 to 30 seconds. Now, switch your arms so that the arm that was on top is now on the bottom. Give yourself another hug, and hold for 15 to 30 seconds. You can do this while you are sitting or standing.

Stretching the Chest Muscles

Your chest muscles can become shortened by poor posture, such as hunching forward. Stretching the chest can help you breathe better as well as improve your posture. To stretch your chest muscles, interlock your fingers and place your hands behind your head. Press your elbows back so that they are wide apart. Avoid arching your back. Hold this stretch 15 to 30 seconds.

Stretching the Neck Muscles

Our neck muscles also carry a lot of stress. To relieve stress and relax your neck, lean your head toward your left shoulder. Hold this stretch for 15 seconds. Now, drop your head to the center in front of you. Hold this stretch for 15 seconds. Now, lean your head to your right shoulder. Hold this stretch for 15 seconds. You may also add little micromovements in all these directions, which are just little gentle movements that massage the edge of your stretching range. These gentle movements will extend your range of motion, or ability to stretch a little further, by helping you relax into the stretch. The head can roll gently forward from one shoulder to another, as well. You may repeat these stretches if you like.

WHERE TO FIND HELP AND SUPPORT

Now you have some ideas about the types of exercise you can do, how much and how often you might exercise, which exercises will help strengthen your muscles and what stretches will help promote flexibility. For more detailed information, you may need to get personal help. If you have heart disease, or numerous risk factors, the best choice for you would probably be a cardiac rehabilitation program. These can be found throughout the world, and have the advantage of being staffed by dietitians, nurses, exercise physiologists, and cardiologists who have a special interest in heart disease. Although most cardiac rehabilitation programs are still teaching 30 percent fat guidelines, and will thus not produce as impressive results as the nutrition plans outlined in this book, they will at least offer you a safe and instructive place to exercise, the comradery of others with similar problems and challenges, and may offer emotional support groups and/or therapy. Ask your doctor for recommendations.

Few diagnoses limit patients' confidence in their physical abilities as much as a heart attack or stroke, so it is of utmost importance—not only physically, but emotionally—for patients to return (or begin) to exercise as soon as their physicians give you the O.K. Cardiac rehabilitation programs are great for providing not only a medically trained staff to help deal with any fears, but also a supportive environment of peers who have literally walked through the same challenges. For a decade, I have watched cardiac rehabilitation participants reclaim their confidence and self-esteem, as well as a more positive perception of their health and prognosis. There is nothing like an encounter with another heart patient who has gone on to run a marathon to raise expectations and dissolve fears. This example is not to suggest that marathon distances should be your exercise goal, but to inspire you to realize that there is life after heart disease or stroke.

YMCAs have excellent programs and generally follow a standard practice of exercise prescription. If you are looking into personal trainers, gyms, or health spas, check for staff certifications by the American College of Sports Medicine (ACSM), American Council on Exercise (ACE), International Fitness Institute, National Academy of Sports Medicine, and the National Strength and Conditioning Association (NSCA). Also, the staff should be CPR (Cardio-Pulmonary Resuscitation) certified.

To locate certified fitness professionals in your area, you may call ACE at 1-800-529-8227 or the NSCA at 712-632-6722. Also, for fitness consumer pamphlets, call IDEA—International Association of Fitness Professionals at 1-800-999-4332.

Try not to be seduced by "perfect," hard bodies. Just because someone looks beautiful by some standards does not mean that their workout will work for you. That is the problem with model and celebrity videos. These folks are genetically destined to be models and celebs. We are not all like them. Most of us won't dunk a basketball like Michael Jordan or do a *Sports Illustrated* swimsuit layout, so the workouts of these stars may not work for you. Moreover, their workouts could be dangerous to you.

So find a workout that seems sensible for your lifestyle and abilities. Find people who work to help average folks be the healthiest that they can be. Most important, listen to your body and move.

10

HEALING YOUR HEART THROUGH EMOTIONAL AND SPIRITUAL RENEWAL

The emotional and spiritual aspect of the Heal Your Heart Program encompasses a wide variety of paths for every spiritual affinity and personality type. Each path can lead to a deeper understanding of yourself, thus a clearer awareness of what you would be happiest, most fulfilled, and most effective at doing with your life. I will refer to this seeking of your optimal path or choices in life as pursuing your "higher calling." My experience, and that of many others, has been that if enough meditative or introspective time is spent alone (via one of the many paths we will discuss) we will become increasingly more clear about what choices are best for us. By committing to one or more of these spiritual disciplines, you will not only feel more confident in how to proceed but you will be more joyful and fulfilled in the process. This chapter will guide you through choosing the right healer, and which spiritual paths to pursue, as well as finding the best support groups and stress management instruction.

CHOOSING A HEALER

One of the keys to healing physically, emotionally, and spiritually is choosing the right healer—a physician or therapist you like, who believes that you can be healed. When I had severe joint pain, I went to a rheumatologist who told me I had arthritis and gave me larger and larger doses of anti-inflammatory drugs. It finally dawned on me that I needed a physician who truly believed I could recover, or at least that I needed fewer medications, not more. Since I began suffering from allergies at about the same time the arthritis-like symptoms crippled me, I consulted an allergist, who asked me lifestyle questions for almost an hour. When I asked his opinion on the connection between the allergies and my arthritislike condition, he declared, "You do not have arthritis, you have stress-induced joint pain. And if you do not slow down you will be in a wheelchair by forty." He prescribed two hours of counting squirrels on the Eno River per day! Although my home overlooked the Eno River, I broke down in tears, terrified by the fact that I knew I would not be able to "waste" that much time each day. Although I have yet to reach two hours of uninterrupted meditative squirrel counting, I got his point and began to seek emotional and spiritual inner healing. It took some time, but I am now free from my dependence upon anti-inflammatory medications. This physician was key to my recovery. He also assisted me in selecting a therapist who helped me get in touch with, and begin to let go of, my need to be in complete control.

So, if you do not at first succeed in selecting an effective physician or therapist, continue to seek one who feels right for you. In addition to the healer having hope for your recovery, it is important that he or she tells you what you *need* to hear, which is not always what you may *want* to hear. The therapists who helped me most were the ones who were willing to confront me about my addictive behavior. Initially, I was angered by what I thought was their judging me, but as my healing progressed, I began to appreciate the power of their spoken truths and the healing power of bringing my darker side into the light.

The most significant part of my healing and my success at choosing the right healers to guide me, was in learning to "let go" (of my perceived control) "and let God." The Twelve Step practitioners call it surrendering to a power greater than ourselves. Since I believe that seeking or surrendering to this Higher Power on some level is key for all healings, I want to offer you a structure that not only has helped me personally, but has helped me in assisting others in finding their path(s) to healing.

PATHS TO EMOTIONAL AND SPIRITUAL RECOVERY

From my personal and professional experience with healing, I have found that choosing a healer and commiting to a spiritual discipline is most effectively done through a commitment to prayer. Attending to our emotional and spiritual selves inevitably involves developing a relationship with our Higher Power. Prayer not only assists the development of this relationship, it becomes a manifestation of the relationship as well. Prayer is communication or communion with our Higher Power, and, like any relationship, it doesn't evolve without regular practice.

How do you get started if you weren't raised with a particular religion? The most fulfilling way for you depends on your personality and gifts. Urban Holmes presented a helpful diagram for understanding different approaches to spiritual life. His diagram of a circle illustrates the possibilities for spiritual practice. The top of the circle represents a *speculative* spirituality that focuses on the illumination of the mind, and the bottom of the circle represents an *affective* spirituality that focuses on the illumination of the heart. He goes on to suggest that there are two means toward those ends: a *direct way of knowing,* in which our relationship with God is not mediated, practiced by an *emptying* technique of meditation; and an *indirect way of knowing,* in which our relationship with God is mediated, practiced by an *imaginal* technique of meditation.

In a spiritual formation course at Duke University's Divinity School, Dr. John Westerhoff introduced me to these four schools of spirituality (although I have renamed them to make them a bit easier to understand): *speculative-imaginal, affective-imaginal, affective-emptying,* and *speculative-emptying* (see Figure 14.1). He wisely shared his recommendation that priests, preachers, or spiritual directors needed to familiarize themselves with these different schools, as people of all these types would be seeking their spiritual guidance. He described how he tried to regularly attend retreats offered by practitioners of these four schools of spirituality, so that he would have first-hand information to share.

Because I am a visual learner, the diagram helped me affirm my natural tendencies towards seeking direction and communion with God. It also helped me gain appreciation for the different paths that others choose. In Dr. Westerhoff's book, *Spiritual Life: The Foundation for Preaching and Teaching* (Westminster John Knox Press, 1994), he expounded on Holmes's spiritual schools. He identified the *speculative-imaginal* school as sacramental, and as a *thinking* spirituality, with its primary aim to aid people in fulfilling their vocation in the world. This school is dominated by mental prayer or meditation, engaging the senses in reflecting on a poem, musical piece, or scripture. Long before the printed word, the Jewish people enjoyed the tradition of repeating the Psalms and the Torah. Most leaders of Judaism would be associated with this school. One of the most famous Jewish examples, Moses Maimonides, was a physician as well as renowned scholar of Judaism. The rosary is a type of mental prayer common to this school, from the Catholic tradition, where scriptural or familiar prayers are repeated to lead you into a deeper experience with your Higher Power. Christians who would exemplify this school include Ignatius of Loyola, Martin Luther, and

Speculative

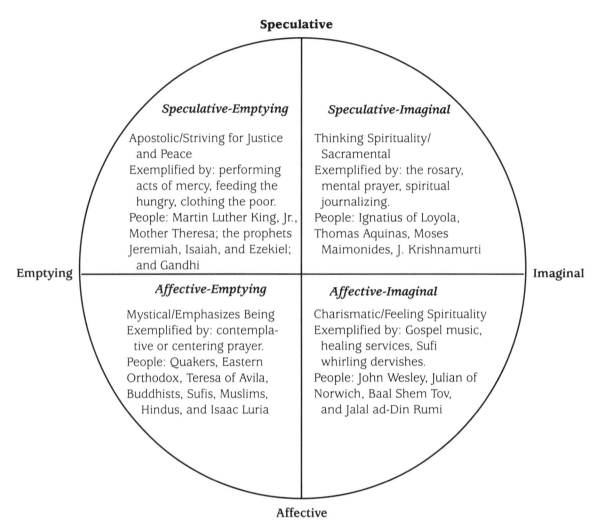

Speculative-Emptying

Apostolic/Striving for Justice
 and Peace
Exemplified by: performing
 acts of mercy, feeding the
 hungry, clothing the poor.
People: Martin Luther King, Jr.,
 Mother Theresa; the prophets
 Jeremiah, Isaiah, and Ezekiel;
 and Gandhi

Speculative-Imaginal

Thinking Spirituality/
 Sacramental
Exemplified by: the rosary,
 mental prayer, spiritual
 journalizing.
People: Ignatius of Loyola,
 Thomas Aquinas, Moses
 Maimonides, J. Krishnamurti

Emptying

Affective-Emptying

Mystical/Emphasizes Being
Exemplified by: contempla-
 tive or centering prayer.
People: Quakers, Eastern
 Orthodox, Teresa of Avila,
 Buddhists, Sufis, Muslims,
 Hindus, and Isaac Luria

Affective-Imaginal

Charismatic/Feeling Spirituality
Exemplified by: Gospel music,
 healing services, Sufi
 whirling dervishes.
People: John Wesley, Julian of
 Norwich, Baal Shem Tov,
 and Jalal ad-Din Rumi

Imaginal

Affective

FIGURE 10.1   Schools of Spirituality

Thomas Aquinas. J. Krishnamurti was one of the more popular contemporary
Hindu scholars in this category.

The *affective-imaginal* school can be defined as charismatic. Its concerns
include seeking an outpouring of the Higher Power's spirit and providing an
experience of this presence in personal and communal life. This path is a
very *feeling* spirituality, where every sense in the body can appreciate God;
prayer can include clapping, dancing, shouting, and a general freedom to
move with the spirit. Popular prayers from this school include chanting of
the Psalms and singing gospel hymns. Historical Christian figures associated

with this approach include Martin Luther King, Jr., John Wesley, George Herbert, and Julian of Norwich. No tradition is richer in emotional language than the devotional literature of the Jews, such as "the joy of the Lord is my strength." Baal Shem Tov, the founder of Hasidic Judaism, would exemplify this school within the Jewish faith. Jalal ad-Din Rumi, the founder of the Sufi Whirling Dervishes, would certainly be described in this school.

The *affective-emptying* school is best described as mystical, a spirituality that emphasizes *being*. This school is primarily practiced through contemplative prayer, or centering prayer, which can occupy and free the mind so that you may commune with God directly, without mundane distractions. This school includes both the Quakers and the Eastern Orthodox, both of whom seek to empty themselves of all distractions so they can be fully receptive to the Higher Power's spirit in their lives. Quakers do this by creating empty, white space where nothing is sought to stimulate the senses. In contrast, the Eastern Orthodox Church uses icons, music, and incense to help people make direct contact with the mystery and essence of God. Christians associated with this school include Teresa of Avila, John of the Cross, Thomas Merton, and George Fox. Isaac Luria, a famous sixteenth century Jewish leader from this school, introduced mysticism into the Jewish ritual. The followers of Eastern religions, such as Sufis, Hindus, Muslims, and Buddhists, primarily practice their spirituality in this school as well. Mandalas, incense, and chants are often used to help tune out the material world and achieve a meditative state. Thich Nhat Hanh, a contemporary teacher of the Buddhist meditation technique of mindfulness, uses a focusing on the breath to bring one into a keener awareness of self. The significant difference between the goals for knowing and emptying oneself in Eastern versus Western religions is that those from the Judeo-Christian experience believe that once the physical distractions are quieted, their Higher Power is invited in.

The *speculative-emptying* school can be described as apostolic. It involves praying through activities, from hiking, drawing, or fasting, to playing music, serving at soup kitchens, and giving alms. This school's primary concerns are witnessing for our Higher Power and striving for justice and peace. Christians in this school include John Calvin, Catherine of Genoa, Dominic, and Mother Theresa. All of the great Jewish prophets had a social ethic as an integral part of their fabric of spirituality: Jeremiah, Isaiah and Ezekiel would be the best known for these concerns. And Gandhi, from the Hindu tradition, was world renowned for his commitment to social justice for spiritual reasons.

Dr. Westerhoff also pointed out that people within any school of spirituality are likely to have some characteristics from other schools, especially their opposite quadrant. This is natural and healthy. Some people, as they spiritually mature, will move from one quadrant to the opposite as their home base or primary affinity. One such example was Dr. Martin Luther King, Jr., who started from the *affective-imaginal,* or charismatic school, but moved toward the *speculative-emptying* school, where he spent most of the last half of his life striving for justice and peace.

Meditation as an "In Road"

My experience has been that regardless of your spiritual orientation (or school), the most powerful tool for emotional and spiritual health and healing is a commitment to a daily practice of meditation and quiet introspective time. You can approach this in a variety of ways, depending on your religion (or lack thereof) and personality.

The basic requirement is that you be alone and not distracted by television, telephones, radio, or other noises. Dr. Kempner, the founder of the Rice Diet Program, used to suggest going for a daily walk, and Dr. Rosati, his successor, added that the walk should be done meditatively—without a Walkman. This initial stress management prescription has since evolved into a much broader offering of introspective paths to explore. For instance, yoga, a breath-focused practice of meditation in motion, is taught. We also offer other meditation techniques and practices such as journalizing courses, inner healing sessions, and a general recommendation to spend at least an hour a day alone in quiet reflection. This meditative practice is more likely to become a habit if it is done at the same time each day, preferrably in the same place.

Many people avoid being alone without interruptions, out of fear that unresolved issues will present themselves. That is the exact reason that I am suggesting that you do so. It is inevitable! If you are not denying your feelings by feeding them with large amounts of food or distracting yourself with everything imaginable, such as excessive work or indiscriminate sex, your true feelings and self-knowledge will surface.

In his research, Dr. Herbert Benson, author of *The Relaxation Response* and *Beyond the Relaxation Response,* used a simplified approach to meditation that incorporated four essential elements: a quiet environment, a mental device such as a word or a phrase that was repeated over and over again, a quiet mind, and a comfortable position. Rather than assign mantras (a secret word, sound, or phase repeated in Eastern meditation) Dr. Benson found that participants were more likely to get a deeper level of the relaxation response if they incorporated their own personal system into their repeated word or phrase.

For example, many Christians often felt comfortable with phrases from the New Testament such as: "Love one another" (John 15:12), "My peace

I give unto you" (John 14:27), "I am the way, the truth, and the life" (John 14:6), "The peace which passes all understanding" (Phil. 4:7), or "We have the mind of Christ" (I Cor. 2:16), or "Nothing can separate us from the love of God" (Romans 8:39).

A Catholic friend of mine uses a centering prayer that comes from the Russian Orthodox Church and is known as the Jesus Prayer or the Breath Prayer. The words are "Lord Jesus Christ, Son of God, have mercy on me, a sinner." To use this, you inhale as you say the first part, "Lord Jesus Christ," then exhale to "Son of God." Inhale again while saying "have mercy on me," and exhale to "a sinner." This prayer is ideally suited to this type of meditation because it corresponds to our body's pattern of breathing. This type of prayer is a natural for those in the *affective-emptying* school.

Jewish people (and many Christians, as well) were comfortable with words or phrases from the Torah or Old Testament in English or in Hebrew, such as: "Shalom" (peace), "Echad" (one), "You shall love the Lord, your God, with all your heart, and all your soul, and all your might" (Deut. 6:5), "Love your neighbor as yourself" (Lev. 19:18), "May God uncover his face to you, and bring you peace" (Numbers 6:26), "Peace be unto you, for your God is with you" (I Chr. 12:18).

If you prefer images to words, focusing on icons, mental pictures, or visualizations may prove more helpful. I have benefited from listening to tapes that lead you into a favorite place of relaxation, bask you in God's healing light, have you imagine your body being healed, or guide you over a bridge or into an adventure that inspires unresolved issues to surface. Others find that quiet inspirational music can help them relax into a more sacred and centered state.

I find that my preferences for meditation methods change over time and that I enjoy a variety of approaches. The only constant is a space to myself. Sometimes I like to be in silence, focusing on my breath and the sensations I feel within my body. Other times I like to repeat a verse of scripture as I inhale and exhale. Be comforted with the fact that almost everyone finds it a challenge to still the mind, but that it does get easier with practice. Try a few of these suggestions, starting with the ones that you are most comfortable with. A meditation group may help you get started and give you ideas for alternative approaches. Try attending a workshop led by someone you respect and trust, who is practiced at leading guided meditations.

The more practiced you get at seeking your Higher Power's lead, the more confident you will get with your spiritual growth and direction, such as how to choose which retreats or groups are best for you. An inner sense of knowing which path is for you will get stronger. You'll get in the habit of asking your Higher Power in a meditative state to reveal from within the answers, rather than expecting yourself or some spiritual leader to have them for you. When you ask for direction in such matters, your Higher Power will not only lead you to the next door, but will confirm and assure you that your choice is the best one for your "higher calling."

Many people tell me they procrastinate or postpone praying because they do not think they are "holy" enough or that they are not perfect enough at praying. It helps to remember that prayer is simply conversation with your Higher Power. Unfortunately, we often feel we need to approach our Higher Power as we do the world—with competence and control rather than by acknowledging our incompetence and surrendering control. Richard Foster, the author of *Celebration of Discipline: The Path to Spiritual Growth* (Harper and Row, 1988) and *Prayer: Finding the Heart's True Home* (Harper, 1992), describes "simple prayer" as coming before God just as we are, warts and all. He reminds us that simple prayer is the most common form of prayer in the Bible. The Old and New Testaments are filled with unpretentious conversations with God where the pray-er simply shared feelings, concerns, and petitions. These prayers ranged from feelings of rage to songs of thanksgiving and praise. God can handle whatever you want to throw at Heaven.

If scripture, formal prayer, or the word "God" turns you off, please realize that the power that created you can meet you where you are. One of my mentor's mentors was Agnes Sanford who, although a Christian herself, was utterly unconcerned about the creed or lack of creed of those to whom she ministered. In her book, *The Healing Light* (Macalester Park Publishing Co., 25th ed., 1961), she tells of introducing a soldier to healing prayer:

> I explained to the suffering soldier boy that there was a healing energy in him that the doctors called "nature," that this same healing life was in the world outside of him too, and that he could receive more of it by asking for it. "Who'll I ask?" Sammy wondered. "Ask God. Because He is the one who made nature and He's in nature and He is nature." "But I don't know anything about God." "You know there's *something* outside of yourself, don't you? After all, you didn't make this world. There's *some* kind of life outside of you." "Oh, sure. When you're scared enough you feel like there must be something." "Well then, ask that Something to come into you. Just say, 'Whoever you are or whatever you are, come into me now and help nature in my body to mend this bone.'"

You don't need to be of any particular faith to receive healing if you seek "the God of your understanding" and prepare to respond. Most people identify "the God of their understanding" with the power of love, and it is this love that heals us, not only physically, but emotionally and spiritually as well.

The Power of Prayer

Most view meditation as listening to God, while prayer is talking to God. For me, there is a very fine line between the two, but I often go from a quieted, meditative state to having a "quickening of my spirit" regarding a particular person or concern. This I think of as prayer. Since I am very visually oriented, I imagine that I am surrounding this person or situation with a healing, white light and then placing the person or situation in God's eternally open arms. I also enjoy a prayer technique that I learned from Rev. Tommy Tyson called "soaking prayer." This approach simply involves imagining the person in need of prayer immersed in a flood of God's healing water or love, and just be with that vision of God soaking them through and through for awhile. But remember that your best approach to prayer, as with meditation, is via whatever route feels and works best for *you*.

Journalizing into Recovery

There are many formats for journalizing, so experiment with a few until you find a style that suits you. For starters, use the forms provided in Appendix C and Appendix D. You'll find the Food Journal with Feelings form especially useful if you are struggling with overeating or more severe eating disorders. With it, you will be able to understand what feelings may be causing your unhealthy food habits. This understanding can, in turn, inspire a transformation in your relationship with food. In addition to writing about your food intake, spend some time each day recording facts and feelings. If you do not find an emotional connection after a few weeks of this and are more interested in pursuing an understanding of food allowances, use the Food Journal with Allowances form. Either way, it is of utmost importance to record general facts and feelings each day.

Morton Kelsey is the most profound teacher I have found for those interested in journalizing, meditation, and dreams from a Christian perspective. In addition to forty-five years of personal journalizing experience, he has studied with Carl Jung, taught at the University of Notre Dame for decades, served as an Episcopalian priest, and written prolifically on the relations between the insights of depth psychology and religious experience. I recommend his books, *Adventure Inward* (Augsburg Publishing House, 1980) on journalizing; *The Other Side of Silence* (Paulist Press, 1976) on meditation; and *Dreams: A Way to Listen to God* (Paulist Press, 1978), if you are interested in these approaches to exploring your inner self.

Other good resources for journalizing are Ira Progoff's *At a Journal Workshop* (Dialogue House Library, 1992); *The Power of the Other Hand* (Newcastle Publishing Co., Inc., 1988) by Lucia Cappachione; and *The Twelve-Steps: A*

Spiritual Journey (Recovery Publications, Inc., 1988) and *The Twelve Steps: A Way Out* (Recovery Publications, Inc., 1988).

For practical advice on dream interpretation for psychological and spiritual revelation, I highly recommend Ira Progoff's Intensive Journal process. Although I will share from my experience with this process, it would be more revealing to read Ira Progoff's *At a Journal Workshop* (Dialogue House Library, 1992), or better yet, take the course, which is taught throughout the world by facilitators trained by Ira Progoff. They offer numerous courses, but you must take a two-day workshop to get to the dream work, which is a deeper level of processing. To enter into a deeper understanding of your dreams you need to go to sleep with an expectancy to recall your dreams upon waking. Everyone has dreams, but some people are not in the habit of recalling them. As another signal to your subconscious, prepare yourself with a dream notebook and pen beside your bed to make it convenient to successfully record dreams without disturbing yourself much when you awake. Dream recall, journalizing, and interpretation are like all of the other spiritual disciplines in that you get better with practice.

When you awake with your dream, quickly begin writing about it in your notebook. Give your dream a title. Recall whatever senses or fragments that come to your mind if the dream does not feel complete or intact. After documenting the dream, list all words of images vertically down the left margin of your page. Don't worry if there are many, or if this takes a significant amount of time. Then, to the right of each word, free-associate— write the first three words that come to mind when you repeat that key word or dream image. After doing this for every word on the left, go back and highlight the free-associated words that resonate the most for you. Then simply read down the list of highlighted words and the dream's true meaning will be apparent! This may seem too simplistic to believe, but you must try it for yourself to know. The results have been profound most of the times I have used this method. Obviously, if you are recalling your dreams every morning you may not have the time to interpret them in this detailed a fashion, but you will start to feel or discern which dreams are more important and worthy of the time commitment. So ideally, try to journalize all your dreams, then give detailed analytic attention to those you feel inspired to explore. Journalizing your dreams is a very productive way to identify and examine your inner healing needs.

Interpreting Your Dreams

Dreams, and their accompanying revelations, are as significant a source of spiritual direction today as they were in biblical times. Once, when I excitedly shared a prophetic dream that was more real than any previous encounter

I had had with God, Rev. Tommy Tyson helped me back to earth with a loving and humorous comment. He said, "If you won't give God sufficient alone time to communicate with you when you are awake, God will come to you when you are asleep!"

Dreams, and our recollections and interpretations of them, can be a powerful guide for us. They are a manifestation of the subconscious, and thus can reveal to us insights that we are not aware of. The first morning of a dream workshop with Morton Kelsey, I awoke with some great material. My dream was filled with the most horrific and delightful images I had ever retained from a dream state. During the morning break, I shared a few of the more grotesque segments with Morton and asked him what on earth could have inspired such a dream. He smiled with more compassion, grace, and acceptance than I had ever witnessed and said that he thought it was an invitation from God to explore my darker side. I told him I didn't think I had a darker side. He again smiled in a very loving way before breaking the news to me that we all have a darker side and that a good therapist can often help us explore it and learn more about ourselves. The next week I met a wonderful therapist who proved his words to be true.

So dreams are simply another wonderful path to explore on our journey to knowing ourselves. The healing and learning potential of paying attention to our dreams is really beyond our imagination. Dreams can be blatantly prophetic to prepare us for something to come. They can also open the door to healers like Morton Kelsey. He not only educated me on the physical, emotional, and spiritual healing potential of dreams, but also helped open my mind to my readiness for psychotherapy. This turned out to be the next leg of my spiritual journey. In my experience, healers from many arenas come to you when you are receptive to healing, and your best choices of healers will be apparent when you have spent time seeking God's will or "higher calling" for you.

Confessing Your Sins

Identifying blockages in your mind, emotions, or spirit is the core and essence of confession. When you get into your quiet, meditative time, ask your Higher Power what is blocking the flow of health and light being manifested in you. Confession is also relevant for such specific concerns as your nutritional blocks. Getting honest during one of your alone times, and admitting your feelings (of shame, frustration, guilt, anger) with respect to your food struggle (sugar binges, weight gain, or sodium and blood pressure increases), has powerful healing potential. One of the great advantages of a spiritual discipline, or an inner journey, is to have these blocks, and their roots, revealed to us.

Inner awarenesses of blocks and their origins also occur for those who are not disciplined with a confessional practice, just as Sammy was healed through Agnes Sanford's relationship with a loving God without his having a particular religion. But being more spiritually aware and disciplined makes you more able to discern the best way for you to pursue and enjoy wholeness, or your "higher calling," more often.

So the first step of confession is spending alone time with your Higher Power, so that your blocks and their roots are revealed. This can occur through meditation, prayer, or by journalizing thoughts, feelings, and dreams. As we gain more consciousness during this alone time, it inevitably makes us more conscious during our time in community.

Then we start to see ways and means for us to act on our "higher calling," which we previously may have dismissed as fortunate coincidences. As we really make a serious commitment to "the God of our understanding" and start to pay more attention to who we are, and what we are to do to realize our "higher calling," we will quite naturally flow into the second aspect of confession, which is sharing our blocks, or our darker side, with someone trustworthy. Most people find that when they are ready to verbally confess these blocks, and their roots, the best person to truly hear you and help you will become apparent. These little miracles will start to become more obvious to you the more you seek your Higher Power's lead, rather than relying on your own devices to control everything.

The third basic aspect of confession, after confessing our blocks to another, is following this with our commitment to obey the call that has been given, or the truth that has been realized. There is a great temptation to accept knowledge as a substitute for obedience. Coming to the knowledge of the blocks, and their roots, must be expressed by definite acts of obedience. Reading all the self-help and nutrition books that have ever been written, and then not responding, is making a mockery of the truth revealed. When people see the truth, and give themselves to obey it, they discover they need a power beyond themselves to obey the highest that has been given to them.

Although confessors and people to support you in pursuing your new-found truth obediently can be found anywhere, from golf courses to synagogues, many throughout the world are finding this quality of spiritual support from Twelve Step Anonymous Programs.

The Twelve Step Programs

The Twelve Step Programs began as a result of Carl Jung telling an alcoholic, whom he had been unsuccessfully treating for years, that true recovery in cases as serious as his were rare. Although Jung himself was not religious, his parting remark to his patient was that he had never seen true healing with such an affliction without a religious conversion experience. To make a long and wonderful story short and sweet, the man had a conversion, then shared this prescription with a friend who also succeeded, and this friend shared this advice with another friend. This last friend was a man named Bill Wilson, whose healing and conversion expraince led to the birth of Alcoholics Anonymous.

I find it miraculous and uplifting that the Twelve Step Anonymous groups have succeeded in providing the most effective therapy for addictions in the history of the world without one paid health or church professional controlling the helm. Now there are countless anonymous groups that help people who struggle with every addiction imaginable. Overeater's Anonymous (see Appendix B) may be a group you would like to investigate, as would the Adult Children of Alcoholics (ACOA) group, which accepts anyone who knows an alcoholic (which is virtually everyone). Groups vary dramatically, so patiently try numerous groups before you make a commitment to one or give up. For instance, when I was trying to find a nice confidential group in which to share, I went to one group and felt that they spent an excessive amount of time trying to "fix" one of the members. Refraining from offering free advice to someone sharing is usually a well-respected rule in all Anonymous groups, so at the end of the meeting I simply asked if their responses to the person were typical for the group. I nicely explained that I was looking for a group to commit with, but did not feel comfortable with that degree of assisting. They agreed that their group did allow for more of that than most groups because they had all been meeting for so long that they felt confident that their advice was being appreciated. I politely thanked them for the time together, but admitted that I would be visiting other groups rather than staying with theirs. My discernment was affirmed the next week when a friend asked if I was the Kitty who had come to a specifically named Twelve Step group that her boyfriend was in. I was initially angry that a member present that night had broken the confidentiality rule, which is usually widely honored. But, I soon allowed my anger to be replaced by an appreciation that I had trusted my feeling that the group was not right for me.

You are more likely to find the best group naturally if you spend the meditative alone time with God. Open yourself to your Higher Power's choice for the optimal Twelve Step group for you; then keep your eyes and ears open for the next path to unfold. You may even begin to feel a flutter or quickening of your heart when you sense your inner voice say "yes" to an open door.

Support Groups

At the Rice Diet Clinic and Heart Disease Reversal Program we have a unique advantage of offering a supportive environment for healing every day, fifty-two weeks a year. With some type of introspective activity offered six days per week, there is plenty of opportunity for those ready for inner healing. Our continuity groups are safe, confidential gatherings, where participants know they can come and share from their hearts. Here we practice unconditional love by truly listening to others, without offering judgment or free advice. Most people find it very refreshing to be really heard. The healing power of simply sharing our stories—our truths, our fears and our faiths—is quite frankly beyond description.

There are many different types of groups available, and also unlimited potential to create our own. I have seen heart disease reversal patients do this quite successfully when their cardiac rehabilitation programs did not meet their needs. For starters, I would suggest checking your local paper for existing support groups. The variety of confidential support groups today is vast. If none of these interest you, and if you don't have a group of friends that you think would be interested in this kind of group (or with whom you would want to share that intimately with), consult the *Self Help Source Book: Finding and Forming Mutual Aid Self Help Groups* (American Self Help Clearing House. See Appendix B for more information). Group support enriches our concern and caring for others, and offers us new insights on the true meaning and purpose in life. We seek and realize a whole healing of body, soul, and spirit that we really do need to heal not only individually, but collectively.

Stress Management

Although I believe that all people's answers lie within themselves, and that God will lead us into the realization of all the truths we will need, stress management techniques may also help us cope in the process. Cardiac rehabilitation groups and other organizations offer stress management seminars, which vary from behavior modification strategies such as biofeedback, to combinations of coping strategies, which may include introductions into many of the spiritual paths we have briefly explored. Remember that meditative exercises, such as yoga and tai chi, as well as massage or body work can be very effective stress management disciplines. Again, check your newspaper and your local hospital for such opportunities.

Many people stumble in their health promotion/disease prevention plans because a stressful incident disrupts their newly acquired healthy lifestyle. Stress management practices, and the emotional stability and peace they can provide, will greatly enhance your ability to reach your health goals, and then to maintain them.

THE PATH YOU TAKE MUST BE YOUR OWN

Everyone's path is different, and the joy and adventure is in finding your own. Research on the health advantages of spiritual growth has concluded that the spiritual dimension is related to meaning and purpose in life, concern and caring for others, and commitment to a Higher Power. Although the commitment to a Higher Power is not always specifically defined, when people honor a practice of solitary meditation they almost always come to the realization that they need help to reach their "higher calling" and thus seek guidance from a Higher Power to do so.

This concept of opening to the experience and assistance of a Higher Power may go against all of your independent, self-sufficient tendencies and training, but it has worked for millions of others, and I invite you to try it. It is free, with no risks! Seeking a spiritual director, a meditation teacher, or a renewal retreat that is right for you may include *asking* your friends, whose spirituality you respect, if they have any recommendations. Make your own judgment of their recommendation by observing the fruits of their spiritual endeavors. Are they "walking their walk?" Journalizing on your spiritual needs is a way to access your subconscious feedback, which can inspire answers through your dreams. Gleaning from your soul's wisdom, or being mindful of and resourceful with your emotions, mind, subconscious, and will (heart's desire) can also help lead you to your "higher calling."

Seeking spiritual growth is a natural process, and like all other lifestyle changes, choosing to prioritize it in your life is the first key step. As with exercise and dietary changes, your desire and will to grow and change in this arena is really all that is required for success. And as with the other lifestyle changes, your persistance and determination will be the added insurance you need. If at first try a path is not found to be rewarding, then try another that feels right for you. Remember that you will be best equipped to discern and pursue your spiritual path if meditation is a daily commitment. Enjoy your spiritual journey; your answers are all awaiting within you.

PART FOUR

HEAL YOUR HEART FOODS AND RECIPES WITH RESULTS

❖ ❖ ❖

11

SELECTING HEART-HEALTHY FOODS

Most people admit they would eat more healthily if it were convenient. It is your responsibility to yourself to ensure that it is! Keeping the following staples and snacks available makes life a lot easier here in Durham, North Carolina. You will probably find many of them where you live. If not, try writing or calling the distributor for them directly. (See Appendix A for information on acquiring the products mentioned in this book that interest you.)

STOCKING THE HEART-HEALTHY PANTRY

Beans and Peas (Legumes)

Dried beans and peas are an excellent substitute for meat as they offer similar nutritional value and satiety. They are impressive sources of protein, iron, zinc, and potassium. Enjoy experimenting with the potential of beans. They are great in pasta or grain salads, bean dips, and even breads. The following sources for beans are listed in the order of preference:

❖ Dried beans and peas, any variety (They are less expensive when bought in bulk from food cooperatives.)

❖ Frozen beans and peas, no salt or fat added

❖ Canned beans, no salt or fat added (Walnut Acres and Eden products can be found in health food stores)

❖   Soy products: tofu (soy cheese), tempeh (cultured or fermented soybeans), or TVP (texturized vegetable protein). Read the ingredients to insure you are buying the varieties with no added salt or fat. Most health food stores carry these. If TVP is not available in your area, call Harvest Direct for their unflavored (no-salt) varieties. (See Appendix A.)

Beverages

The most popular beverages are loaded with caffeine, sodium, fat, sugar, and/or artificial sweeteners. All of these can be potentially harmful. Even the decaffeinated beverages have some potentially adverse effects. Decaffeinated coffee and tea have been shown to aggravate hiatal hernias and inhibit the absorption of iron. If you do desire some decaffeinated coffee, look for the "naturally decaffeinated" coffee, which is slightly better for you. But better yet, try my favorite coffee substitute, Dacopa. (See Appendix A if not locally available.)

If you are allowed dairy products, use nonfat dry powdered milk or evaporated skim milk instead of the partially hydrogenated nondairy creamers.

However, there are many healthier beverage choices to stock:

❖   Water: good well, bottled spring, or distilled water. No-salt seltzer water is great when mixed with 100 percent fruit juice.

❖   Herbal teas (decaffeinated). But limit comfrey, sassafras, and licorice, which reportedly can cause numerous adverse effects if consumed regularly.

❖   Fruit juices, unsweetened (check ingredients to confirm fruit juice only), or fruit juice and seltzer water blends.

❖   Vegetable juices. Unsalted is great if you add lemon, lime, or other salt and fat-free condiments, such as fresh or no-salt horseradish. R. W. Knudsen's Very Veggie, Low Sodium Natural Vegetable Cocktail is delicious "straight-up."

❖   Coffee substitutes. Postum, Cafix, and Pero are found in most chain grocery stores; Dacopa (my favorite) is roasted dahlia root and is found in some health food stores.

❖   Nonalcoholic malt beverages, such as Metbrau or Moussy.

❖   Milk (if allowed). Use skim, $\frac{1}{2}$ percent or soy milk—the brand lowest in fat and sodium is presently Health Valley Soy Moo.

Grains and Grain Products

Breads, Crackers, and Cookies

Most breads or starchy snacks have more than 100 milligrams of sodium per slice or serving, which is too high in sodium for someone with hypertension or kidney disease. In addition, almost all commercially available grain products, except for those made at health food bakeries, contain partially hydrogenated fat. Look for the following choices which can be found without any added sodium or saturated fat.

❖ Corn tortillas containing only corn, lime, and water. (Wheat flour tortillas usually have hydrogenated fat and salt added.)

❖ Cracottes, no-salt variety

❖ Edward and Son's Baked Brown Rice Snaps

❖ Buckwheat, no salt

❖ Hain Natural Crackers, no-salt varieties

❖ Matzos or whole wheat pita bread, no-salt added variety

❖ Rice cakes, no-fat and no-salt varieties

❖ Snyder's Sourdough Pretzels or Harry's Whole Wheat Honeys, no-salt varieties

❖ Baked Tostitos, Smart Temptations, or Guiltless Gourmet no fat or salt corn chips. The former two are thinner and crispier and thus, preferable.

Cold Cereals

Most cereals contain partially hydrogenated fats and 200 to 300 milligrams of sodium. The following have no added fat or sodium and 6 grams or less of added sugar or sucrose, making them superior choices to the majority of cereals sold in chain grocery stores:

❖ Shredded Wheat or Frosted Mini Wheats (if the sugar doesn't trigger binge eating)

❖ Raisin Squares

❖ Puffed Rice and Puffed Wheat

The following cereals are found in a growing number of health food sections in the larger chain grocery stores. Of course, health food stores or cooperatives would have the largest selection:

❖ Grainfield cereals

❖ Health Valley cereals

❖ Kolln cereals

❖ Most of New Morning cereals

❖ Kashi (a brand name for a 7-grain mixture that is puffed)

Hot Cereals
Excellent choices for hot cereals are:

❖ Cream of Rice

❖ Wheat and Rye Farina

❖ grits

❖ Kashi (a brand name for a 7-grain and sesame seed mixed cereal)

❖ oat bran

❖ oatmeal

❖ buckwheat groats

❖ Wheatena

Most health food stores have numerous other hot and cold cereals. Take care to read the ingredients and choose one without added sodium or fat. The nutritional analysis should read no more than 2 grams of fat, 10 milligrams of sodium, and 6 grams of added sugar.

Whole, and Slightly Processed, Grains
The ultimate cereal is the whole grain itself before it has been puffed, flaked, or processed in any way. Most refined products have half the fiber content and significantly less nutrients than the original whole grain. The following can be found at most health food stores and a growing number of chain groceries:

❖ Barley (Hulled is less processed, thus better, than pearled, flaked, or barley flour.)

❖ Whole wheat kernels or bulgur (cracked wheat)

❖ Couscous and pasta (more processed than wheat kernels or bulgur)

❖ Kasha (roasted buckwheat groats)

❖ Millet

❖ Oat groats

❖ Polenta

❖ Popcorn, hot-air-popped or microwaved from scratch with no oil or salt

❖ Quinoa (a South American grain that is relatively new to the United States; it has a great crunch!)

❖ Rice. Brown, wild, Basmati, or any type that does not contain added fat and sodium.

❖ Rye-berries (less processed, thus better, than flakes or flour)

❖ Oat groats, and steel cut oats, also called Scottish or Irish oatmeal

❖ Wheat berries, wheat germ, and wheat bran. (The latter two are the inner and outer fractions of the whole berry, respectively.)

Condiments

The ultimate condiments to substitute for the traditional salt- and fat-laden ones are herbs, spices, lemon, lime, and chili peppers. But the following condiments are also convenient and are usually available in chain grocery stores.

❖ Vinegar. Balsamic and fruit- or herb-flavored varieties are delightful; beware of the few with added sodium and most white vinegars. (Heinz advertises they are "the only white vinegar that is not a petroleum product," but is made from corn.)

❖ Conserves or "fruit only" jams and jellies

❖ Enrico's No-Salt Salsa (my favorite)

❖ Hot Cha Cha! salsa, no-salt

❖ Featherweight condiments (no-sodium/no-fat): BBQ sauce, catsup, chili sauce, mustard, etc.

❖ Molasses, honey, and fruit syrups should be limited because of their concentrated calories. Molasses is the only sweetener with any significant nutritional value.

❖ Mrs. Dash

❖ Robbie's no-salt/no-fat condiments. (The garlic sauce is great!)

❖ Mustard and horseradish, fresh or no-fat/no-salt varieties

❖ Mr. Spice Sauces from Lang Naturals (eight different varieties of no-salt, no-fat sauces; Tangy Bangy is their popular hot sauce)

❖ Wines, except for cooking wines, are usually low enough in sodium

Convenience Foods

As you may have noticed, many products advertise low or no fat, sodium, or sugar but rarely are they clean of all three! The following convenience foods are free of or very low in all of these concerns:

❖ Salt-free spaghetti sauce produced by Enrico, Prego, Tree of Life, or Pritikin

❖ Bearitos Vegetarian Refried Beans, no-salt

❖ Frozen vegetables for quick stir-fries

❖ Hain soups, no-salt

❖ Health Valley no-salt added products. (My favorite is their Vegetarian Chili.)

❖ Most Pritikin products are no-salt-added—inspect labels.

❖ Tabatchnick no-salt frozen soups

❖ Better Than Burger? by Naturally Tofu is great if you prepare it as instructed in *The Best "Burger" Out!* (See Chapter 14)

❖ Boca Burger. Their "original vegan" Boca Burger is the best ready-made vegetarian, no-salt- or fat-added burger on the market.

Remember when using convenience foods that have no added salt or fat to use a little imagination in preparing them. See *15-Minute Meals* recipes in Chapter 14 for specific ideas.

Dairy Products

All dairy products are fairly high in sodium and protein, averaging 126 milligrams of sodium and 8 grams of protein per cup of skim milk. If you are allowed that much sodium and protein, the following products are your best low-fat, low-sodium choices:

❖ Skim milk

❖ Breakstone ½ percent dry curd cottage cheese (less than 65 milligrams of sodium per ½ cup). Moisten with nonfat yogurt for improved consistency.

❖ Nonfat plain yogurt with *live* or *active yogurt cultures*. Beware that most fruit-filled types are loaded with excessive sugar or artificial sweeteners.

❖ Light 'n Lively nonfat sour cream alternative

❖ Sorrento Fat-Free Ricotta

Fruits and Vegetables

Fresh, organic, locally grown fruits and vegetables are always the preferred choice. But when fruits and vegetables are not looking all that fresh, you may be better off nutritionally with frozen ones. Be sure to check the ingredients list to avoid any products with added fat or salt. Or better yet, during the summer buy your fresh fruits and vegetables direct from a farmer's market, and freeze enough for the year. There is something really wonderful about meeting the farmer who picked your produce early that morning! And, you will certainly thank yourself next winter when you are enjoying an interesting variety of delicious produce. Many people appreciate the convenience of frozen vegetable medleys. Keeping yourself stocked with a variety of your favorite frozen vegetables, like spinach, kale, collards, turnip greens, and artichoke hearts, may also help you enjoy them more often than you would if you had to clean and prepare them from "scratch."

The no-salt-added canned vegetables would be the least preferred, since the canning process destroys significant amounts of potassium. (The average American consumes less than optimal amounts of potassium, and a higher potassium *and* a lower sodium intake means a lower blood pressure.) Canned un-salted tomatoes are really the only justifiable canned vegetable purchase, as they are the only commonly eaten vegetable that is not available frozen and un-salted.

Research and experience has shown that creating menu plans and shopping lists helps people seeking to lose weight do so more successfully. Anyone would have an easier time making healthier choices if such choices were readily within reach. Reduce your excuses and improve your odds: stock you home, car, and office with many of your favorite foods from this chapter.

DIMINISHING THE DINING-OUT DILEMMA

Although many people on a low-fat, low-sodium, and low-sugar diet think that dining away from home is inevitably a hopeless situation, it does not have to be. Granted, choices low in all these factors do not dominate restaurant menus, but they can usually be acquired if you are persistent. This is especially important if you frequently eat outside your home, since fat-, sodium-, and sugar-rich restaurant foods can significantly increase your risk for most chronic diseases. The following tips should help you in your challenge to enjoy dining out while also pursuing a healthier lifestyle.

❖   Contact the restaurant in advance to insure that it will be able to honor a low-fat and low-sodium request. It is best to be specific, since the employee answering the phone may know very little about this subject. For instance, ask if they have a fresh seafood or vegetarian dish that can be prepared without added dairy, fat, and salt.

❖   When you get to the restaurant, ask if they have a heart-healthy menu. You may then want to ask your server for any suggestions about ordering a very-low-fat and low-sodium meal. Most of the more expensive restaurants will cook a very-low-fat and low-sodium vegetarian or seafood entree for you upon request. The important thing to remember is that you do not know that a healthy choice is out of the question until you ask for it! As a general rule, baked potato/salad bars, Chinese restaurants, and Mediterranean gourmet restaurants are the easiest places to achieve your low-fat, no-salt requests.

❖   If you are still having problems ordering, scan the menu for dishes that use methods of preparation that are generally lowest in fat. Look for foods that are steamed, broiled, roasted, grilled, or poached. Ask that the chef not add fat (except for a teaspoon of olive oil if you like) or sodium (including salt, broth, monosodium glutamate, and soy sauce) to your food and to flavor it with wine, lemon, lime, vinegar, and/or herbs. Avoid foods that are buttered, fried, creamed, in cream sauce, with gravy or hollandaise, au gratin, or pickled.

❖   If you are struggling with a tendency to overeat, you may find it is easier to ask what fresh vegetables and seafood choices are available instead of looking at the menu and being tempted by the many items that are less than appropriate. For instance, in a nice Mediterranean restaurant, it is often easier to ask, "What fresh vegetables do you have today?" If they say, "We have sweet red and yellow peppers, portabello mushrooms, Roma tomatoes, asparagus, and carrots," then you could respond, "Great, I would like all of those stir-fryed in wine with extra garlic, onion, basil, and red pepper flakes, served on a bed of pasta, with no cheese, oil or salt added." This is absolutely delicious!

❖   Remember to specify every item with low-fat and low-sodium instructions, otherwise you may be served inappropriate side dishes. For instance, "May I please have fresh grilled tuna with one teaspoon of olive oil, garlic, and lemon and no added salt; a baked potato with no topping; and a tossed salad with olive oil and vinegar on the side."

❖   For buffet dining it is always smart to walk completely around the table before starting to make your choices. By knowing all of the food choices, you are then equipped to make the lowest fat and sodium selections.

❖   The best dessert choice is fresh fruit with nothing added. Other possibilities are ices, sorbet, gelatin, or angel food cake. But typically, the lower the fat content of frozen desserts, the higher the sugar and calories, so be aware of portions and frequency of consumption if weight loss and/or diabetes are concerns.

12

COOKING HEART-HEALTHY RICE, GRAINS, AND BEANS

Many people in developed nations or affluent societies know little about what the majority of the world considers the staples of life: grains and beans. The majority of the world's population are basically vegetarian by necessity; they simply cannot afford the animal products that those of us with chronic diseases are eating in excess. The center of their plate typically holds a generous portion of grains and beans. Those of us seeking to reverse or prevent heart disease would benefit from a paradigm shift in this direction, from a meat-centered consciousness to a grain-and-bean–centered one.

ALL YOU NEED TO KNOW ABOUT RICE

Rice is the favorite grain of the Rice Diet Program. Dr. Kempner initially chose it as the staple grain for his patients because of its high-quality protein. In the treatment of people with kidney disease, congestive heart failure, and heart disease and its risk factors, it was not only important to serve patients low sodium, but also low animal protein. Thus, the protein that they did eat had to come from a grain with high-quality protein, with an impressive amino acid distribution. Rice fits this bill.

Although we serve numerous types of rice at the Rice Diet Program, it would be impossible to introduce more than a tiny fraction of the thousands of different varieties. Considering the many varieties and its international popularity, it is surprising how few Americans eat rice regularly. It is grown on every continent except Antarctica. China, India, Indonesia, Thailand, Vietnam, and Burma grow the most rice in the world. Americans have always been more interested in exporting rice than consuming it. Today the United States ranks as the twelfth largest producer worldwide and the second largest exporter of rice, exporting about half of all the rice we grow.

Here is a brief summary of the major types and varieties of rice:

❖ *Brown rice* is what all rice starts out as. Only the inedible outer hull or husk is removed. The color is tan, the flavor is nutty, and the texture is slightly chewy. It has twice as much fiber as white rice, five times the vitamin E, and three times the magnesium. It is available in long, medium, and short grain. The shorter grain contains more of the starchy substance called glutin (not to be confused with gluten in wheat, which is absent in rice), so the main difference between short- and long-grain rice, besides size, is that short-grain rice cooks up sticky and long-grain rice comes out fluffy.

❖ *Rose rice,* or short-grain rice, is considered short-grain if the length is less than two times its width. When cooked, short-grain rice is softer and stickier than medium-grain rice, thus popularly called "sticky" rice. In Japan it is also known as sushi rice. Medium- and short-grain rice require slightly less water; 1 cup of rice to $1\frac{1}{2}$ cups of water.

❖ *White rice* has had the hull, bran, and germ removed. After almost all of its nutritive value is stripped away during this process, 90 percent of all American-grown rice is enriched with thiamin, niacin, iron, and in some instances riboflavin, vitamin D, and calcium. Enriched white rice may have more iron and thiamin than brown rice, but it is nutritionally inferior to brown rice in most respects. White pigments, such as chalk or talc, and preservatives may be added to white rice. White rice has a rather bland flavor when compared with brown, but it is popular in America because it takes only 12 to 25 minutes to cook, rather than the 45 minutes required for brown rice.

❖ *Parboiled or converted rice* falls approximately midway between brown and white rice in terms of nutrition. This rice variety is steamed before being dried and is then polished to make it white. The steam pressure treatment done before milling forces many of the B vitamins and minerals into the endosperm (inner layer) from the bran and germ (outer layers). The rice is firm-textured and separate when cooked, the way most Americans like it. The term "converted" is a trademark of Uncle Ben's rice.

❖ *Precooked, quick, or instant rice* has been milled, completely cooked, and dried. Generally speaking, what is gained in cooking time is lost in texture and flavor, but a new quick-cooking brown rice successfully retains much of the nutty flavor and chewiness of its unprocessed counterpart.

❖   *Aromatic rice* is a term given to numerous varieties of rice identified by a pronounced nutty aroma and a flavor similar to popcorn. This aroma is due to a much higher proportion of 2-acetyl-1-pyrrole, a naturally occurring compound found in all rice.

❖   *Basmati rice* is an aromatic rice grown primarily in India and Pakistan. *Basmati* means "queen of fragrance." This title is well deserved, as anyone will agree who has smelled its sweet, popcornlike aroma. Although Indians usually eat rice twice a day, basmati is a high-quality luxury food typically eaten only on special occasions. Trimati (also called Texmati) is a cross between basmati and domestic long-grain and may be erroneously labeled as basmati.

❖   *Jasmine rice* is an aromatic long-grain rice originally grown in Thailand and now being grown quite successfully in the United States. It is distinguished by its sweet, popcorn-like fragrance, and grains that are silken to the touch due to a water milling process.

❖   *Glutinous rice,* also known as sticky, waxy, or sweet rice, is most often used in desserts. The grains can be either round or long and have a high percentage of amylopectin, a starch that makes the grains stick together.

❖   *Italian rice* predominates the European market. Arborio, vialone nano, padano, and carnaroli are the most popular rices from the Piedmont and Lombardy regions of Italy. These varieties are used to make risotto. They have a large central core that cooks firm to the bite, or *al dente.*

❖   *Rice bran* is the nutty-tasting outer bran layer of rice, which can be added to baked goods and cereals. High in soluble fiber, it has been found to lower cholesterol impressively.

❖   *Brown rice flour* is made from ground short-grain brown rice. It can replace up to 15 percent of the wheat flour in recipes and yields a drier, crispier texture.

❖   *Wild rice* may look like rice, but it is not even in the same botanical family. As its name implies, it is a wild crop that is grown in northern Minnesota, the Wisconsin lake country, and southern Canada. But much of the wild rice available today is domesticated. Since the 1960s, "paddy wild rice" has been seeded, cultivated, and mechanically harvested.

Cooking Rice

In a Rice Cooker

Using a rice cooker is the ultimate way to cook rice. If you have ever tasted rice cooked in a rice cooker, you will have a hard time not buying one. Besides making better-tasting rice and being more convenient and efficient, it has the added advantage of keeping the rice warm and ready to eat—all day long! Follow the manufacturer's directions, which usually suggest $\frac{1}{4}$ to $\frac{1}{2}$ cup less water than conventional cooking methods.

Conventional Stove-Top Method

Brown rice takes a little longer to cook, but it is worth the effort. One cup of regular brown rice cooks in 2 cups of liquid in about 45 minutes; parboiled or converted rice requires slightly more water. If you want to reduce the cooking time by 20 minutes, soak 1 cup of brown rice in 2 cups of water overnight. The next day, drain the remaining water from the rice into a measuring cup, and add enough fresh water to equal $2\frac{1}{2}$ cups. Boil rice in this water, covered, for about 25 minutes. (I always turn the temperature down for the last five minutes of cooking to reduce the odds of scorching the rice!)

The general rule of thumb for cooking white rice is 2 cups of water for 1 cup of rice to yield moist, soft rice. For firmer, more separate grains, $1\frac{3}{4}$ cups of water may suffice. Do not stir rice until you think it is done. When rice cooks, little passageways form to allow it to cook evenly, so disturbing this network produces a gummy, sticky texture.

COOKING WHOLE GRAINS

Most of the foods that we traditionally call whole grains are the edible seeds of plants of the grass family. Packed with nutrients, they have provided the basis of the human diet for millennia. Whole grains refers to these seeds in the unprocessed form, including all four of its given parts: the hull, bran, germ, and endosperm. The hull is the outer husk, a hard, protective covering that is removed by grinding or threshing. The bran is beneath the husk and provides an excellent source of minerals, B vitamins, and fiber. The germ is beneath the bran. Since it contains the lifeforce of the kernel, it is rich in protein, enzymes, vitamins, and oils. The endosperm is the starchy center of the grain and is basically carbohydrate. Endosperm is the primary ingredient of processed grains, or the white, lighter starches that most of us were fed as children. Whole grains are much more nutritious than their refined counterparts even after the enrichment process, and provide twice the fiber.

Unlike refined grains which have been cleaned as part of the refining process, whole grains must be rinsed thoroughly to remove dust and natural coatings that can leave a bitter taste. Whole grains bought in bulk may need more cleaning than those that are already cleaned before packaging. Rinse only the amount of grain that you plan to cook. Usually it is easier to pour the desired amount into a strainer and rinse it under running water until the water runs clear.

Pre-toasting grains before cooking them is an option that many feel improves the flavor of the grain. Browning brings out the nutty flavor of grains by opening their pores, allowing the grains to absorb liquid more readily and to cook more evenly. Although toasting a cup or two of grains takes only 10 to 15 minutes, it does not seem worth the effort to me except in the case of millet. Not only is the flavor of millet improved by pre-toasting, but the texture becomes fluffier as well. To toast grains, heat a large, heavy skillet over medium heat. Add the rinsed grain and stir with a wooden spoon until all the moisture has evaporated. Lower the heat and continue to stir until the grains begin to pop, smell roasted (like popcorn), and start to darken a little.

Soaking grains overnight can reduce the cooking time by approximately 30 percent to 40 percent. This is worth doing for some of the longer-cooking grains like hulled barley, oat groats, wheat berries, rye berries, and triticale. If you want to cook any of these grains in combination with brown rice, soak them overnight so their cooking time will be the same as the rice. The end result provides a textural contrast since the pre-soaked grains will be chewier, except for the oat groats which are a bit mushy.

In the interests of time and energy efficiency, it is most practical to cook several times more whole grains and beans than you need for a meal. Although leftovers are not quite as nutritious as freshly prepared foods, they are definitely more convenient, and having them will inspire you to eat healthily more frequently. If bulk quantities assist us in eating a variety of whole grains, beans, fruits, and vegetables, then the overall nutritional gain will far outweigh the small amount of nutrient loss. If you plan to cook a significant portion of your meals at home, a rice steamer is a purchase well worth your money. If grain is not being held at a hot temperature, it should be refrigerated after cooling. Grain leftovers can be safely kept in the refrigerator for up to a week. Although refrigeration will dry out and harden the grains somewhat, microwaving a cup of grain with a tablespoon or two of water for a minute usually restores the grain to its optimal texture and moisture. If you do not have a microwave, you can place grain in a heatproof bowl and set the bowl on a rack in a pot over a few inches of boiling water. Cover with a lid and steam for 3 to 4 minutes, stirring once or twice to insure that the grains are rehydrated and heated through.

Although whole grains are heavier and chewier than the more familiar refined grains (such as white rice, white bread, and pasta), they are more nutritious and time-consuming to chew. The latter point may seem humorous until you realize how much more slowly thin people eat than do those who are overweight. Learning to eat whole foods more slowly and savoring their

❖ TABLE 12.1   BASIC GUIDELINES FOR PREPARING GRAINS ❖

GRAIN (1 CUP DRY)	WATER (CUPS)	COOKING TIME	YIELD
Amaranth	2	20 minutes	2 cups
Arborio rice	2	25 minutes	$2\frac{1}{2}$ cups
Barley (hulled)	3	1.5 hours + 10 minutes standing	$3\frac{1}{2}$ cups
Barley (pearled)	3	50 minutes + 10 minutes standing	$3\frac{1}{2}$ cups
Basmati rice	$2\frac{1}{2}$	20 minutes	3 cups
Brown rice	2	45 minutes	3 cups
Buckwheat groats (kasha)*	2	30 minutes	3 cups
Bulgur wheat	2	20 minutes + 5 minutes standing	$2\frac{3}{4}$ cups
Couscous	2	1 minute + 5–10 minutes standing	3 cups
Millet*	$2\frac{1}{2}$	25 minutes + 5 minutes standing	$3\frac{1}{2}$ cups
Oat groats	$2\frac{1}{4}$	1 hour + 10 minutes standing	$2\frac{1}{2}$ cups
Polenta	4	25 minutes, or 5 minute type	3 cups
Quinoa	2	15 minutes + 5 minutes standing	3 cups
Rye berries	3	1 hour	$2\frac{1}{2}$ cups
Spelt	3	2 hours + 15 minutes standing	$2\frac{1}{4}$ cups
Triticale	3	1.75 hours + 10 minutes standing	$2-2\frac{1}{2}$ cups
Wild rice	3	1 hour	$3\frac{1}{2}$ cups
Whole grain wheat berries	3	2 hours	$2\frac{1}{2}$ cups

true flavor and texture is an important lifestyle change to be enjoyed. Exploring a wide variety of new and interesting whole grains can greatly enhance your appreciation of a lower fat and sodium nutrition plan!

With the exception of the following grains, Table 12.1 summarizes the amount of boiling water and cooking time required to cook various rinsed, whole grains. The asterisk (*) indicates that guidelines for millet and buckwheat groats are based on pre-toasting recommendations.

Wheat berries, triticale, and whole rye are the only grains listed which should be combined with water *before* being brought to a boil. After the 2-

---

* Toast before boiling or add 10 to 20 minutes to suggested cooking time.

hour cooking period, remove from the heat and pour off any excess liquid that remains.

Quinoa is one of the few grains that needs additional instructions. Quinoa in its natural state is coated with a bitter substance called saponin, an insect repellent. Most packaged quinoa has already been cleaned, but it is important to do so (in a very fine mesh strainer) unless the package states otherwise.

COOKING DRIED BEANS AND PEAS

Since beans are usually minimally sorted, it is important to pick over and wash beans carefully to remove any foreign substances, such as small stones or stems. With the exception of split peas and lentils, dried beans and peas should be soaked for at least 4 hours, and preferably overnight, before cooking. Rinse them a few times before you go to bed and once again before you cook them the next day. A good rule of thumb is to use three parts water to one part beans to soak, and use bottled water if yours is very hard. Soak, and later cook, in a pot that is significantly greater than the volume of beans, as beans will double in size while soaking and bubble up approximately one-third higher than the level of the beans and water while cooking. After covered beans are boiling, reduce heat, and simmer for 45 minutes to an hour. See specific times below. Of course, beans are always good cooked with garlic, onions, and herbs.

If you forget to soak your beans or do not have time, you can use a quicker method. Bring the beans to a boil, then remove them from the heat and let them sit for one hour. Then rinse the beans, and they will be at the stage they would have been had you soaked them overnight. Cover with fresh water and follow cooking times recommended for soaked beans.

Rinsing the beans a few times during the soaking process and before cooking will reduce the gassy effect that beans may have on your digestive system. This is because rinsing limits the sugars that your body is not accustomed to handling. But, if you ease into eating beans ($\frac{1}{4}$ cup today, $\frac{1}{3}$ cup tomorrow, and so on) you will eventually develop the enzymes needed to break down these discomforting sugars. Although rinsing does slightly reduce the beans' nutritional content, it is well worth the loss if it encourages you to eat them more frequently. They will still offer you more nutrients and fiber than most other foods. Beans are high in potassium, protein, and iron, and contain about five times the fiber of most other high-fiber foods. In particular, they are very high in soluble fiber, which lowers cholesterol and minimizes blood sugar swings. Smaller legumes like split peas and lentils are often easier to digest. The soaking process also significantly reduces the cooking time.

Although scientific research has not documented the following anecdotal advice, it seems to work for people, and therefore bears repeating. A piece of kombu or a slice of fresh ginger root added to the beans as they cook also reportedly helps reduce the gaseousness of beans. Kombu, a sea vegetable found in most health food stores and Asian markets, also provides nice flavor and many minerals. Baking soda is often mentioned as a cure for bloating, but it is not recommended because of its excessive sodium content. In Mexico and the Southwest, the most popular gas preventive additive for beans is a green tea or herb called epizote. A new product called Beano is reportedly effective at digesting the sugar that inspires the gaseousness, but ask your doctor before using it, as it should not be used by people with diabetes or certain other health problems.

Cooking Times and Tidbits
Since no two batches of beans are grown or stored under the exact same conditions, cooking times are approximate. The older the beans the longer

❖ TABLE 12.2   BASIC GUIDELINES FOR PREPARING DRIED BEANS AND PEAS

LEGUMES (1 CUP DRY)	WATER (CUPS)	COOKING TIMES IN HOURS		YIELD (CUPS)
		SOAKED	UNSOAKED	
Anasazi	3	$1\frac{1}{2}$–2	2–3	$2\frac{1}{4}$
Adzuki beans	3	1–$1\frac{1}{2}$	2–3	2
Black (turtle) beans	4	$1\frac{1}{2}$–2	2–3	2
Black-eyed (cow) peas	3	$\frac{1}{2}$	$\frac{3}{4}$–1	2–$2\frac{1}{4}$
Cannellini	3	1–$1\frac{1}{2}$	$1\frac{1}{2}$–2	2
Chick-peas (garbanzos)	4	$1\frac{1}{2}$–2	3	$2\frac{1}{2}$
Cranberry beans	3	1–$1\frac{1}{2}$	$1\frac{1}{2}$–2	$2\frac{1}{2}$
Fava beans	3	$1\frac{1}{2}$–2	2–3	2
Great Northern beans	$3\frac{1}{2}$	1–$1\frac{1}{2}$	2–3	2–$2\frac{1}{4}$
Kidney beans	3	1	$1\frac{1}{2}$	2
Lentils	3	—	$\frac{1}{2}$–$\frac{3}{4}$	2–$2\frac{1}{4}$
Lima beans	2	$\frac{3}{4}$–1	$1\frac{1}{2}$	2
Navy beans	3	$1\frac{1}{2}$–2	2	2
Pinto beans	3	$1\frac{1}{2}$–2	2–3	2–$2\frac{1}{4}$
Red beans	3	$1\frac{1}{2}$–2	2–3	2
Split peas	3	—	$\frac{3}{4}$	2–$2\frac{1}{4}$

they will take to cook, so you may want to note the date of purchase on their storage container. Beans are cooked sufficiently when you can smash one fairly easily between your tongue and the roof of your mouth. For firmer cooked beans to be used in salads, check them for doneness at the minimum time indicated in Table 12.2. You would obviously want to cook beans "well done" for dips and spreads. But, in general, beans should be well done to facilitate easy digestion.

Whether you are concerned with your sodium intake or not, it is best not to cook beans with salt or any acid (like tomatoes or vinegar) as this toughens their skins and prevents them from cooking properly. As the recipes in this book suggest, cook beans until they are done, then add cooked tomato or other acidic ingredients later. You may also note that the bean recipes are usually for large portions. Cooked beans will last in the refrigerator for at least five days and retain their good flavor for four months frozen, so why not make large quantities and save time, money, and energy?

Pressure Cooking

Although pressure cookers can be a real time and energy saver, be aware that the jiggle-top pressure cookers require 1 to 2 tablespoons of oil for each cup of dried beans to reduce the chance of a bean skin getting caught in the vent. Ellen Buchman Ewald, in her book *Recipes for a Small Planet* (1985), reported that beans could be safely cooked in a pressure cooker without fat to control the foaming by pouring 2 cups of water into the cooker, placing beans in a 2-quart stainless-steel bowl and covering them with 2 inches of water, then lowering the bowl into the cooker with the aid of a foil strip and setting the bowl directly on the bottom of the cooker. (A foil strip is simply a 2-foot-long strip of aluminum foil doubled twice lengthwise. The bowl should be placed in the center and lowered into the cooker. Loosely fold the ends of the foil strip over the bowl). Lock the lid in place, bring to high pressure, then lower the heat just enough to maintain a high pressure. Although this method takes approximately three times longer to cook than the traditional pressure cooker method with oil, it is still less than half the time and energy of a standard stovetop method.

13

FLAVORING YOUR HEART-HEALTHY FOODS WITH HERBS AND SPICES

Herbs and spices will enhance not only the flavor of various foods but also your enjoyment of a lifestyle with no added salt and little fat. Basically, a herb is defined as a plant useful to humankind by its leaf, flower, stem, or root. Spices are the dried berries, seeds, or bark of certain trees and bushes, such as black pepper, cinnamon, nutmeg, allspice, and mustard.

The following suggestions for herb and food combinations and recipes of herb and spice blends should prove to be a valuable crash course in their use, especially if you are unsure about experimenting on your own with foods. Try the blends in small test amounts. If you really like their flavor, make a bigger batch the next time. Having these herb and spice blends prepared in advance can make 15-minute meals a reality. For example, I like combining practically any of these blends (except, of course, *Sensual Cider Spices* and *Apple Pie Spice* which are designed for dessert use) and mixing them in equal parts with oat bran or flour and corn meal for a fish batter. Then I cook as directed in the recipe for *Blastin' Blackened Red Snapper*. As dried herbs and spices will keep their flavors for at least three months, make a good-sized batch of the blends that you like and save yourself some time!

Remember that herbs are always more flavorful fresh, rather than frozen or dried, so if you can grow just a few of your favorites, you will be glad that you did. Generally speaking, to convert a recipe that asks for fresh herbs into dried herbs, divide the fresh herb volume by two because the flavor of the dried herb is twice as potent as the fresh herb (2 teaspoons fresh parsley = 1 teaspoon dried parsley). As there are some exceptions to this rule, learn to trust your taste preferences by adding the herbs at the end of the cooking time, tasting the dish, and adding more if desired. If you are planning for leftovers, be forewarned that herb and spice flavors will taste stronger the next day. Obviously it is more prudent to err on the safe side, as you can always add more herbs or spices but you cannot take them away.

ARE HERBS AND SPICES SAFE FOR EVERYONE?

Note that historically, Dr. Kempner did not permit his patients to use herbs and spices while on the Rice Diet Program, although they were allowed to do so with discretion at home. This was because herbs and spices do make foods taste better, and few patients needed an appetite stimulant. Also, spices were thought to be stronger than herbs and more likely to irritate the gut or cause some other health problem. In fact, very few people have any allergic and digestive problems with such seasonings. Chili powder is the only spice that has been consistently shown to aggravate ulcer patients.

Tracking your reactions to seasonings is another good reason to keep a food record. If you are recording your food intake, you will soon be able to tell if any foods or spices are creating a physical problem for you, or are encouraging you to eat too much or too often. Be aware of what the addition of herbs and spices does for your quantity of consumption. If you are losing two pounds of weight per week consuming simply prepared grains, beans, fruits, and vegetables, then find that you plateau when you start eating more spicy foods, read the clues. This is a red flag that you need to return to very plain cuisine until your weight goal is reached or until you feel you are further into your recovery from overeating. The Food Journal with Feelings (Appendix D) has a space for stating your "plan of abstinence." An example entry could be: "I will avoid refined sugar and wheat products. I will enjoy a low-fat and no-salt vegetarian nutrition plan, with unlimited use of spices if I can continue to lose 1 pound per week. If I do not lose with this plan, I will go back to the basics, without spices, to help limit my intake."

Enjoy your herbs and spices—with awareness! See Appendix A for mail order information.

HERBS AND THEIR USES

❖ *Basil* is probably my favorite for dishes with tomato, but it is also very good with most vegetables, fish, and eggs. The purple variety makes the best vinegar.

❖ *Chervil* has a subtle flavor with hints of anise, tarragon, and cucumber. Great in salads or added at the last minute to sauces, soups, and egg dishes.

❖ *Chives* are great anywhere onions would be used, such as in soups, sauces, and dips. Especially nice with tomatoes, potatoes, eggs, green salads, vinegar, carrots, and fish. The lovely lavender blossoms are both beautiful to view and delicious to eat when scattered over a green salad.

❖ *Cilantro* is my favorite herb! Be forewarned that people usually really like it or really do not. Used extensively in Mexican and Asian cooking, it is often referred to as "Mexican parsley" or "Chinese parsley." Although typically used in these cuisines, I like to substitute it for parsley in almost any recipe. It is a must for salsa, chili, refried beans, and egg dishes. (The leaves are called cilantro, and the seeds are ground to make the spice called coriander.)

❖ *Dill* is delicious in breads, fish, egg dishes, potatoes, carrots, tomatoes, and vinegars. It cooks satisfactorily, but it has a stronger flavor when raw.

❖ *Lavender* is probably the all-time favorite fragrant herb. Its fragrant leaves and blossoms are most frequently used for sachets and potpourri, but are also used in fish dishes, vinegars, jellies, and desserts.

❖ *Lovage* has a flavor reminiscent of celery, and it has the unusual characteristic of giving a yeasty, almost meatlike flavor to other ingredients. Its a good addition to potatoes, root vegetables, soups, and whole-grain breads. Ancient Greeks and Romans chewed on lovage seeds to aid digestion, and legend tells of seeds put in potions to conjure up love spells, thus its name of lovage, or love parsley. Consumption of large amounts can harm the kidney. Lovage should not be used during pregnancy.

❖ *Marjoram* is delicious with tomato, fish, pasta, and egg dishes. Its leaves contain thymol, which is a powerful antiseptic, and the delicious flavor of the herb is akin to thyme, yet spicier.

❖ *Mint.* The distinctive essential oil in the plant is menthol, and its refreshing flavor has made mint popular throughout the world. From the yogurt mint drinks of India to tabouli and rice dishes from the Middle East, mint is the "coolest" of herbs. It is absolutely wonderful in fruit salads. Spearmint is the mint meant when recipes call for "mint," and it is my favorite of the countless varieties presently available.

❖ *Oregano* has a pungent flavor similar to but stronger than marjoram. Great with most Mediterranean dishes, it's especially nice with tomatoes, salad dressings, bean, and seafood dishes.

❖ *Parsley* is probably the most popular herb in America, but as a garnish is often left uneaten on the plate. While the curly variety is more decorative, the Italian flat-leaf variety has much more flavor and nutrition. Use it to flavor virtually all foods—soups, sauces, vegetables, and fish.

❖   *Roquette, or arugula,* although officially a fresh salad herb, is eaten by the bowlfuls in Italy. This strong mustard-tasting green is my favorite tossed salad ingredient, but the Italian desire for quantities, sauteed in garlic and olive oil, is understandable!

❖   *Rosemary* is known as the "Queen of Herbs." The highly aromatic leaves give a delightful flavor to honey and syrups, vinegars, breads, and vegetables such as potatoes, garlic, beets, cabbage, beans, spinach, zucchini, and carrots. It also imparts a fine flavor to grilled food if sprigs of it are burning in the charcoal.

❖   *Sage* is another Italian favorite. It is superb in lentil soup, and a must for stuffings.

❖   *Savory.* Winter savory, with a nice peppery taste, is basic to salt substitutes. Known as the "bean herb," it is also good in any soups, stuffings, fish, or vegetable dishes.

❖   *Sorrel.* Its lemony, tart flavor is a delicious surprise in any mixed tossed salad. If using it cooked, add at the last minute. The citruslike sharpness makes sorrel an admirable partner to fatty fish such as salmon, mackerel, or trout, and egg dishes.

❖   *Tarragon,* the "King of Herbs," has a mild licorice flavor that is nice with fruit, marinades, salad dressings, egg dishes, and vinegars.

❖   *Thyme* is another native of the Mediterranean that is delicious in marinades, soups, stews, vinegars, fruits, vegetables, and Creole dishes. Lemon thyme is superb on fish.

NOTE: Hardier leaves such as thyme, sage, and oregano may keep as long as two weeks when refrigerated in small zip-closure bags. The more delicate herbs like cilantro, basil, and dill should be refrigerated with stems in water and leaves loosely covered with a plastic bag. As moist herbs rot quickly, do not wash them until you are ready to use them. If they are wet, wrap in a paper towel or dry at room temperature.

Herb and Spice Delights

Bouquet Garni

Add this "herb bouquet" to stews, soups, and sauces, and remove it just before serving. The essential oils in the herbs provide a subtle flavor and aroma.

1 bay leaf
4 sprigs fresh parsley
½ teaspoon dried thyme or chervil
¼ teaspoon crushed red pepper
Fresh celery and rosemary, optional

If fresh herbs are used, you can bunch them together with a string and tie the end of the string to the pot handle to make the removal easy. Dried herbs can be contained in a cheesecloth bag. Of course you may add other seasonings to suit your taste.

Fines Herbes

Unlike *Bouquet Garni, Fines Herbes* are left in the dish to add color as well as flavor.

1 tablespoon basil
2 teaspoons chervil
2 teaspoons chives
1 teaspoon marjoram
½ teaspoon tarragon
½ teaspoon thyme

Mince the above ingredients and add to sauce or omelet at the end of cooking.

To enhance your enjoyment of food (while avoiding sodium-rich ingredients) try creating your own salt substitutes. You can literally fill your old salt shaker with dried herbs. The combinations are unlimited. Experiment with a variety of dried herb leaves and seeds, spices like ground cloves or ginger, orange or lemon peel, and various peppers.

Herb Seasoning

¼ cup dried parsley
¼ cup dried savory
¼ cup dried thyme
2 tablespoons dried marjoram

Grind with a mortar and pestle or mix ingredients together in a blender.

Spicy Herb Seasoning

3 tablespoons dried basil
3 tablespoons dried marjoram
3 tablespoons dried parsley
3 tablespoons dried thyme
4½ teaspoons dried chives
2½ teaspoons paprika
2½ teaspoons dried rosemary
2½ teaspoons onion powder

Grind ingredients together with a mortar and pestle or mix well in a blender.

Homemade Curry Powder

½ tablespoon cardamom
⅛ teaspoon cayenne
½ tablespoon cloves
6 tablespoons coriander
1½ tablespoons cumin
1 tablespoon fenugreek
1½ teaspoons turmeric

Combine all ingredients and use in stir-frying or in marinades, soups, or sauces.

Garlicked and Herbed Olive Oil (not Butter!)

We keep garlicked olive oil around at all times, varying the fresh herbs as the spirit moves us!

10 cloves garlic, chopped
1 cup extra virgin olive oil
½ cup minced fresh parsley
½ cup minced fresh lovage (or 1 tablespoon celery seed)
1½ teaspoons minced fresh thyme
½ teaspoon minced fresh sage
½ teaspoon minced fresh marjoram
¼ teaspoon freshly ground black pepper (or gourmet blend of green, red and black peppercorns)

Wash and spin dry herbs thoroughly. Mix ingredients together and enjoy on just about anything!

Saltless Seasoning Blends

The following seasoning blends can be created with proportions you prefer. Of course, as with all use of herbs and spices, be guided by your own taste preferences. Each seasoning blend should be mixed well and stored in an airtight container to retain freshness.

Sensual Cider Spices

This blend is delicious simmered in hot apple cider, or used to jazz up fruity herbed teas.

1 tablespoon cinnamon
2 teaspoons allspice
1 teaspoon dried orange peel
1 teaspoon dried lemon peel
½ teaspoon nutmeg
¼ teaspoon star anise
¼ teaspoon whole cloves
¼ teaspoon fenugreek
¼ teaspoon ginger

Apple Pie Spice

A good blend for apple pie or similar desserts.

1 tablespoon cinnamon
1 teaspoon fenugreek
1 teaspoon dried lemon peel
½ teaspoon ginger
¼ teaspoon ground cloves
¼ teaspoon nutmeg

Barbecue Seasoning

Sprinkle on this blend before grilling any main-course meatlike item, such as slices of extra-firm tofu or tempeh, or fish steaks. Or add some to a little water or Basic Veggie Stock and spoon over grilling vegetables, such as potatoes or onions.

1 tablespoon dried, ground chili peppers
2 teaspoons dehydrated garlic
2 teaspoons nutritional yeast
1 teaspoon dehydrated onion
$\frac{1}{2}$ teaspoon paprika
$\frac{1}{4}$ teaspoon black pepper
$\frac{1}{4}$ teaspoon cumin
$\frac{1}{8}$ teaspoon nutmeg
$\frac{1}{8}$ teaspoon cayenne pepper
dash of hickory smoke, optional

Garlic 'n Herb

This is a good blend to enhance a quick salad dressing or vegetable dip.

1 tablespoon sesame seeds
2 teaspoons freshly ground black pepper
2 teaspoons dehydrated garlic
2 teaspoons dried chives
1 teaspoon dried lemon peel
$\frac{1}{2}$ teaspoon citric acid

Italian Seasoning

This blend is great to have on hand for a quick salad dressing or dip, or to season any stir-fry or grilling medley.

1 tablespoon oregano
2 teaspoons marjoram
2 teaspoons thyme
1 teaspoon rosemary
1 teaspoon basil
$\frac{1}{4}$ teaspoon sage

Mexican Seasoning

A tasty blend to sprinkle on Latin dishes, which might include roasted or grilled potatoes, onions, peppers, fish, or tempeh.

1 tablespoon chili peppers
2 teaspoons dehydrated garlic
2 teaspoons dehydrated onion
1 teaspoon paprika
1 teaspoon cumin
1 teaspoon celery seed
1 teaspoon oregano
$\frac{1}{4}$ teaspoon cayenne pepper
$\frac{1}{4}$ teaspoon crushed bay leaf

Oriental Seasoning

This is a delicious blend to have ready for your next salad dressing or vegetable stir-fry.

2 tablespoons toasted sesame seeds
1 tablespoon dehydrated onion
1 tablespoon dehydrated garlic
1 teaspoon freshly ground black pepper
1 teaspoon celery seed
1 teaspoon dried lemon rind
1 teaspoon dry mustard
1 tablespoon dehydrated red bell pepper, optional
1 tablespoon dehydrated green bell pepper, optional

Jamaican

When you want a Caribbean touch to your meal, try this blend on grilled, roasted, or stir-fried vegetables, fish, or tempeh. Or add it to cooking rice.

2 teaspoons dehydrated onion
2 teaspoons dehydrated garlic
½ teaspoon cayenne pepper
½ teaspoon allspice
½ teaspoon black pepper
½ teaspoon ginger
½ teaspoon cinnamon
½ teaspoon fructose
½ teaspoon chives
⅛ teaspoon nutmeg
⅛ teaspoon crushed bay leaves
1½ teaspoons dried tomato, optional

Thai Touch

Use this blend to impart Thai flavors to grilled or stir-fryed vegetables, fish, or tempeh. Also good for flavoring grains, salad dressings, or dips.

1 tablespoon dehydrated garlic
1 tablespoon dehydrated onion
1 teaspoon coriander
1 teaspoon dried tomato
1 teaspoon dried lemon peel
½ teaspoon citric acid
½ teaspoon paprika
½ teaspoon cilantro
¼ teaspoon cayenne pepper
¼ teaspoon black pepper
¼ teaspoon dried basil
¼ teaspoon white pepper

Cajun Blend for Blackened Fish

Blackened fish is a breeze. Simply sprinkle this blend on a plate, and coat both sides of fish before pan-frying or grilling.

1 tablespoon dehydrated onion
1 teaspoon dried red or yellow bell pepper
1 teaspoon ground dried chili peppers
1 teaspoon paprika
1 teaspoon dehydrated garlic
1 teaspoon thyme
1 teaspoon fennel seed
1 teaspoon dried lemon peel
1 teaspoon oregano
1 teaspoon citric acid, optional

Cookin' Cajun

A great blend for some Cajun flair. Add to marinades for grilled fish, tempeh, and vegetables. You could also add it to grains or bread dough before cooking.

1 tablespoon paprika
2½ teaspoons dehydrated onion
2 teaspoons dehydrated garlic
1½ teaspoons thyme
1 teaspoon marjoram
½ teaspoon fennel
½ teaspoon cumin
½ teaspoon cayenne pepper

Homemade Chili Powder

Great in quick coleslaws, salad dressings, or on grilled fish and vegetables.

1 tablespoon dried/ground chili peppers
2 teaspoons cumin
1 teaspoon oregano
1 teaspoon dehydrated garlic

Chili Powder Cha Cha

Cook with beans, grains, or vegetables for a nice Latin "kick."

1 tablespoon dried/ground chili peppers
2 teaspoons cumin
2 teaspoons dehydrated garlic
1 teaspoon oregano
$\frac{1}{2}$ teaspoon coriander
$\frac{1}{4}$ teaspoon allspice
$\frac{1}{8}$ teaspoon ground cloves

Seafood Boil

Great to boil with any seafood, without all the sodium found in commercially prepared alternatives.

1 tablespoon mustard seed
2 teaspoons dill seed
1 teaspoon ginger
1 teaspoon crushed dried chilis
1 teaspoon crushed bay leaf
$\frac{1}{2}$ teaspoon allspice
$\frac{1}{2}$ teaspoon celery seed
$\frac{1}{4}$ teaspoon cinnamon
$\frac{1}{4}$ teaspoon black pepper

Seafood Seasoning Surprise

A nice and tasty addition to any seafood dish or salad.

1 tablespoon dill weed
1 tablespoon sesame seed
2 teaspoons dried lemon peel
2 teaspoons basil
1 teaspoon tarragon
$\frac{1}{2}$ teaspoon celery seed or dried celery leaf

Cajun Kickin' Popcorn Seasoning

Who wants commercially prepared microwave popcorn loaded with fat and/or sodium when you can microwave plain popcorn kernels (coated with a teaspoon of olive oil) in a paper bag, then sprinkle with this healthier seasoning blend?

1 tablespoon paprika
1 tablespoon nutritional yeast
1 tablespoon dehydrated onion
1 tablespoon dehydrated garlic
2 teaspoons thyme
2 teaspoons cumin
1 teaspoon fennel
1 teaspoon marjoram
$\frac{1}{2}$ teaspoon cayenne pepper

Indian Curry Blend

This is a delicious addition to stir-fried vegetables and rice.

1 tablespoon turmeric
1 tablespoon coriander
2 teaspoons paprika
1 teaspoon fenugreek
1 teaspoon black pepper
1 teaspoon cumin
1 teaspoon ginger
$\frac{1}{2}$ teaspoon cloves
$\frac{1}{2}$ teaspoon celery seed
$\frac{1}{2}$ teaspoon caraway seed
$\frac{1}{4}$ teaspoon cayenne pepper

14

RECIPES WITH RESULTS

The recipes in this section are designed to taste good as well as produce results bordering on the miraculous. During ten years of private practice, I have often seen these recipes (when used in conjunction with the rest of the Heal Your Heart Program) inspire cholesterol drops of 100 points within a three-week period. Each is accompanied by a nutritional analysis of calories, protein, fat, carbohydrate, cholesterol, sodium, percent of calories coming from fat and allowances. With the exception of a few salad dressing and salmon recipes, each provides less than 20 percent of calories coming from fat. Otherwise they contain only small amounts of justifiable oil (usually a bit of olive oil to help prevent the reduction of HDL the "good cholesterol") and no added sodium or refined sugar. The small amounts of honey, molasses, or fruit juice used for sweetening can be safely enjoyed by anyone, including diabetics, because these sweeteners are used in combination with soluble-fiber-rich ingredients (such as oats, beans, or barley) which slow blood sugar absorption. For example, it is amazing how effective the pureed lima beans in the pumpkin bread are at slowing one's blood sugar response. By including pureed limas in the batter of sweet breads, even a diabetic can enjoy dessert without guilt, while stabilizing their blood sugars and lowering their cholesterols!

Until you make the shift into thinking about your meals as being centered around whole grains and beans rather than meat, you may be somewhat confused by the organization of the recipes. For instance, the average American would view *Southern Succotash* or *Bayou Baked Bourbon Beans* as vegetable side dishes, rather than as *main* dishes. I cannot in good conscience place them anywhere but where they are—in Main Dishes. When you grow into viewing most of your meals as combinations of whole grains, beans, fruits, and vegetables, you will find the main dishes simply need an additional fruit or vegetable.

You may also note that the recipes are inspired by many international cuisines. I find that patients who continue to explore new and unique recipes tend to stay more interested in their very low-fat and low-sodium nutrition plans. Plus, many of these cuisines are conducive to the use of healthy herbs, spices, and flavorings.

For instance, Italian cuisine is quite receptive to extra garlic, parsley, and peppers, while Chinese cuisine readily accepts extra ginger, garlic, rice wine, and vinegar. Who misses the traditional fat and salt in Mexican food when you can add extra onions, garlic, jalapeños, cilantro, and chipotle? If you are asking "What is a chipotle?," About Ingredients, which follows, is provided to insure that this adventure into healthy eating is fun.

For those who live where unusual ingredients are not readily available, substitutes are suggested. Mail order sources for Health Foods (Appendix A) may also prove helpful.

About Ingredients

Anaheim peppers tend to be slightly hotter than sweet bell peppers but considerably less hot than jalapeño peppers. (Substitute: bell peppers with extra chili powder or cayenne.)

Baking powder, low sodium is made by Calumet and Featherweight. They are usually found in the baking or dietetic section of chain grocery stores. The label states that $1\frac{1}{2}$ times the amount specified in a recipe should be used, but in the recipes in this book, the amount stated is the amount to be used. In traditional recipes that also use baking *soda,* I usually double the low-sodium baking powder and add an egg white to substitute for the baking soda, reducing sodium dramatically.

Barley is not nearly as popular in the United States as elsewhere but has much undiscovered potential. It has a wonderful chewy texture, which is important for many new vegetarians who miss chewier foods. Chain grocery stores typically carry the pearled varieties. Health food stores often carry unhulled barley, which is even higher in soluble (cholesterol-lowering) fiber.

Canned products are rarely my first choice, but when pushed for time it is easy to justify canned beans, tomatoes, and seafood with no salt or fat added. All other products can be found fresh or frozen, which is nutritionally superior to canned items. Try to find these canned staples salt-free. **All**

canned ingredients used in the recipes in this book are the no-salt-added type, and the nutritional analyses reflect their use.

Carob powder may be used as a cocoa or chocolate substitute, but it is best to serve it without that introduction. Most people would like it if they did not compare it to chocolate. Made from the dried pods of the carob tree, it is very high in minerals but, unfortunately, like many healthy whole foods, it is processed into products containing hydrogenated fat, sugar, and salt. Beware of "carob-covered" anything!

Chayote squash ranges from cream to dark green in color and is about the same shape and size as a somewhat flattened pear. The flavor is like a combination of cucumber and zucchini with a slight citrus taste. It was cultivated in pre-Columbian times in Central America and is native to the Southwest where it is typically used in Latin or Southwestern dishes. It is good raw in salads, stuffed, or sautéed with a little olive oil.

Chilis have been used in Mexico and in the American Southwest for more than 10,000 years. Connoisseurs agree that New Mexican chilis are the best, except for those connoisseurs living in Texas who, of course, know that theirs are!

Chilis are rated on a scale from 1 to 120 for hotness. To put their potential heat into perspective, a jalapeño is only 15! But, it is difficult to answer the oft-asked question of which pepper is hottest because this depends upon not only the variety of the chili but on the conditions under which it was grown and the timing of the harvest. Although the heat of the chili is supposedly in the fleshy veins that hold the seeds in place (rather than in the seeds), it is generally recommended that the seeds be removed as well. You may regret it for days if you fail to do so.

It is easy to understand why people who eat chili peppers habitually do so. Green chili when eaten produces endorphins, which are a morphine-like substance that makes you feel good! If you do not want to order the New Mexican green chilis, you can substitute with fresh poblano chilis or the milder Anaheim with a jalapeño pepper for additional heat. Canned chilis are not recommended, as they are usually mushy in texture, inferior in flavor, and loaded with sodium. If New Mexico chili powder is not available, you can use ground ancho chili in its place. Double check any commercial chili powder for salt or other undesirable ingredients. See Appendix A for mail order companies that offer large varieties of chili peppers.

To roast New Mexican, Anaheim, or Poblano chilis, place them under a broiler and broil, turning them until most of the skin is blistered. (Jalapeños and serrano chilis are used with their skins on, so this process is not necessary for them.) Then place the chilis in a plastic bag or a bowl of ice water to loosen the skin. The skin can then be removed easily with a paper towel. Cut off the stem and slice the pepper length-wise. Remove the seeds and the veins, which are the hottest part. Be careful to avoid touching your eyes or other sensitive parts of your body. In fact, it's best to wear thin rubber gloves when you handle chilis.

Chipotle peppers are smoked jalapeño peppers. Dried, salt-free chipotles can be purchased in gourmet or health food stores. The dried type can be softened (or reconstituted) in a heated liquid such as wine. Add one or two to a pot of beans or soup, and an "okay" dish becomes incredible. Try one before adding two, as they are quite hot.

Chips are now available without salt or fat, but be careful to read the fine print to ensure the exclusion of both. Baked Tostitos and Smart Temptations are the thinnest and crispiest no-fat, no-salt corn chips, but Guiltless Gourmet is also good. They are wonderful with a salt-free, fat-free salsa or bean dip. Potato chips are also now made without fat or salt.

Epazote is known as Mexican tea, wormseed, stinkweed, goosefoot, and Jerusalem oak. Epazote grows wild in the Americas and in parts of Europe, but it is most easily found in potted form from nurseries. Be forewarned that it propagates with abandon and can take over a garden if not contained. Do not be concerned with this herb's unusual aroma, which is somewhat reminiscent of kerosene. It has an untamed flavor but many people love it. It is a natural in stews, beans, and seafood dishes. It is especially useful with beans of all types because of its ability to reduce their gaseousness. Epazote is also popular as a tea in Mexico and a tisane in Europe.

Filé is powdered sassafras leaves and is a staple of Creole cooking. It is a must for gumbo—the spice jars are often marked "gumbo filé."

Frozen vegetables, with no added fat or sodium, are the next best choice to fresh ones. In fact, if the fresh vegetables at your market look old or limp, frozen ones may be nutritionally superior. **All frozen vegetables used in the recipes in this book are the no-added-fat-or-sodium type, and the nutritional analyses reflect their use.**

Greens: Chicory comes in a variety of types. The two most common types are the broad-leaf type called **escarole,** and leafy chicory, which is also known as **curly endive.** The broad-leaf type is sweeter, while the frilly type has a pleasantly bitter taste. **Radicchio,** or red chicory, is primarily used in salads for its maroon or purple color. It has a slightly bitter flavor, thus it can be used sparingly. Although it is very expensive, one head of it can jazz up salads and last for approximately two weeks. In Italy it is popular grilled as a vegetable with garlic, olive oil, herbs, and balsamic vinegar.

Jicama is a brown-skinned, beet-shaped root vegetable with crisp white flesh. It has the texture of a radish but tastes somewhere between a potato and a water chestnut (for which it may be substituted). In the Southwest it is usually peeled and eaten raw in salads. It is also good seasoned with chili powder and citrus juice.

Oriental staples are often difficult to find except in Oriental food stores. Most Oriental stores stock the following: golden needles (tiger lily buds), rice noodles, tapioca starch (cornstarch will work as a substitute, but tapioca makes food glisten more), rice wine, rice wine vinegar, black vinegar (made from fermented rice), tree ears (a type of dried Chinese mushroom), lily flowers, bamboo shoots, cellophane noodles (made from mung beans), black mushrooms, bean sprouts, five-spice powder (a popular Chinese spice blend containing star anise, Szechuan peppercorns, cinnamon, cloves, and fennel), jasmine tea, chili oil, bean sheets (made from mung beans), rose rice, wasabi powder (horseradish powder), and nori sheets (pressed and dried seaweed for wrapping sushi).

Polenta is an Italian "mush" made of barley, chestnut meal, or cornmeal. Cornmeal is by far the most popular today. Traditionally, it is served with a lot of cheese and butter but is also typically served with a vegetarian spaghetti sauce. (Substitute: grits without salt or fat.)

Postum, Pero, Dacopa, and **Cafix** are brand names of commonly available coffee substitutes. Decopa is presently my favorite, but it must be purchased in a health food store. As with carob for a chocolate substitute, you will be more successful if you do not approach it as a "fake coffee." Use 1 teaspoon in a cup of boiling water with 1 teaspoon honey and 2 tablespoons soy or skim milk. This is a delicious way to ease off an addiction to coffee.

Quinoa is an ancient Aztec grain that has a delightful crunch to it. The mouth-feel is similar to the subtle crunch of caviar but without the sodium. The Incas considered quinoa a sacred grain, and called it "the Mother Grain." Although it is a tiny grain, no larger than a mustard seed, it once fed an ancient civilization that stretched from the seacoast of Chili to the peaks of the Peruvian Andes. Quinoa has flourished in cultivation for over 5,000 years but has only recently been made commercially available in the United States. It is found in health food stores and some chain grocery stores.

It is great topped with grilled vegetables and barbecued tempeh, or made into a pudding with raisins and cinnamon. It is especially nice in the summer since it is a very light grain. (Substitute: nothing is close, but you could use brown rice.)

Tahini is sesame seed butter—sesame seeds ground into a paste the way peanuts are ground into peanut butter. While peanut butter is very atherogenic (or plaque-causing), tahini has a lower saturated fat content and a better effect on cholesterol. Two teaspoons can be considered a fat exchange and are a delicious substitute for butter or margarine. Try it on bagels or English muffins, then top with no-sugar jelly. Yummy!

Tempeh is a "cultured" soy product, which is made by cooking cracked soybeans, draining the water, and inoculating them with a culture called

Rhizopus Oligosporus. One should be warned that it looks fairly weird, like a molded cake of pressed soybeans. But it is no weirder than eating spoiled milk as cheese, yogurt, sour cream, or buttermilk! In Western cultures people are familiar with cultured dairy products. In Indonesia people enjoy tempeh as much as most Americans do meat. Enjoy the tempeh within a few days of purchase as its flavor gets stronger with time. It freezes beautifully if you do not plan to use it soon. Ignore the black spots as this sporulation is natural to the product. Indonesian tempeh is one of the few vegetarian foods that has appreciable amounts of vitamin B_{12}, but the more sterile American production methods do not usually produce tempeh with reliably high amounts of this vitamin. Tempeh is usually just soybeans and culture, but some contains other grains. These blends are fine, but read the ingredients to avoid the newer tempeh products now adulterated with salt, cheese, or other undesirables.

Texturized vegetable protein or **TVP** is another soy product that is an excellent meat substitute. In fact, most people ask what kind of meat is in the spaghetti sauce when this is used. It is available in most health food stores and looks very much like a beige version of Grapenuts cereal. Simply pour an equal part of boiling water over TVP to reconstitute for 10 to 15 minutes. Drain and use anywhere you would use ground hamburger. Tempeh could be substituted, but TVP is even closer to the ground beef consistency. TVP is good for replacing meat in sauces and casseroles, while tempeh is best grilled. There is also now a chunkier version of TVP that can be substituted for beef chunks or strips in stir-fried dishes.

Tofu is a soybean cheese found in most chain grocery stores. It is called a cheese because its method of manufacture is similar to dairy cheese. Tofu will keep refrigerated for about 10 days if it is stored in fresh water and rinsed every other day. It can be frozen, but the texture changes radically. (The texture of frozen and thawed tofu resembles ground beef.) Tofu can be used in many recipes in place of meat. Soft tofu is good for blending into dressings and desserts.

Tomatillos look like small green tomatoes enclosed in an easily removable papery brown husk. Their tart flavor marries beautifully with serrano chilis, garlic, and cilantro. Next to the tomato, tomatillo is the most widely used salsa ingredient, and it forms the basis of many Mexican green sauces.

Vegetable bouillon with no fat or salt added is hard to find. Look for it at health food stores.

Vegetable cooking spray, used in many recipes in this book, should be the nonaerosol type, which does not contain propellants harmful to the environment. Pan Max brand, which contains only canola oil and lecithin, is more expensive than others, but comes in a refillable container, making it doubly environment-friendly. If you cannot find this product, simply use 1 teaspoon of olive or canola oil to coat your cookware.

WonderSlim is a product that can replace fat in homemade baked goods. Like applesauce or other pureed fruits, it helps produce moist fat-free (or fat-reduced) results. Look for it in health food stores, or order by mail (see Appendix A).

BREAKFASTS AND BREADS

Cream of Something, Sweetened

$\frac{1}{3}$ cup oat bran, bits of barley, or cream of wheat, rice or other grain
$\frac{3}{4}$ cup water, approximate
2 tablespoons raisins
1 tablespoon maple syrup
Cinnamon to taste
Banana, optional

Cook the grain in water as directed on the package. Stir in the raisins approximately one minute before the grain is cooked; then cook for another minute. Add the remaining ingredients.

Yield: 1 serving

Depending upon the type of cereal you use, each serving contains approximately:
■ Calories: 210 (8% from fat); Protein: 4 gms; Fat: 1–2 gms; Carbohydrate: 45 gms; Cholesterol: 0; Sodium: 14 mgs; Allowances: 2 starches + 1 fruit

Heart Healthy Hotcakes

$1\frac{1}{2}$ cups skim milk
$\frac{3}{4}$ cup regular rolled oats
6 tablespoons oat bran
$\frac{3}{4}$ cup plus 2 tablespoons whole wheat flour
$\frac{1}{2}$ cup all-purpose flour
2 teaspoons low-sodium baking powder

$\frac{3}{4}$ teaspoon ground cinnamon
$\frac{1}{2}$ teaspoon ground ginger
6 egg whites, beaten
1 teaspoon canola or olive oil
$\frac{1}{4}$ cup WonderSlim or applesauce
Sliced fruit, optional
Vegetable cooking spray

Heat milk in medium-size pan over low heat until hot, stirring occasionally. Remove from heat, stir in oats, and let stand for 5 minutes. Combine the oat bran, flours, baking powder, cinnamon, and ginger in a large bowl. In a separate bowl, combine beaten egg whites, oil, "WonderSlim" or applesauce, and sliced fruit if using, and then stir into oat mixture. Add oat mixture to flour mixture and stir until combined.

Spray a griddle or skillet with vegetable cooking spray and heat over medium heat. Pour on $\frac{1}{4}$ cup batter. When pancake surface is bubbly, edges are slightly dry, and underneath is golden brown (approximately 1 to 2 minutes), turn to cook the second side.

Yield: 16 3-inch pancakes ■ Each pancake contains approximately: Calories: 79 (11% from fat); Protein: 4 gms; Fat: 1 gm; Carbohydrate: 14 gms; Cholesterol: .4 mg; Sodium: 32 mgs; Allowances: $\frac{3}{4}$ starch + $\frac{1}{4}$ protein

Wonderful Waffle or Pancake Topping

Vegetable cooking spray, nonaerosol type
4 pears (or any firm fruit), thinly sliced
½ cup unsweetened apple or pear juice
¼ teaspoon cinnamon
¼ teaspoon vanilla extract
1 tablespoon chopped walnuts

Spray skillet or saucepan with vegetable cooking spray, and place over medium-high heat. Add the remaining ingredients and sauté for 5 to 10 minutes. Remove from heat and mash with a potato masher until the mixture achieves a texture you like.

Yield: 5 servings; serving size ½ cup ∎
Each serving contains approximately: Calories: 88 (14% from fat); Protein: 1 gm; Fat: 1.4 gms; Carbohydrate: 21 gms; Cholesterol: 0; Sodium: 2 mgs; Allowances: 1¼ fruits + ¼ fat

Cheese and Fruit Topping for Pancakes

2 cups blueberries
1 cup ½% dry curd cottage cheese
1 teaspoon honey
2 tablespoons fresh orange juice

Wash blueberries and set aside 1 cup. Put remaining cup of berries and the other ingredients in a blender, blend well, and pour into a bowl. Mix in the reserved blueberries.

Yield: 5 servings ∎ Each serving contains approximately: Calories: 52 (5% from fat); Protein: 3 gms; Fat: .29 gm; Carbohydrate: 10 gms; Cholesterol: 0; Sodium: 6 mgs; Allowances: ½ protein + ½ fruit

Berry-Barley Fruited Salad

1½ cups oat groats
1½ cups pearled barley or hulled barley
1½ cups chopped dried fruit (see note)
½ cup sherry
1 tablespoon fresh lemon juice
2 tablespoons toasted sesame or canola oil
3 tablespoons raspberry vinegar
¾ cup finely minced fresh chives or scallions
2½ teaspoons minced fresh mint leaves (about 15 large leaves)
5 firm ripe red plums, sliced
2 Granny Smith apples, sliced

Note: I like ½ cup pitted prunes, ½ cup peaches, ¼ cup pears, and ¼ cup mangoes, but the choice of dried fruits is up to you.

Place oat groats in 4 cups of water, cover, and bring to a boil. Reduce heat and simmer for 1 hour or more until tender, adding more water if needed. Wash barley until the rinse water looks clear. Add barley to 4¼ cups of water, and bring to a boil. Reduce heat and simmer for 30 minutes for pearled barley, 45 minutes for hulled barley.

Place dried fruit and put in a bowl with sherry. Marinate from 15 minutes to overnight, as convenient.

Combine cooked grains and marinated dried fruit, and stir in all of the remaining ingredients, except for the fresh fruit. Cover and chill. Add fresh fruit just before serving. The grain mixture will keep for a week or more, and the mixture of fresh fruit can simply be added when desired.

Yield: 15 cups, or 30 servings; serving size $\frac{1}{2}$ cup. ■ Each serving contains approximately: Calories: 128 (14% from fat); Protein: 2 gms; Fat: 2 gms; Carbohydrate: 17 gms; Cholesterol: 0; Sodium: 5 mgs; Allowances: 1 starch + $\frac{1}{2}$ fruit + $\frac{1}{2}$ fat

Basic Whole Wheat Bread
by Dr. Robert Rosati

$1\frac{1}{2}$ cups lukewarm water (105 to 115 degrees)
2 teaspoons regular dry yeast
2 teaspoons fast-acting dry yeast
3 tablespoons honey
3 cups 100% stone-ground whole wheat flour
6 tablespoons wheat gluten (sold at health food stores)

Bread by Hand

Place the lukewarm water in a small bowl. Sprinkle the yeast on top of the water, add honey, and let stand until dissolved and foamy, about 10 minutes. Mix the flour and wheat gluten in a large bowl. Make a well in the center of the dry ingredients. Pour the dissolved yeast and honey into the well, and with a fork, gradually work in the flour until all of it is absorbed. Knead the dough until it is smooth and soft, about 5 minutes. Shape

the dough into a ball; lightly flour the ball and cover with plastic wrap. Let rise at room temperature until doubled in bulk, about 2 hours.

Turn the dough out onto a floured work surface. Punch down the dough and divide it in half. Shape each half into a loaf. Lightly dust a baking sheet with flour and place the loaves on it. Let rise at room temperature until doubled in size, about 30 minutes. Meanwhile, preheat oven to 400 degrees. Bake until golden brown, about 30 minutes. Remove from oven and let cool completely on a wire rack before slicing.

Bread Machine Method

Mix the whole wheat flour and gluten in a mixing bowl. (If they have been stored in the freezer, bring to room temperature first.) Pour lukewarm water into bread machine pan. Sprinkle the yeast into the water, then add honey. Next add the premixed dry ingredients into the bread pan. Turn the flour mixture once with a large spoon in each corner of the bread pan.

Place the bread pan immediately into the home bakery. Select BREAD menu, LIGHT or MEDIUM color; then press START button and LOCK button. My Hatachi Bread Machine bakes this in 4 hours and 10 minutes. Remove bread from machine when ready.

Yield: 18 slices. ■ Each serving contains approximately: Calories: 87 (5% from fat); Protein: 4 gms; Fat: .5 gm; Carbohydrate: 18 gms; Cholesterol: 0; Sodium: 1 mg; Allowances: 1 starch + $\frac{1}{10}$ fruit

Pane Paesano

by Dr. Robert Rosati

Although baking bread the old-fashioned way is time-consuming, it is also very thera-peutic—good for the soul as well as the tastebuds! Covering the loaves with a floured towel, placing water beneath the loaves, and turning the loaves upside down are Old World tricks that guarantee the best crust and texture you have ever tasted. You can bake the bread on either baking sheets, pizza stones, or bread bricks, which can be found in any gourmet culinary shop. This bread is also wonderful with $\frac{1}{2}$ cup chopped fresh sage, 1 tablespoon freshly ground black pepper, and $\frac{1}{4}$ cup walnuts (if allowed) added to the batter.

2 packages fast-rising dry yeast
$2\frac{1}{2}$ cups tepid water (about 110 degrees)
$6\frac{1}{2}$ cups unbleached white bread flour (do not use all-purpose flour)
$\frac{1}{8}$ cup cornmeal or semolina flour (to flour the board)

Dissolve the yeast in the water and let stand 5 minutes. Add 4 cups of the flour to make a batter, stirring to help it dis-solve. Beat for 10 minutes with the pad-dle of an electric mixer or until it pulls away from the sides of the mixing bowl. Or mix by hand if you prefer. Add the re-maining flour and knead for 5 minutes in a machine using a dough hook or approxi-mately 15 minutes by hand. The corn-meal or semolina flour can be used as needed to dust your kneading surface. You may need to add more water to get a moist elastic dough.

Leave the dough on a piece of plastic wrap, and cover with a large metal bowl.

Allow the dough to rise until doubled, which will take 1 to 2 hours. Punch down the dough with your fists, folding it over a few times into a nice mound, and let rise for another $1\frac{1}{2}$ hours.

Punch down again, then cut dough into three sections, molding them into loaves. Place the loaves on a floured cotton towel, dust them with a little more flour, then cover with another floured cotton towel. Preheat the oven to 450 degrees and place a pan of hot water on the bot-tom shelf. When the loaves have doubled in volume again, place them in the upper third of the oven, upside down, where the bottom is now the top and vice versa. Bake for approximately 25 minutes or un-til the crust is slightly browned and the loaves sound hollow when thumped. Cool on a rack before slicing.

Yield: 40 slices. ■ Each serving contains approximately: Calories: 84 (3% from fat); Protein: 3 gms; Fat: .25 gms; Carbo-hydrate: 17 gm; Cholesterol: 0; Sodium: 1 mg; Allowances: 1 starch

D'Liteful Cornbread

with Joy Nelson

3 cups yellow cornmeal
$2\frac{1}{4}$ cups all-purpose flour
3 tablespoons low-sodium baking powder
12 beaten egg whites or $1\frac{1}{2}$ cups egg sub-stitute
6 tablespoons honey or 3 tablespoons honey and 3 tablespoons molasses
1 tablespoon WonderSlim or 1 extra egg white
3 cups skim milk
Vegetable cooking spray

Preheat oven to 350 degrees.

Combine the dry ingredients and mix well. Set aside. Then combine wet ingredients and mix well. Pour the wet ingredients into the dry mixture. Mix only until the dry ingredients are moistened. Do not overmix.

Spray muffin tins with vegetable cooking spray. Bake for 15 to 20 minutes. Or use a $13\frac{1}{2} \times 8\frac{3}{4} \times 1\frac{3}{4}$ baking pan; bake for 25 to 30 minutes and cut into 24 or 36 pieces.

Yield: 24 or 36 servings. ∎ Each serving contains approximately: *If 24 muffins:* Calories: 144 (2% from fat); Protein: 5 gms; Fat .39 gm; Carbohydrate: 30 gms; Cholesterol: 0; Sodium: 37 mgs; Allowances: $1\frac{1}{2}$ starches + $\frac{1}{8}$ protein + $\frac{1}{8}$ dairy. *If 36 muffins:* Calories: 96 (2% from fat); Protein: 3 gms; Fat: .26 gm; Carbohydrate: 20 gms; Cholesterol: 0; Sodium: 24 mgs; Allowances: 1 starch + $\frac{1}{10}$ protein + $\frac{1}{12}$ dairy

No Salt Challah
by Judy Ladner

$3\frac{1}{2}$ ounces skim milk
2 tablespoons honey
2 teaspoons dry yeast
$3\frac{3}{8}$ cups (1 pound) bread flour (see note)
$1\frac{1}{2}$ tablespoons nonfat dry powdered milk
$1\frac{1}{2}$ tablespoons olive oil
1 cup Egg Beaters or 8 egg whites
Vegetable cooking spray

Glaze:
$\frac{1}{4}$ cup Egg Beaters
1 teaspoon skim milk

Note: If whole wheat flour is used, double the yeast.

Heat milk until 110 to 115 degrees, add honey and stir, then add yeast. Let stand 10 minutes. Combine yeast mixture with remaining ingredients and knead for 10 minutes. Coat a large bowl with vegetable cooking spray. Place dough in bowl, cover with a damp cloth, and allow to rise until doubled in bulk. Punch down. For finer texture, allow to rise again.

Divide dough into 3 equal portions. Roll each into a long rope, slightly tapered at the ends. Braid the 3 ropes and press ends together. Cover with cloth and allow to rise until doubled. Combine the glaze ingredients and brush surface of bread. Bake for 35 to 40 minutes until golden.

Yield: 18 slices. ∎ Each slice contains approximately: Calories: 105 (15% from fat); Protein: 4 gms; Fat: 1.7 gms; Carbohydrate: 18 gms; Cholesterol: .3 mg; Sodium: 30 mgs; Allowances: 1 starch + $\frac{1}{8}$ protein + $\frac{1}{4}$ fat

Banana Barley Bread

3 cups barley flour
4 teaspoons low-sodium baking powder
3 ripe bananas
$\frac{1}{2}$ cup honey
$\frac{1}{4}$ cup molasses
3 tablespoons Wonderslim (if unavailable use 2 tablespoons of applesauce and 1 more egg white)
5 egg whites, beaten
1 teaspoon grated lemon peel
$1\frac{1}{2}$ teaspoons fresh lemon juice
$\frac{1}{2}$ cup chopped walnuts, optional
Vegetable cooking spray

Preheat oven to 350 degrees.

Sift together the barley flour and baking powder. In a food processor blend bananas, honey, molasses, and Wonder-Slim. Pour into a large bowl, then mix in beaten egg whites, lemon peel, and lemon juice. Fold dry mixture into the liquid mixture, blending well. Add chopped nuts if desired.

Spray two $8\frac{1}{4} \times 4\frac{1}{2}$-inch loaf pans with vegetable cooking spray and lightly flour them. Pour batter into prepared pans. Bake for 35 to 40 minutes. Cut each loaf into 13 slices.

Yield: 26 servings; serving size 1 slice. ■ Each serving contains approximately: *Without walnuts:* Calories: 79 (4% from fat); Protein: 2 gms; Fat: .3 gm; Carbohydrate: 20 gms; Cholesterol: 0; Sodium: 11 mgs; Allowances: $\frac{1}{2}$ starch + $\frac{1}{2}$ fruit + $\frac{1}{13}$ protein. *With walnuts:* Calories: 86 (10% from fat); Protein: 2 gms; Fat: 1 gm; Carbohydrate: 20 gms; Cholesterol: 0; Sodium: 11 mgs; Allowances: $\frac{1}{2}$ starch + $\frac{1}{2}$ fruit + $\frac{1}{13}$ protein + $\frac{1}{6}$ fat

Fat-Free Oat Bran Muffins

$2\frac{1}{4}$ cups oat bran
5 teaspoons cinnamon
$\frac{1}{4}$ teaspoon ground cloves
$\frac{1}{2}$ teaspoon ground nutmeg
2 tablespoons low-sodium baking powder
1 cup chopped pitted dates
1 cup unsweetened applesauce
1 tablespoon vanilla extract
3 tablespoons plain nonfat yogurt
1 cup raisins
12 egg whites
Vegetable cooking spray

Preheat oven to 400 degrees.

Sift together the oat bran, cinnamon, cloves, nutmeg, and baking powder in a large bowl. Put the dates, applesauce, vanilla, yogurt and $\frac{1}{2}$ cup of the raisins in a food processor and purée. Combine with the oat bran mixture and stir in the remaining $\frac{1}{2}$ cup of raisins. Beat egg whites, then fold into mixture. Stir as little as possible to blend the ingredients. Spray muffin tins with vegetable cooking spray. Spoon batter into muffin tins almost to top (batter will not rise much). The tins will be approximately $\frac{3}{4}$ full if you plan on making 18.

Bake 20 minutes, or until a knife can enter the muffin and come out fairly clean.

Yield: 16 or 18 muffins. ■ Each muffin contains approximately: *If 16 muffins:* Calories: 132 (8% from fat); Protein: 6 gms; Fat: 1 gm; Carbohydrate: 26 gms; Cholesterol: 0; Sodium: 42 mgs; Allowances: $\frac{4}{5}$ starch + $1\frac{1}{10}$ fruits + $\frac{1}{3}$ protein. *If 18 muffins:* Calories: 118 (8% from fat); Protein: 5 gms; Fat: 1 gm; Carbohydrate: 23 gms; Cholesterol: 0; Sodium: 38 mgs; Allowances: $\frac{1}{2}$ starch + 1 fruit + $\frac{1}{4}$ protein

Pumpkin Bean Bread

This surprising bread is delicious for breakfast or as dessert. People who claim they hate any type of beans love this, and are none the wiser!

$\frac{1}{2}$ cup dried baby lima beans (1 cup cooked and mashed)
$1\frac{3}{4}$ cups whole wheat flour
1 cup oat bran
1 tablespoon low-sodium baking powder
$\frac{1}{2}$ cup chopped walnuts, optional

1 16-ounce can pumpkin
2½ teaspoons plus ½ teaspoon canola or olive oil
⅓ cup molasses
6 egg whites
1½ teaspoons vanilla extract
2 teaspoons pumpkin pie spice

Soak baby limas overnight, rinsing a few times, then cook for approximately 55 minutes. Drain and mash or put through a food processor.

Preheat oven to 350 degrees.

Mix all dry ingredients together, then combine with remaining ingredients (except the ½ teaspoon canola oil). Stir only enough to blend.

Coat two 5 × 9 × 3-inch loaf pans with the remaining canola oil and pour in batter.

Bake at 350° 60 to 70 minutes, or until a toothpick inserted in the bread emerges clean. Let cool in pans for 5 minutes and then remove bread to a rack to cool. Cut each loaf into 12 slices. Toast before serving, and top with a few tablespoons of plain nonfat yogurt plus a teaspoon of maple syrup.

Yield: 12 servings; service size 1 slice. ■
Each slice contains approximately: *With walnuts:* Calories: 84 (19% from fat); Protein: 4 gms; Fat: 1.8 gms; Carbohydrate: 14 gms; Cholesterol: 0; Sodium: 15 mgs; Allowances: 1⅓ starches + ⅓ vegetable + ⅓ fruit + ½ fat. *Without walnuts:* Calories: 80 (12% from fat); Protein: 4 gms; Fat: 1.1 gms; Carbohydrate: 14 gms; Cholesterol: 0; Sodium: 15 mgs; Allowances: 1⅓ starches + ⅓ vegetable + ⅓ fruit + ⅛ fat

Appetizers

Roasted Garlic

Use this absolutely delicious sweet garlic spread in place of butter or margarine. It can also be used to enhance the flavor of sauces, dips, or soups. Even those unfortunate few who do not like garlic tend to love this! Keeps for weeks in the refrigerator.

3 heads garlic (preferably not the large elephant garlic, which is very mild)
½ teaspoon extra virgin olive oil
1 teaspoon freshly chopped Italian herb blend (rosemary, oregano, basil, and/or thyme), optional

Preheat oven to 450 degrees.

Peel most of the thin layers of papery skin from the garlic heads, but keep the garlic heads intact. Slice approximately ⅛ inch off the smaller end of each garlic head. Pour the olive oil in the palm of your hand, then coat the outside of the garlic heads with the oil. Sprinkle the oiled heads with the fresh herbs, if using, then wrap them together in a piece of aluminum foil. (Although gourmet stores sell garlic roasters, they tend to be too small to contain more than one head. If I am going to heat an oven for this long, I'm going to cook a few garlic heads along with a half dozen sweet potatoes!)

Bake for 1 hour. Cool for a few minutes before separating the cloves, then squeeze the fatter end of each clove. If you have sliced the tips of the bulbs sufficiently, the brown garlic paste will easily exude from the tips of the cloves.

Yield: approximately 7½ tablespoons, or 11 servings; serving size 2 teaspoons. ■ Each serving contains approximately: Calories: 18 (9% from fat); Protein: 1 gm; Fat: .18 gm; Carbohydrate: 3 gms; Cholesterol: 0; Sodium: 2 mgs; Allowances: ⅔ vegetable

Sushi, Vegetarian Style

2 cups short-grain rice (Rose rice)
2 baby cucumbers, thinly sliced
¼ cup shredded red pepper or carrots
1 teaspoon grated ginger root
2 tablespoons honey
4 tablespoons rice vinegar
2 tablespoons rice wine
3 tablespoons water
5 nori sheets
1 teaspoon extra virgin olive oil
2 tablespoons sesame seeds
2 egg whites, beaten
2 tablespoons wasabi powder

Cook rice. Combine the cucumber, red pepper or carrots, and ginger in a small bowl. In a small saucepan combine honey, rice vinegar, rice wine, and 2 tablespoons water over medium-high heat, stirring until honey is dissolved. When warm, add ⅔ of this cooked sauce to the cooked rice, and blend the remaining sauce into the vegetable-ginger mixture.

Lightly toast the nori sheets in a wok over medium heat, turning each sheet a few times. Remove and set aside. Place sesame seeds in the wok and toast until

lightly browned and set aside. With a paper towel, coat the wok with a teaspoon of olive oil. Heat the wok over medium heat, then pour in ⅓ of the beaten egg whites. Tilt and rotate the wok to form a thin layer, and continue to cook over medium heat until the egg is set. Turn the egg sheet over and cook for 15 seconds more. Make 3 egg sheets, then shred them into small pieces. Add 1 tablespoon water to wasabi powder to make a wasabi paste about the consistency of mustard and set aside.

To make the sushi, first wet your hands with water, then spread about 1 cup of the rice on a toasted nori sheet, leaving a margin of approximately ½ inch (on one side) free from rice or other toppings, so that when it is rolled the ingredients will remain within. Spread ⅕ of the cucumber mixture, wasabi paste, and toasted sesame seeds down the center of the rice. With the nori sheet placed on a bamboo mat and with the uncovered edge of the nori sheet away from your body, roll the nori sheet away from you to enclose the filling. Then wrap the bamboo mat completely around the sushi roll and press firmly.

Remove the sushi roll from the bamboo mat, and cut into ½-inch pieces. Repeat this process four more times.

Yield: 5 sushi rolls, or appetizers for 5 people. ■ Each serving contains approximately: Calories: 197 (9% from fat); Protein: 5 gms; Fat: 1.9 gms; Carbohydrate: 39 gms; Cholesterol: 0; Sodium: 23 mgs; Allowances: 2 starches + 1½ vegetables

Skordalia

In Detroit's Greek Town this dish is made with so much garlic it burns your mouth! Of course the raw garlic is much more potent than the roasted, which is almost sweet in its subtleness. Add garlic as desired, while remembering that tomorrow it will taste significantly stronger!

4 cups cooked white beans (Great Northerns or baby limas) or potatoes
2 heads of *Roasted Garlic* (see page 243) or 4–6 cloves of raw garlic, pushed through a press
4 teaspoons extra virgin olive oil (preferably *Lemon-Zested Olive Oil,* see page 263) or ¼ cup walnuts
6 tablespoons fresh lemon juice (less if using *Lemon-Zested Olive Oil*)
10–12 tablespoons bean cooking liquid or *Basic Veggie Stock* (see page 249)
¼ cup finely chopped fresh parsley or basil, as garnish

Purée all ingredients, except for the parsley, in a food processor. Add chopped parsley, mix and refrigerate. This dip is best the second day, after the flavors have had a chance to blend. Enjoy on bread or as a vegetable dip.

Yield: 5 cups or 10 servings; serving size ½ cup. ■ Each serving contains approximately: Calories: 121 (17% from fat); Protein: 7 gms; Fat: 2.3 gms; Carbohydrate: 19 gms; Cholesterol: 0; Sodium: 2 mgs; Allowances: 1¼ starches + ½ fat

Chahine's Eggplant Spread

2 large eggplants
6 garlic cloves, minced

3 tablespoons *Basic Veggie Stock* (see page 249), plus 1 teaspoon olive oil, if allowed
1 cup chopped tomato
Juice of 1 lemon
Freshly ground black pepper to taste
Freshly chopped basil to taste
Dash of ground cumin, optional

Pierce each eggplant all over (5 to 10 times) with a fork. Microwave for 10 minutes; turn, then microwave another 10 minutes, or until eggplant is quite soft. If using a conventional oven, bake on a cookie sheet at 400 degrees for 45 minutes. Sauté garlic in vegetable stock, adding olive oil if fat is allowed. Scoop cooked eggplant out of skin, chop into small pieces, then add with tomatoes to garlic and stir-fry for 5 minutes. Stir in remaining ingredients. Serve on no-fat/no-salt whole wheat bread, corn chips, or as a vegetable dip.

Yield: 5 cups or 10 servings; serving size ½ cup. ■ Each serving contains approximately: *With olive oil:* Calories: 24 (23% from fat); Protein: 1 gm; Fat: .6 gm; Carbohydrate: 5 gms; Cholesterol: 0; Sodium: 5 mgs; Allowances: 1 vegetable (fat is too insignificant to count). *Without olive oil:* Calories: 19 (7% from fat); Protein: 1 gm; Fat: .16 gm; Carbohydrate: 5 gms; Cholesterol: 0; Sodium: 5 mgs; Allowances: 1 vegetable (fat is too insignificant to count)

High-Five Hummus

2 15-ounce cans no-salt garbanzo beans
1 cup chopped onion
⅔ cup tomato purée
2–3 garlic cloves, minced

3 tablespoons fresh lemon juice
1 teaspoon ground cumin
$\frac{1}{8}$ teaspoon cayenne
$\frac{1}{4}$ teaspoon paprika
$\frac{1}{4}$ teaspoon freshly ground black pepper
$\frac{1}{2}$ chipotle pepper, reconstituted in $\frac{1}{4}$ cup heated wine and minced, or $\frac{1}{4}$ teaspoon chili powder
$\frac{1}{4}$ cup freshly minced cilantro, basil, Italian parsley, or mint, for garnish

Place all ingredients except garnish in a food processor, and blend until very smooth. Sprinkle garnish on top. Serve with no-fat/no-salt corn tortillas or chips.

Yield: $3\frac{1}{2}$ cups, or 7 servings; serving size $\frac{1}{2}$ cup. ■ Each serving contains approximately: Calories: 100 (9% from fat); Protein: 6 gms; Fat: 1 gm; Carbohydrate: 22 gms; Cholesterol: 0; Sodium: 15 mgs; Allowances: 1 starch + 1 vegetable

My Favorite Thistle, the Artichoke

Although artichokes have typically been cooked by immersing them in lots of boiling water, steaming them in just a little water will retain more of their nutrients and flavor. You can preserve even more nutrients—and reduce the cooking time further—by cooking them in a microwave oven.

4 artichokes
3 tablespoons fresh lemon juice

Wash artichokes, and cut off about $\frac{3}{4}$ inch from the top leaves. To prevent discoloration, dip the cut edges immediately in lemon juice. Cut the stem off at the base of the globe so that the artichoke will sit upright when served. Then trim off the hard prickly tips of the exposed whole leaves. The artichoke is then ready for your choice of cooking methods.

To *steam:* Put approximately 1 inch of water in a large pot. Add 2 tablespoons of fresh lemon juice, and stand artichokes upright in the water. Cover the pot, bring to a boil, then reduce heat to medium-low. After 25 minutes, test the artichokes for doneness by tugging a leaf gently. If it fails to pull free, cook 5 minutes more, then retest. When leaf comes off easily, remove the artichokes from the pot, and stand them upside down to drain.

To *microwave:* Wrap artichokes while still slightly moist from washing in heavy-duty plastic wrap. Place each one upside down in a glass custard cup, and microwave on high. Allow 4 to 7 minutes cooking time for one artichoke; add approximately 3 minutes for each additional artichoke. Halfway through the cooking time, rotate each one 180 degrees to ensure even cooking. Let the cooked artichokes remain wrapped for 5 minutes before serving them.

Yield: 4 servings. ■ Each serving contains approximately: Calories: 55 (4% from fat); Protein: 3 gms; Fat: .22 gm; Carbohydrate: 13 gms; Cholesterol: 0; Sodium: 79 mgs; Allowances: 2 vegetables

Yogurt and Pimiento Sauce for Artichokes

4 artichokes, trimmed, cooked, and chilled
$\frac{2}{3}$ cup plain nonfat yogurt

1 teaspoon no-salt prepared mustard
3 ounces Marinated Roasted Peppers, finely chopped (see page 270)
2 teaspoons skim milk
1 teaspoon extra virgin olive oil
1 garlic clove, finely minced
1 teaspoon fresh lemon juice

Prepare artichokes as described in *My Favorite Thistle, the Artichoke,* on page 246.

In a bowl blend the yogurt and mustard together with a whisk. Then whisk in the remaining ingredients. Refrigerate for 1 hour or more. Serve artichokes on a plate with the sauce in a small bowl on the side.

Yield: 4 servings. ■ Each serving contains approximately: Calories: 84 (13% from fat); Protein: 5 gms; Fat: 1.2 gms; Carbohydrate: 13 gms; Cholesterol: 2 mgs; Sodium: 62 mgs; Allowances: 2 vegetables + $\frac{1}{8}$ dairy + $\frac{1}{4}$ fat

Shrimp-Spiraled Artichokes

4 small to medium artichokes
1 lemon, quartered
$1\frac{1}{2}$ cups water
$\frac{1}{2}$ pound medium shrimp, unpeeled
8 ounces plain nonfat yogurt
2 tablespoons minced fresh dill
2 tablespoons no-fat/no-salt Dijon mustard
$\frac{1}{2}$ teaspoon grated lemon rind
1 teaspoon freshly ground horseradish or full-strength no-fat/no-salt prepared horseradish
$\frac{1}{8}$ teaspoon freshly ground black pepper
$\frac{1}{8}$ teaspoon molasses, or to taste

Prepare artichokes, as described in *My Favorite Thistle, the Artichoke,* on page 246. When artichoke is cool, gently spread the leaves apart and scoop out the fuzzy thistle center. Discard the splintery center, and place the artichokes in the refrigerator to chill.

In a saucepan, boil $1\frac{1}{2}$ cups of water, then add the shrimp. Reduce heat and cook for $2\frac{1}{2}$ minutes. Drain, rinse with cold water, and chill. Peel and de-vein the shrimp when cool.

Combine yogurt with remaining ingredients in a bowl, and stir well. Spoon approximately $\frac{1}{4}$ cup of yogurt mixture into each artichoke center. Distribute the shrimp evenly among the artichokes, hanging the shrimp along the outside edge of the artichoke tops. Garnish with additional dill.

Yield: 4 servings. ■ Each stuffed artichoke contains approximately: Calories: 127 (11% from fat); Protein: 16 gms; Fat: .2 gm; Carbohydrate: 16 gms; Cholesterol: 84 mgs; Sodium: 157 mgs; Allowances: 1 vegetable + $1\frac{1}{2}$ proteins + $\frac{1}{4}$ dairy

Yogurt Cheese

The uses of yogurt cheese are endless! Try it anywhere you previously might have used diet mayonnaise, cream cheese, or sour cream such as on baked potatoes or bean burritos, in tuna or salmon salads. One of my favorite ways to use it is to add a few tablespoons of sugar-free jelly and use it instead of cream cheese on bagels. If you cook with yogurt cheese, add about 1 tablespoon of cornstarch to 1 cup of yogurt cheese to prevent it from separating.

4 cups plain nonfat yogurt (use a brand that does not contain gelatin or carrageenan)

Line a funnel or colander with a large paper coffee filter or at least three layers of cheesecloth and place it in a large bowl or pan. Spoon yogurt into the filter. Cover and refrigerate for 8 to 14 hours—the longer it is allowed to drip, the thicker the product will be. Discard the whey that drips into the bowl, and transfer the yogurt cheese from the filter to a covered container.

Yield: approximately $1\frac{1}{4}$ cups, or 10 servings; serving size 2 tablespoons. ■ Each serving contains approximately: Calories: 29 (2% from fat); Protein: 4 gms; Fat: .08 gm; Carbohydrate: 2 gms; Cholesterol: 2 mgs; Sodium: 25 mgs; Allowances: $\frac{1}{3}$ dairy

Yogurt Cheese Fruit Dip

Taking this dip with you to pot lucks or parties will enhance your appetizer choices!

$\frac{3}{4}$ cup *Yogurt Cheese* (see page 247)
2 bananas
1 tablespoon currants or raisins
2 tablespoons chopped apricot
2 tablespoons chopped prune
$\frac{1}{8}$ teaspoon cinnamon
Dash of vanilla extract

Blend *Yogurt Cheese* and bananas until smooth. Add remaining ingredients and enjoy as a dip for fruit or nonfat crackers.

Yield: 2 cups, or 8 servings; serving size $\frac{1}{4}$ cup. ■ Each serving contains approximately: Calories: 60 (4% from fat); Protein: 3 gms; Fat: .24 gm; Carbohydrate: 12 gms; Cholesterol: 1.5 mgs; Sodium: 19 mgs; Allowances: $\frac{1}{2}$ fruit $+$ $\frac{1}{3}$ dairy

Yogurt Cheese Veggie Dip

$\frac{3}{4}$ cup *Yogurt Cheese* (see page 247)
2 tablespoons chopped green onion
2 tablespoons grated carrot
2 tablespoons sliced radish
$\frac{1}{4}$ cup diced tomato
1 teaspoon no-salt prepared mustard
1 tablespoon fresh lime juice
$\frac{1}{2}$ teaspoon honey
2 teaspoons freshly chopped cilantro
$\frac{1}{4}$ cup $\frac{1}{2}$% dry curd cottage cheese
2 teaspoons orange juice

Combine all ingredients and enjoy as a dip for vegetables or crackers.

Yield: $1\frac{1}{4}$ cups, or 5 servings; serving size $\frac{1}{4}$ cup. ■ Each serving contains approximately: Calories: 51 (4% from fat); Protein: 7 gms; Fat: .2 gm; Carbohydrate: 5 gms; Cholesterol: 3 mgs; Sodium: 37 mgs; Allowances: $\frac{1}{2}$ vegetable $+$ $\frac{2}{5}$ dairy

Soups

Basic Veggie Stock

10–20 cups of vegetable scraps that you have saved in a plastic bag in the freezer. A good blend could include:

Skins, peelings, and/or ends from potatoes, onions, carrots, celery, tomatoes, and garlic

Stems from asparagus, greens, lettuce, mushrooms, parsley, etc.

Bay leaf, freshly ground black pepper, or fresh herbs—as desired

Water to cover

Note: Some people prefer to avoid the stronger-flavored vegetables of the cabbage family, such as broccoli, cauliflower, turnips, rutabagas, and kohlrabi. Vegetables with bleeding colors (such as beets, red cabbage, and greens) should not be added if stock could be used in a lighter-colored soup. Take care not to use much green pepper and eggplant as these can make the stock bitter. And remember not to add lots of tomatoes or other acidic vegetables if the stock will be used with dairy products that could curdle.

If you have not been saving vegetable scraps, add 2 gallons of water to:

4 large unpeeled potatoes, quartered
4 large carrots, peeled and thickly sliced
2 celery stalks, chopped
2 large onions, peeled, quartered, and sliced
1½ cups fresh corn kernels (3 ears)
1 pound mushroom stems, trimmed
1 apple, seeded and quartered
1 pear, seeded and quartered

5 heads of garlic, cut in half horizontally
6 bay leaves
25 peppercorns
1 teaspoon each chopped fresh basil, thyme, tarragon, oregano, parsley, and chives

Place all ingredients in a large pot and simmer for 1 to 2 hours. Pour through a colander or sieve and discard vegetable solids. The stock can be frozen in quart containers for future use as soup stock or frozen in ice cube trays for smaller needs such as stir-frying (using 1 or 2 cubes rather than oil).

The nutritional analysis is negligible for calories and fat. Sodium could be excessive if many high-sodium vegetables such as green leafy vegetables and tomatoes, are used. Generally speaking, kidney and hypertensive patients are the only ones who should be concerned with limiting their consumption of naturally occurring sodium.

My Favorite Lentil Soup

This delicious, hearty soup is a meal in itself, great accompanied by *Pane Paesano,* page 240, and a fresh salad.

3 cups raw lentils
12 cups water or *Basic Veggie Stock* (see this page)
10–15 garlic cloves, minced
2 large onions, chopped
2 large carrots, chopped
1 large bunch spinach, chopped

1 large bunch red chard, chopped
1 large bunch beet greens, chopped
4 tablespoons dry red wine
Juice of 1 large lemon
6 ounces no-salt tomato juice
2 12-ounce cans no-salt plum tomatoes, chopped
2 tablespoons blackstrap molasses
2 tablespoons wine vinegar
Freshly ground black pepper to taste
Chopped fresh herbs (such as thyme, oregano, or basil) to taste

Start boiling stock and add lentils. While lentils are cooking, sauté garlic, onion, carrots, and greens in the wine, lemon juice, and tomato juice. When vegetables are cooked al dente, add to lentils (which should be fairly well done).

Although this soup can be thrown together in less than 30 minutes, it is best if the soup is allowed to simmer for 2 to 3 hours. About 30 minutes before serving, add the tomatoes, molasses, vinegar, pepper, and fresh herbs.

Yield: 17 servings; serving size 1 cup ■
Each serving contains approximately: Calories: 145 (6% from fat); Protein: 9 gms; Fat: 1 gm; Carbohydrate: 28 gms; Cholesterol: 0; Sodium: 78 mgs; Allowances: $1\frac{2}{3}$ starches + 1 vegetable

The Ultimate Vegetable Soup

I usually double this recipe on cold, rainy, or snowy days. It is fun to give a quart to a friend in need!

3 large carrots, sliced
3 large onions, chopped
2 large red potatoes, chopped (do not peel)

$\frac{1}{2}$ head cauliflower, chopped
2 stalks broccoli, chopped
$\frac{1}{2}$ yellow pepper, chopped
$\frac{1}{2}$ sweet red pepper, chopped
$\frac{1}{4}$ head cabbage, chopped
5 ounces frozen lima beans
8 ounces frozen corn
5 ounces frozen peas
$2\frac{1}{4}$ cups green beans, de-stemmed, de-veined, and snapped
14 ounces no-salt crushed tomatoes
1 12-ounce can no-salt tomatoes or 6 fresh tomatoes
5 ounces spinach ($\frac{1}{2}$ bag)
8 cups *Basic Veggie Stock* (see page 249)

Combine all ingredients and simmer for 30 to 60 minutes, depending upon how tender you like your vegetables.

Yield: 14 servings; serving size 1 cup ■
Each serving contains approximately: Calories: 100 (5% from fat); Protein: 5 gms; Fat: .6 gm; Carbohydrate: 20 gms; Cholesterol: 0; Sodium: 26 mgs; Allowances: $\frac{1}{2}$ starch + $\frac{8}{9}$ vegetable

Borscht Beautiful

This is the best borscht I have ever had. I truthfully did not think I liked borscht before trying this recipe! It is wonderful with a dollop of nonfat yogurt on top and with *Basic Whole Wheat Bread,* page 239.

2 teaspoons olive oil
2 garlic cloves, minced
1 medium onion, chopped
2 tablespoons whole wheat flour
5 cups *Basic Veggie Stock* (see page 249)
1 bunch of beets with greens, chopped (approximately 3 large or 6 small)
1 large carrot, chopped

1 large red potato, chopped
1 large stalk celery, chopped
$\frac{1}{2}$ head small to medium cabbage, shredded
4 canned plum tomatoes, chopped (no salt, if canned)
1 teaspoon honey
1 bay leaf
$\frac{1}{4}$ teaspoon freshly ground black pepper

Heat olive oil and sauté garlic and onion. When almost opaque, stir in flour and cook for about a minute. Add *Basic Veggie Stock,* as needed, to prevent scorching. Then add the remaining stock and bring to a boil.

Wash all vegetables carefully with a bristled brush, trimming off rough ends but saving the beet leaves. Chop beets, carrot, potato, and celery fairly thin; add to soup base. These can simmer as you shred the cabbage and chop the tomatoes and beet leaves into small pieces. Add these with the remaining ingredients to the stock and simmer until all vegetables reach desired tenderness. Some people prefer this soup puréed, while some like it very chunky. I really like it best with about half of the soup blenderized or food processed, and the other half of it "as is." That way the stock is very rich and flavorful, and there is also some good texture for contrast.

Yield: 11 servings; serving size 1 cup ■
Each serving contains approximately: Calories: 47 (18% from fat); Protein: 15 gms; Fat: less than 1 gm; Carbohydrate: 8 gms; Cholesterol: 0; Sodium: 16 mgs; Allowances: $\frac{1}{4}$ starch + $\frac{3}{4}$ vegetable + $\frac{1}{5}$ fat

Dutch Split Pea Soup

This hearty soup freezes beautifully.

1 tablespoon olive oil
2 garlic cloves, minced
2 large leeks, finely chopped
1 sweet Spanish onion, finely chopped
1 cup finely chopped celery
1$\frac{1}{2}$ cups chopped bell pepper
2 cups chopped carrots
$\frac{1}{2}$ teaspoon thyme
2 cups dried green split peas
7 cups *Basic Veggie Stock* (see page 249)
1 bay leaf
2 tablespoons chopped fresh parsley
2 large potatoes, cubed
Freshly ground pepper to taste

Heat olive oil, and sauté the garlic, leeks, onion, celery, bell pepper, carrots, and thyme until the onions are translucent. Stir in the peas until they are well mixed with the other vegetables.

Add the stock and bay leaf, stirring well. Bring to a boil, then reduce heat. Cover and simmer for 30 minutes.

Add the parsley, potatoes, and pepper. Simmer for another 30 to 35 minutes until the potatoes and peas are tender.

Yield: 22 servings; serving size $\frac{1}{2}$ cup ■
Each serving contains approximately: Calories: 77 (10% from fat); Protein: 4 gms; Fat: .9 gm; Carbohydrate: 15 gms; Cholesterol: 0; Sodium: 22 mgs; Allowances: $\frac{5}{6}$ starch + $\frac{1}{3}$ vegetable + $\frac{1}{10}$ fat

Adesse Hamod (Sour Lentil Soup)
by Farida Gindi

This is absolutely delicious served with whole grain bread, roasted peppers, and a fresh salad.

6 cups water or *Basic Veggie Stock* (see page 249)
2 cups red lentils
2 tablespoons coriander, freshly ground from seeds (or 1 tablespoon dried coriander)
2 teaspoons olive oil
6 large garlic cloves, minced
5 tablespoons fresh lemon juice
Pinch of crushed red pepper
1 teaspoon cumin seeds, freshly ground (or $\frac{1}{2}$ teaspoon dried cumin)

Rinse lentils and then boil in 6 cups of water or stock. Simmer uncovered for 15 to 20 minutes, until tender. If using fresh whole coriander seeds, bake the seeds for about 10 minutes at 300 degrees, or until they turn pink. Grind coriander seeds with mortar and pestle and then sauté in olive oil with garlic, lemon juice, and red pepper. Grind cumin seeds and add to lentils with sautéed mixture. Purée the soup in a food processor or blender.

Yield: 6 servings; serving size 1 cup ■
Each serving contains approximately:
Calories: 175 (11% from fat); Protein: 12 gms; Fat: 2.2 gms; Carbohydrate: 29 gms; Cholesterol: 0; Sodium: 4 mgs; Allowances: 2 starches + $\frac{1}{3}$ fat

Roasted Eggplant and Pimiento Soup

Roasting the eggplant and pimiento (sweet red peppers) lends a wonderful smoky flavor to this unique soup.

1 cup dried baby lima beans
6 cups *Basic Veggie Stock* (see page 249)
2 sweet red peppers
2 medium eggplants
2 large leeks
2 teaspoons olive oil
1 teaspoon vinegar or fresh lemon juice
Dash of ground allspice
Minced fresh cilantro or basil (for garnish)

Rinse the lima beans, cover with a generous amount of water, and soak overnight. Drain the beans, and place beans and stock in a large saucepan. Bring to a boil, then reduce heat. Cover and simmer for 30 minutes.

Turn oven on broil. Perforate the skin of the eggplants with a few fork pricks. While beans are cooking, place the eggplants and red peppers on a rack set in a broiling pan 3 to 4 inches from the broiler. Broil the vegetables 15 to 20 minutes, turning them every 5 minutes, until their skin is thoroughly charred.

When the peppers are sufficiently charred, their skin will bubble and they will have softened. Remove them from oven, and put them in a paper bag for 10 minutes to sweat. This will make it easier to remove the skin from the fleshy part. You save much flavor by using a damp paper towel to remove the charred skin (rather than removing skin under running water, as many recipes suggest). Remove and discard the seeds and stems.

While waiting for the peppers to sweat, cut the eggplants in half and scoop out the pulp into a medium bowl. Coarsely chop the eggplants, dice the peppers, and set aside.

Cut the leeks in half length-wise, and trim off the tougher green tops (discarding about ½ of the dark green tops). Spread the leek open under running water to remove all dirt hidden within the leaves. Chop the leeks finely, then sauté in olive oil until slightly browned.

Add leeks, eggplants, and peppers to the partially cooked beans. Return to a boil and then reduce heat. Cover and simmer for about an hour longer, or until the beans are tender.

Stir in the vinegar or lemon juice and allspice. Add more water or stock to make 11 cups of soup. Serve garnished with the minced cilantro.

Yield: 11 servings; serving size 1 cup ■ Each serving contains approximately: Calories: 49 (16% from fat); Fat: .8 gm; Carbohydrate: 8 gms; Cholesterol: 0; Sodium: 6 mgs; Allowances: ⅓ starch + ½ vegetable + ½ fat

Barley Soup at Its Best

10 cups *Basic Veggie Stock* (see page 249)
1¼ cups pearled barley
1½ teaspoons olive oil
6 large garlic cloves, minced
1 large onion, chopped
3 stalks celery, chopped
5 cups sliced mushrooms (1 pound of portobello and shittake mushrooms)
2 cups shredded carrots
3 tablespoons dried basil
1 teaspoon freshly ground black pepper, or to taste
¼ cup balsamic vinegar

Start stock boiling before washing and preparing the vegetables. Add barley to boiling stock. Heat oil and sauté garlic and onions for 2 to 3 minutes. Then add celery, mushrooms, carrots, basil, pepper, and vinegar and cook another few minutes.

After barley has cooked 40 minutes or so, add sautéed vegetables and simmer another 25 minutes.

Yield: 13 servings; serving size 1 cup ■ Each serving contains approximately: Calories: 101 (5% from fat); Protein: 3 gms; Fat: 1 gm; Carbohydrate: 21 gms; Cholesterol: 0; Sodium: 17 mgs; Allowances: ⅘ starch + 1 vegetable + ⅛ fat

Escarole Bean Stew

3 pounds fresh escarole (3 large heads)
2 cups *Basic Veggie Stock* (see page 249), or water
1 head garlic, or 8 large cloves, minced
2 15-ounce cans no-salt navy beans (or Cannelini beans, if you care to cook them)
½ teaspoon freshly ground black pepper, or more to taste
¼ teaspoon crushed red pepper, or more to taste
Juice of 1 lemon, or more to taste

Wash and drain escarole. Chop escarole leaves in 2-inch pieces, lengthwise. Boil stock or water in a 6-quart pot. When liquid has come to a boil, add escarole. Cook approximately 45 minutes or until al dente.

Heat the juice from the canned beans in a 2-quart pot, and sauté the garlic for 1 to 2 minutes on medium. Add beans and pepper, and bring to a boil. Add heated beans and lemon juice to escarole. Stir well and heat thoroughly.

Yield: 9 servings; serving size 1 cup ■
Each serving contains approximately: Calories: 62 (3% from fat); Protein: 7 gms; Fat: .18 gm; Carbohydrate: 16 gms; Cholesterol: 0; Sodium: 34 mgs; Allowances: $\frac{1}{2}$ starch + 1 vegetable

Bean Barley Soup

1 cup pinto beans
1 cup small white beans
8 cups *Basic Veggie Stock* (see page 249)
$\frac{1}{2}$ cup red or white wine
1 large red onion, chopped
1 bell pepper, chopped
1 cup chopped carrots
$\frac{1}{4}$ cup chopped fresh parsley
1 dried red chili or 1–2 dried and reconstituted chipotle peppers, minced
$\frac{1}{4}$ cup split peas, yellow or green
$\frac{1}{4}$ cup lentils
$\frac{1}{2}$ cup pearled barley
2 teaspoons no-salt prepared mustard
Juice of $\frac{1}{2}$ lime
1 teaspoon molasses
1 teaspoon balsamic vinegar

Soak pinto and white beans overnight in water, rinsing a few times to reduce gaseous compounds. Drain well. Then cover beans with stock and cook for 30 minutes. Wash and chop the vegetables, then sauté in the wine with parsley and minced chili for 10 minutes. After beans have cooked for 30 minutes, add the split peas, lentils, and barley and simmer for another 30 minutes. Then add the sautéed vegetables, mustard, lime juice, molasses, and vinegar for the last 5 minutes of cooking.

Yield: 12 servings; serving size 1 cup ■
Each serving contains approximately: Calories: 92 (2% from fat); Protein: 5 gms; Fat: .2 gm; Carbohydrate: 20 gms; Cholesterol: 0; Sodium: 38 mgs; Allowances: 1 starch + $\frac{1}{2}$ vegetable

Maria's Great Northern Bean Soup
by Maria Zagorianos

1 pound Great Northern beans
2 medium onions, chopped
$\frac{1}{2}$ head garlic, minced
2 stalks celery, sliced
2 carrots, sliced
2 tablespoons minced fresh dill
1$\frac{1}{2}$ teaspoons freshly ground black pepper
1 16-ounce can no-salt tomatoes, chopped
1 6-ounce can no-salt tomato paste
1 tablespoon extra virgin olive oil
Juice of 1 lemon

Boil the Great Northern beans for approximately 30 minutes, drain, and place in a pot with $\frac{1}{2}$ gallon of cold water. Add remaining ingredients except lemon juice, and cook until tender, probably another 45 to 60 minutes. Top with the lemon juice as desired.

Yield: 17 servings; serving size 1 cup ■
Each serving contains approximately: Calories: 106 (11% from fat); Protein: 6 gms; Fat: 1.3 gms; Carbohydrate: 19 gms; Cholesterol: 0; Sodium: 20 mgs; Allowances: 1 starch + $\frac{3}{4}$ vegetable + $\frac{1}{6}$ fat

Fresh Fruit Soup

6 tablespoons instant tapioca
5 cups water
1 12-ounce can frozen unsweetened fruit
  juice
6 cups mixed fresh fruit (pineapple,
  mango, bananas, blueberries, seedless
  green grapes, etc.)
2 tablespoons chopped fresh spearmint

Combine tapioca and 2 cups of the water.
Bring to a boil, then simmer for 3 to 4 minutes, stirring periodically. Add fruit juice
and blend well. Add remaining 3 cups water. Pour into an airtight container and refrigerate until thoroughly chilled. Cut the
fruit into bite-size pieces and add to the
chilled soup.

Serve in well-chilled mugs or bowls and
garnish with fresh spearmint.

Yield: 8 servings; serving size $6\frac{3}{4}$ ounces
of soup with $\frac{3}{4}$ cup of fruit ■ Each serving
contains approximately:
Calories: 170 (4% from fat); Protein:
2 gms; Fat: .7 gm; Carbohydrate:
41 gms; Cholesterol: 0; Sodium: 9 mgs;
Allowances: $2\frac{4}{5}$ fruits

Salads, Dressings, Condiments, and Sauces

My Favorite Vegetable Salad

Besides being a delicious start to any
meal, salad is the smartest weight loss or
maintenance strategy I know. You can enjoy a lot of chewing satisfaction for very few
calories and then feel satisfied with smaller
servings of the higher calorie dishes that
follow.

16 cherry tomatoes
1 cup romaine lettuce, torn
1 cup leaf lettuce, torn
1 cup arugula, torn
1 cup radicchio, torn
1 cup Belgian endive, torn
1 large carrot, julienned
$\frac{1}{2}$ cup sliced mushrooms
$\frac{1}{2}$ large red bell pepper, sliced
$\frac{1}{2}$ large yellow pepper, sliced

Wash and prep all ingredients and toss.
Top with *Dijon Yogurt Vinaigrette* on page
262.

Yield: 4 very generous servings. Leftovers
can be enjoyed the next day if stored
without dressing in an airtight container. ■
Each serving contains approximately: Calories: 48 (9% from fat); Protein:
3 gms; Fat: .5 gm; Carbohydrate: 10 gms;
Cholesterol: 0; Sodium: 24 mgs; Allowances: 2 vegetables

An Italian Finale Salad

In Italy, salad is usually eaten after the
main course, and radicchio and arugula are
as common there as iceberg lettuce is in the
United States. My family enjoys this salad as
a first course. Consuming a large vegetable
serving at the beginning of the meal helps
reduce your caloric intake. But if you prefer
to go Italian and eat it last, what a way to
cleanse the palate!

2 tablespoons balsamic vinegar
1 tablespoon extra virgin olive oil, optional
1 tablespoon no-fat/no-salt Dijon mustard
Freshly ground black pepper to taste
3 cups Boston or Bibb lettuce, washed, dried, and torn
3 cups arugula, washed, dried, and torn
1 head radicchio, washed, dried, and thinly sliced into julienne strips
1 fennel bulb

Whisk together the vinegar, oil, mustard, and pepper. The dressing can be made ahead and stored for 3 days if necessary.

Wash and prep the leafy vegetables. Trim off the tough outer layer of the fennel bulb. To prevent stringy pieces, it is best to peel the outer surface with a vegetable peeler, then core out the tough base. Then cut the bulb in half lengthwise, and slice it thinly. Soak the fennel in a bowl of cold water for 10 minutes. Drain fennel and toss with radicchio. Toss other leafy vegetables, then top with fennel, radicchio, and dressing.

Yield: 6 servings ■ Each serving contains approximately: Calories: 35 (62% from fat, 9% if olive oil is omitted); Protein: 1 gm; Fat: 2.4 gms; Carbohydrate: 2 gms; Cholesterol: 0; Sodium: 4 mgs; Allowances: $\frac{1}{2}$ vegetable + $\frac{1}{2}$ fat (insignificant fat if olive oil is omitted)

Grecian Potato Salad

5-6 medium potatoes, boiled and cut into bite-size pieces
4 scallions, chopped
$\frac{1}{2}$ red pepper, chopped
$\frac{1}{2}$ green pepper, chopped

1 carrot, grated
1 cup finely shredded red cabbage, optional

Dressing:
1 tablespoon extra virgin olive oil
1 tablespoon fresh lemon juice
2 tablespoons red wine vinegar
2 tablespoons minced fresh parsley
$\frac{1}{4}$ cup plain nonfat yogurt
Freshly ground black pepper to taste

Combine all the vegetables in a large salad bowl. Combine the dressing ingredients in a separate bowl, mixing well. Pour over the salad and toss together gently.

Yield: 16 servings; serving size $\frac{1}{2}$ cup ■ Each serving contains approximately: Calories: 55 (15% from fat); Protein: 1 gm; Fat: .9 gm; Carbohydrate: 11 gms; Cholesterol: trace; Sodium: 5 mgs; Allowances: $\frac{1}{2}$ starch + $\frac{1}{4}$ vegetable + $\frac{1}{5}$ fat

Tabbouleh

Enjoy this quick and easy cold salad with a cold bean salad or dip and a slice of nice crusty, whole-grain bread.

$2\frac{3}{4}$ cups water
$1\frac{1}{2}$ cups bulgur wheat
3 tomatoes, chopped
1 medium red onion, diced
2 large garlic cloves, minced
3 tablespoons minced fresh parsley
6 tablespoons minced fresh mint
5 tablespoons fresh lemon juice
Freshly ground black pepper, to taste
2 teaspoons extra virgin olive oil, optional

Bring the water to a boil, add the bulgur, and stir. Remove from heat, cover with an airtight lid and let stand for 1 to 2 hours before opening. Drain off any excess water and toss the bulgur with remaining ingredients.

Yield: 9 servings; serving size 1 cup ■ Each serving contains approximately: *With olive oil:* Calories: 102 (13% from fat); Protein: 3 gms; Fat: 1.5 gms; Carbohydrates: 20 gms; Cholesterol: 0; Sodium: 6 mgs; Allowances: 1 starch + $\frac{1}{2}$ vegetable + $\frac{1}{2}$ fat. *Without olive oil:* Calories: 93 (4% from fat); Protein: 3 gms; Fat: .5 gm; Carbohydrate: 20 gms; Cholesterol: 0; Sodium: 6 mgs; Allowances: 1 starch + $\frac{1}{2}$ vegetable

Broccoli Salad

1 large bunch broccoli (2 large stalks)
1 small onion, chopped
2 medium tomatoes, chopped
Juice of 1 lemon
$\frac{1}{4}$ cup plain nonfat yogurt
2 tablespoons no-salt mustard

Steam broccoli for 5 to 10 minutes or until al dente, slightly crisp. Prepare and mix the remaining ingredients. When broccoli has cooled somewhat, cut the stalk into thin slices and the flowerets into small bite-size pieces. Toss with the other ingredients, and refrigerate until cool.

Yield: 7 servings; serving size 1 cup ■ Each serving contains approximately: Calories: 48 (9% from fat); Protein: 4 gms; Fat: .5 gm; Carbohydrate: 6 gms; Cholesterol: 0; Sodium: 18 mgs; Allowances: 2 vegetables

Brown Rice and Mixed Fruit Salad with Jalapeño Cilantro Dressing

Dressing:
$\frac{3}{4}$ cup plain nonfat yogurt
1 tablespoon chopped fresh cilantro
2 teaspoons chopped fresh jalapeño

1 cup uncooked brown basmati rice
1 medium mango, peeled and diced
1 cup blueberries
1 cup strawberries, hulled and cut into $\frac{1}{2}$-inch pieces
1 medium banana, sliced
$\frac{1}{4}$ cup minced onion
2 tablespoons chopped fresh parsley
1 tablespoon extra virgin olive oil
3 tablespoons fresh lime juice
4 springs fresh cilantro

Combine the dressing ingredients and set aside. Steam or boil rice for 45 minutes, or until tender, and set aside, uncovered, to cool. Combine the remaining ingredients, except cilantro. When rice is cool, mix with fruit mixture.

Place fruit/rice salad on plates and top with dressing and cilantro sprig.

Yield: 4 servings. ■ Each serving contains approximately: *With dressing:* Calories: 272 (16% from fat); Protein: 6 gms; Fat: 4.7 gms; Carbohydrate: 54 gms; Cholesterol: 1 mg; Sodium: 39 mgs; Allowances: 1$\frac{1}{2}$ starches + $\frac{1}{5}$ vegetable + 2 fruits + $\frac{1}{4}$ dairy. *Without dressing:* Calories: 244 (17% from fat); Protein: 4 gms; Fat: 4.6 gms; Carbohydrate: 50 gms; Cholesterol: 0; Sodium: 5 mgs; Allowances: 1$\frac{1}{2}$ starches + $\frac{1}{5}$ vegetable + 2 fruits

Orange-Blueberry-Arugula Salad with Tarragon Sauce

8 oranges
1 teaspoon honey
2½ teaspoons no-fat/no-salt Dijon mustard
¼ teaspoon freshly ground black pepper
2½ teaspoons arrowroot dissolved in ¼ cup cold water
2 teaspoons finely chopped fresh tarragon
2 cups blueberries, de-stemmed, washed, and dried
1 pound arugula, de-stemmed, washed, and dried
1 head of Belgian endive
4 radicchio leaves, torn in half
1 kiwi fruit, peeled and sliced widthwise

Squeeze two of the oranges and pour juice into a small saucepan; add honey, mustard, and ground pepper. Bring to a boil over high heat, then whisk in the dissolved arrowroot. Stir just until thickened. Transfer to a small container and place in the freezer until cool. Remove and stir in the tarragon until well blended.

Peel the remaining oranges with a sharp knife, taking care to remove all of the white pith. Carefully slice segments to avoid including any tough fibrous membranes. Combine blueberries with oranges and place on a bed of arugula. Then line the sides of the serving bowl with the alternating colors of Belgian endive and radicchio, and top with artfully placed kiwi slices and tarragon sauce.

Yield: 6 servings; serving size 1 cup ■
Each serving contains approximately: Calories: 104 (4% from fat); Protein: 2 gms; Fat: 3.7 gms; Carbohydrate: 25 gms; Cholesterol: 0; Sodium: 10 mgs; Allowances: ½ vegetable + 1½ fruits

Delicious-Jicama-Chayote Salad

1 Red Delicious apple, cored and julienned
1 small jicama, peeled and julienned
1 chayote, peeled, cored, and julienned
1 mango, peeled and chopped
Juice of 1 lemon or 1½ limes
1 teaspoon toasted sesame oil, optional
1 tablespoon raspberry vinegar
Freshly ground black pepper to taste
2–3 tablespoons chopped fresh spearmint

Combine the ingredients in a large bowl and mix thoroughly. Chill in refrigerator overnight if possible, but it is also delicious if eaten *immediato!*

Yield: 6 servings, serving size 1 cup ■
Each serving contains approximately:
With oil: Calories: 67 (15% from fat); Protein: 1 gm; Fat: 1.1 gms; Carbohydrate: 15 gms; Cholesterol: 0; Sodium: 3 mgs; Allowances: ⅓ starch + ⅙ vegetable + ⅔ fruit + ⅙ fat. *Without oil:* Calories: 60 (6% from fat); Protein: 1 gm; Fat: .4 gm; Carbohydrate: 15 gms; Cholesterol: 0; Sodium: 3 mgs; Allowances: ⅓ starch + ⅙ vegetable + ⅔ fruit

Quinoa Pepper Salad

This dish would be nice served with a cold bean salad or dip.

1½ cups quinoa
3½ cups water

$\frac{1}{2}$ cup currants or raisins
4 tablespoons fresh lime or lemon juice
1 tablespoon orange juice, optional
1 cup chopped orange bell peppers
1 cup chopped yellow bell peppers
$\frac{1}{2}$ cup chopped scallions
$\frac{1}{2}$ cup minced fresh cilantro or parsley
1 tomato, diced
$\frac{3}{4}$ teaspoon freshly ground black pepper or gourmet blend of red, green, and black peppercorns)

Rinse quinoa until water runs clear. Bring $3\frac{1}{2}$ cups of water to a boil. Pour $\frac{1}{2}$ cup boiling water over currants or raisins and set aside for 15 minutes. Add rinsed quinoa to remaining boiling water and simmer, covered, for 15 minutes, then remove from heat and let sit for 5 minutes. Fluff up with a fork, then stir in the raisins and other remaining ingredients. Serve on a bed of lettuce as a light lunch or dinner.

Yield: 13 servings; serving size $\frac{1}{2}$ cup ■
Each serving contains approximately: Calories: 73 (10% from fat); Protein: 3 gms; Fat: .84 gm; Carbohydrate: 15 gms; Cholesterol: 0; Sodium: 4 mgs; Allowances: $\frac{2}{3}$ starch + $\frac{1}{4}$ vegetable + $\frac{1}{4}$ fruit

Fastest Slaw in the West

For *really* fast slaw you can substitute three 16-ounce packages of ready-to-use coleslaw blended vegetables for the first four ingredients.

$\frac{1}{2}$ green cabbage, chopped
$\frac{1}{4}$ red cabbage, sliced
1 carrot, shredded
1 sweet red pepper, diced
1 10-ounce package frozen corn
3 tablespoons honey

$\frac{3}{4}$ cup apple cider vinegar
1 tablespoon sesame oil, optional
2 teaspoons ground cumin
$\frac{1}{2}$ chipotle pepper

As you are preparing the vegetables, cook the frozen corn as directed on package. Combine honey, vinegar, oil, and cumin, and blend well. In a bowl, pour boiling water over dried chipotle pepper and let stand for 15 minutes; discard water and mince pepper finely.

Combine all of the ingredients and refrigerate overnight, if possible. Enjoy with *Bayou Baked Bourbon Beans,* page 286, and *Basic Whole Wheat Bread,* page 239—*salud!*

Yield: 27 servings; serving size $\frac{1}{2}$ cup ■
Each serving contains approximately:
With oil: Calories: 32 (20% from fat); Protein: .7 gm; Fat: .7 gm; Carbohydrate: 7 gms; Cholesterol: 0; Sodium: 7 mgs; Allowances: 1 vegetable + $\frac{1}{9}$ fat. *Without oil:* Calories: 28 (7% from fat); Protein: .7 gm; Fat: .2 gm; Carbohydrate: 7 gms; Cholesterol: 0; Sodium: 7 mgs; Allowances: 1 vegetable

Black Bean Fettuccine Salad

12 ounces spinach fettuccine
1 tablespoon extra virgin olive oil
3 cups cooked black beans or canned no-salt black beans
3 garlic cloves, finely minced
1 small red onion, chopped
2 bell peppers, chopped
$\frac{1}{2}$ cup grated carrot
2 teaspoons ground cumin
Juice of 4 limes

1 tablespoon grated lime or orange rind,
   optional
4 small ripe tomatoes, chopped

Cook spinach fettuccine according to
package directions. Drain and toss with olive oil. Cool. Combine the beans, fettuccine, and remaining ingredients except
for tomatoes. Add tomatoes just before
serving. Toss gently and serve.

Yield: $11\frac{1}{2}$ servings; serving size 1 cup ■
Each serving contains: Calories: 170 (8%
from fat); Protein: 7 gms; Fat: 1.6 gms;
Carbohydrate: 33 gms; Cholesterol: 0; Sodium: 11 mgs; Allowances: 2 starches + $\frac{1}{2}$
vegetable

Rosati's Insalata alla Contadina
by Dr. Robert Rosati

Although this is a labor-intensive salad,
it makes a lot, and it gets better by the day.
You may choose to add the tomatoes just
before serving if you plan to keep it for
more than a few days.

1 pound new potatoes
1 pound string beans, cleaned and
   snapped
3 cups *Basic Black-Eyed Peas* (see page
   286)
3 tomatoes, sliced
1 onion, sliced and separated into rings
1 cup fresh lemon juice
2 tablespoons chopped fresh basil
2–3 garlic cloves, finely minced, optional,
   or use to taste
1 teaspoon dry mustard
1 teaspoon extra virgin olive oil, optional

Start steaming the whole new potatoes
while preparing string beans. Depending
upon the size of the potatoes, add string
beans to steam pot about 15 minutes
later, so that they will be done at approximately the same time. (If you don't have
a multiple-tiered steamer that allows vegetables to be easily removed at different
times, you may choose to steam them
separately.) When the vegetables are
done, but not overcooked, remove them
from the steamer. Slice potatoes into $\frac{1}{8}$- to
$\frac{1}{4}$-inch slices or chunks if preferred. Mix
the potatoes, beans, black-eyed peas, tomatoes, and onion together in a large
bowl. Then blend the remaining ingredients for the vinaigrette dressing, pour
over the salad, and toss.

Yield: 9 servings; serving size $1\frac{1}{2}$ cups ■
Each serving contains approximately:
With oil: Calories: 145 (11% from fat);
Protein: 6 gms; Fat: 1.7 gms; Carbohydrate: 28 gms; Cholesterol: 0; Sodium:
12 mgs; Allowances: $1\frac{1}{2}$ starches + 1 vegetable + $\frac{1}{9}$ fat. *Without oil:* Calories: 141
(7% from fat); Protein: 6 gms; Fat:
1.2 gms; Carbohydrate: 28 gms; Cholesterol: 0; Sodium: 12 mgs; Allowances: $1\frac{1}{2}$
starches + 1 vegetable

Marinated Black-Eyed Peas

This dish keeps for several days, or up
to a week if the tomatoes are added upon
serving.

Marinade:
2 teaspoons extra virgin olive oil
2 tablespoons red wine vinegar
$\frac{1}{4}$ teaspoon oregano
$\frac{1}{4}$ teaspoon basil
$\frac{1}{4}$ teaspoon minced garlic
3 tablespoons cider vinegar

$\frac{1}{4}$ teaspoon mustard powder
$\frac{1}{4}$ teaspoon ground cumin
$\frac{1}{4}$ teaspoon freshly ground black pepper, or
    to taste

3 cups cooked black-eyed peas
$\frac{1}{4}$ cup finely chopped green pepper
$\frac{1}{4}$ cup finely chopped red pepper
$\frac{1}{4}$ cup grated carrot
$\frac{1}{4}$ cup minced red onion
$\frac{1}{4}$ cup chopped fresh parsley
$\frac{1}{4}$ cup sliced radishes
$\frac{1}{2}$ cup diced tomatoes

Combine the marinade ingredients and set aside. In a separate bowl, mix the vegetables together. Pour dressing over bean/vegetable mixture and stir gently. Serve on a bed of lettuce, with whole-grain crackers.

Yield: 5 cups, or about 6 servings ■ Each serving contains approximately: Calories: 114 (18% from fat); Protein: 7 gms; Fat: 2.3 gms; Carbohydrate: 18 gms; Cholesterol: 0; Sodium: 10 mgs; Allowances: $1\frac{1}{8}$ starches + $\frac{1}{3}$ vegetable + $\frac{1}{3}$ fat

Lentil Salad

$\frac{1}{2}$ pound dry lentils
1 small onion
1 whole clove
3 sprigs fresh thyme or $\frac{1}{2}$ teaspoon dried
    thyme
2 bay leaves
Freshly ground black pepper to taste
3–4 cups water
1 tablespoon extra virgin olive oil
5–6 ripe plum tomatoes, cored and
    diced
2 tablespoons chopped fresh parsley
$\frac{1}{2}$ cup finely chopped onions

1 tablespoon minced garlic
2 tablespoons red wine vinegar

Rinse lentils and place in a medium saucepan. Insert clove into onion and add to pan, along with thyme, bay leaves, pepper, water, and oil. Bring to a boil, then reduce heat and simmer for 20 minutes or until lentils are tender, adding water if necessary. Do not overcook. Drain well.

Remove the onion, clove, thyme sprigs, and bay leaves. Place lentils in attractive salad bowl and add the remaining 5 ingredients. Toss well and refrigerate for a couple of hours if possible. Do not worry if time does not permit this; the salad is also wonderful if eaten immediately.

Yield: 10 servings; serving size $\frac{1}{2}$ cup ■ Each serving contains approximately: Calories: 96 (16% from fat); Protein: 6 gms; Fat: 1.7 gms; Carbohydrate: 16 gms; Cholesterol: 0; Sodium: 8 mgs; Allowances: $\frac{3}{4}$ starch + $\frac{3}{4}$ vegetable + $\frac{1}{3}$ fat

Jicama and Citrus Salad
by Carol Ericsson

Delicioso anytime, but especially good with a Southwestern meal.

1 jicama
1 whole grapefruit, skinned, sectioned,
    and juice reserved
2 whole oranges, skinned, sectioned, and
    juice reserved
Juice of $\frac{1}{2}$ large or 1 small lime
1 tablespoon honey
Pinch of cayenne
$\frac{1}{2}$ cup fresh raspberries or pomegranate
    seeds
Small fresh edible flowers (see note)

Note: Johnny Jump-Ups are beautiful in this salad.

Peel and halve jicama. Place halves flat side down and slice thin slices, approximately ⅛-inch-wide. Alternating the citrus fruit and jicama, arrange in a fan-shape design on plate. Blend juice with honey and cayenne and pour over salad. Garnish with raspberries or pomegranate and small edible flowers.

Yield: 6 servings ▪ Each serving contains approximately: Calories: 77 (1% from fat); Protein: 1 gm; Fat: .1 gm; Carbohydrate: 19 gms; Cholesterol: 0; Sodium: 4 mgs; Allowances: ¼ starch + 1 fruit

Carol's Fruit Salad
by Carol Ericsson

1 pint fresh blueberries
1 pint fresh strawberries
1 pint fresh raspberries
3 mangoes, peeled and seeded
Dash of vanilla extract
Chopped fresh mint to taste

Purée mangoes in food processor or blender, and add vanilla. Wash the berries. Stem the blueberries and cap the strawberries. Mix well and top with the mango purée; garnish with mint.

Yield: 8 servings; serving size ¾ cup ▪ Each serving contains approximately: Calories: 93 (6% from fat); Protein: 1 gm; Fat: .7 gm; Carbohydrate: 25 gms; Cholesterol: 0; Sodium: 4 mgs; Allowances: 1½ fruits

Dijon Yogurt Vinaigrette

This dressing is delicious on *My Favorite Vegetable Salad,* page 255, or with any raw vegetables.

5 garlic cloves, minced
4 tablespoons chopped fresh Italian parsley
4 tablespoons chopped fresh basil
4 scallions, chopped, or 2 tablespoons chopped chives
5 teaspoons no-fat/no-salt Dijon mustard
½ cup balsamic vinegar
½ cup plain nonfat yogurt
1 teaspoon molasses or honey

Blend all ingredients together in a blender for approximately 40 seconds.

Yield: 12 servings; serving size 2 tablespoons ▪ Each serving contains approximately: Calories: 12 (7% from fat); Protein: 1 gm; Fat: .1 gm; Carbohydrate: 2 gms; Cholesterol: 0; Sodium: 9 mgs; Allowances: ⅛ vegetable + 1/12 dairy

Joan's Own Balsamic Vinaigrette
by Joan Zipnick

¼ teaspoon freshly ground black pepper
½ teaspoon dry mustard
2 tablespoons dried basil
¼ cup rice wine vinegar
¼ cup water
¾ cup balsamic vinegar
¼ cup extra virgin olive oil
2 large garlic cloves, minced

Combine the first three ingredients in a glass jar or bottle, then add the remaining ones. Cover and shake well. Serve at room temperature on lettuce of your choice. (My favorites are green or red leaf, radicchio, Boston, and endive.)

Yield: approximately 25 servings; serving size 1 tablespoon ■ Each serving contains approximately: Calories: 22 (90% from fat); Protein: 1 gm; Fat: 2.2 gms; Carbohydrate: 1 gm; Cholesterol: 0; Sodium: trace; Allowances: $\frac{1}{4}$ vegetable + $\frac{1}{3}$ fat

Lemon-Zested Olive Oil

This flavored oil is fabulous on vegetable salad or bread, and a teaspoon offers more taste than you can believe.

7 large ripe lemons
4 cups extra virgin olive oil

Wash and dry lemons, then peel with a potato peeler, taking care not to remove any of the bitter white pith with the peel. This should produce a little more than a cup of lemon peel. Refrigerate the peeled lemons until needed for lemon juice.

Place about $\frac{1}{4}$ cup of the olive oil in a mortar along with approximately half the lemon peel. Pound and rub the peel and oil together with the pestle for 1 to 2 minutes. Place in a half-gallon glass jar. Repeat with the remaining lemon peel and another $\frac{1}{4}$ cup of olive oil. Place in the jar and add the remaining olive oil. Allow the lemons and olive oil to marinate at room temperature for 4 days. Then strain the oil and discard the peel. The flavored oil can be stored, covered, at room temperature.

Yield: 4 cups, or 192 servings; serving size 1 teaspoon ■ Each serving contains approximately: Calories: 45 (100% from fat); Protein: 0; Fat: 4.5 gms; Carbohydrate: 0; Cholesterol: 0; Sodium: 0; Allowances: 1 fat

Horseradish Salad Dressing

$\frac{1}{2}$ cup olive oil
1 cup vinegar
1 tomato, peeled
1 heaping tablespoon freshly grated horseradish root
1 teaspoon dry mustard
4 cloves garlic, minced
$\frac{1}{2}$ teaspoon freshly ground black pepper

Blend all ingredients together. Herbs could be added as desired. You might try adding fresh basil, oregano, or thyme, or a dried medley such as *Italian Seasoning Blend*.

Yield: 21 servings; serving size 2 tablespoons ■ Each serving contains approximately: Calories: 50 (94% from fat); Protein: .1 gm; Fat: 5 gms; Carbohydrate: 1 gm; Cholesterol: 0; Sodium: 1 mg; Allowances: $\frac{1}{5}$ vegetable + 1 fat

Horseradish Sauce

You can freeze this sauce in an ice-cube tray, then wrap the cubes in foil and store. It is good with salads, fish, or simply spread on toast or a sandwich.

1 horseradish root
1 apple, chopped
2 carrots, chopped
1 green pepper, chopped

1 large onion, chopped
3 cups cranberries (1 12-ounce package)
Juice of 1 lemon
Honey to taste

Peel and dice the horseradish root and place in a blender with the apple. Blend until smooth. Put aside, then blend the remaining ingredients. Add the horseradish mixture and blend again. Taste it, and add a little honey if you desire.

Yield: 20 servings; serving size $\frac{1}{4}$ cup ■ Each serving contains approximately: Calories: 25 (5% from fat); Protein: .4 gm; Fat: .15 gm; Carbohydrate: 6 gms; Cholesterol: 0; Sodium: 4 mgs; Allowances: $\frac{1}{3}$ vegetable + $\frac{1}{4}$ fruit

Stupendous Cooked Salad Dressing
by Carol Ericsson

1 cup *Basic Veggie Stock* (see page 249)
1 teaspoon potato starch dissolved in $\frac{1}{4}$ cup of cold water
2 tablespoons balsamic vinegar
1 tablespoon apple juice concentrate
$\frac{1}{2}$ tablespoon chopped garlic
2 tablespoons minced green onions
$\frac{1}{2}$ teaspoon Italian Spice Blend (see page 243, in the *Roasted Garlic* ingredient list)

Combine all ingredients and simmer for 3 to 4 minutes. Refrigerate and use within one week.

Yield: 10 servings; serving size 2 tablespoons ■ Each serving contains approximately: Calories: 9 (0% from fat); Protein: trace; Fat: 0; Carbohydrate: 2 gms; Cholesterol: 0; Sodium: 1 mg; Allowances: $\frac{1}{3}$ vegetable

Real Cranberry Relish

This dish can be prepared days in advance, so you, too, can enjoy the holidays!

Last year during the post-holiday leftover time I discovered that this relish was exceptionally good as a topping for *Twice-Baked Garlic Sweet Potatoes,* page 266. It was also very beautiful.

4 cups fresh cranberries
8 large oranges, peeled and chopped
1 pear, chopped (preferably a soft, ripe Bosc pear)
2 tablespoons chopped pecans (approximately $\frac{1}{2}$ ounce)

Grind all the fruit and pecans in a food processor or grinder. Mix well.

Yield: just over 15 servings; serving size $\frac{1}{2}$ cup ■ Each serving contains approximately: Calories: 59 (14% from fat); Protein: 1 gm; Fat: .9 gm; Carbohydrate: 13 gms; Cholesterol: 0; Sodium: trace; Allowances: $\frac{4}{5}$ fruit + $\frac{1}{4}$ fat

Alan's Ginger Garlic Sauce
by Alan B. Sukert

1 quart no-salt chicken or vegetable bouillon, or defatted chicken broth made without salt, or *Basic Veggie Stock* (see page 249)
1$\frac{1}{2}$ teaspoons sesame oil
24 garlic cloves, diced
1 3-inch piece of ginger root, minced
2 scallions, chopped
6 packets Equal or teaspoons of sugar
No Salt to taste, if desired
White rice wine to taste
White pepper to taste
1–2 teaspoons cornstarch dissolved in a few tablespoons of water

Heat chicken or vegetable stock over medium heat. Heat sesame oil in wok on medium-high burner and add garlic, ginger, and half of the chopped scallions. Stir fry, stirring frequently. Add the sautéed vegetables to heated stock. Add the Equal or sugar, No Salt, rice wine, and white pepper. Slowly stir in dissolved cornstarch. Let stand for a few minutes off heat to thicken. Garnish with the remaining chopped scallions. Serve over rice and vegetables.

Yield: 36 servings; serving size 1 ounce ■ Each serving contains approximately: Calories: 6 (32% from fat); Protein: .2 gms; Fat: .2 gms; Carbohydrate: 11 gms; Cholesterol: 0; Sodium: trace; Allowances: $\frac{1}{8}$ vegetable + trace amounts of fat

Mushroom and Onion Gravy

2 teaspoons extra virgin olive oil
6 cups sliced mushrooms (see note)
2 cups chopped onions
1 cup sherry
1 cup *Basic Veggie Stock* (see page 249)
3 tablespoons arrowroot powder
Freshly ground black pepper to taste

Note: Portobello and shittake mushrooms are particularly delicious.

Heat olive oil in wok, then add mushrooms. Sauté for 5 minutes. Add onions and sauté an additional 5 minutes. Combine sherry, *Basic Veggie Stock,* and arrowroot powder until the powder has dissolved. Gradually add this mixture to the mushrooms and onions. Cover and simmer 10 minutes or until desired consistency has been achieved.

Yield: approximately 24 servings; serving size 2 tablespoons ■ Each serving contains approximately: Calories: 15 (19% from fat); Protein: 1 gm; Fat: .32 gm; Carbohydrate: 3 gms; Cholesterol: 0; Sodium: 1 mg; Allowances: $\frac{1}{16}$ starch + $\frac{1}{3}$ vegetable + $\frac{1}{12}$ fat

Vegetables

Carolina Cukes

Enjoy these luscious cukes instead of sodium-loaded pickles.

2 medium to large cucumbers, sliced
1 red onion, sliced
6 ounces balsamic vinegar
2 teaspoons honey
1$\frac{1}{2}$ cups water
Freshly ground black pepper to taste

Place alternating layers of cucumbers and onions in an airtight container. Heat $\frac{1}{2}$ cup of the water and add to the honey. When this has melted the honey, mix with remaining water and vinegar and pour over vegetables.

Marinate overnight if time allows. Container can be turned upside down, then righted periodically, to ensure all the vegetables are equally marinated.

Yield: 6 servings; serving size 1 cup ■
Each serving contains approximately: Calories: 30 (8% from fat); Protein: 1 gm; Fat: .26 gm; Carbohydrate: 7 gms; Cholesterol: 0; Sodium: 3 mgs; Allowances: 1¼ vegetables

Okra and Onions

3 pounds okra, sliced (fresh or no-salt frozen)
1 onion, chopped
2 tomatoes, chopped
1½ cups water or *Basic Veggie Stock* (see page 249)

Place all the ingredients in a saucepan and boil for 10 minutes or until desired tenderness is achieved.

Yield: 10 servings; serving size ¾ cup ■
Each serving contains approximately: Calories: 62 (8% from fat); Protein: 3 gms; Fat: .5 gm; Carbohydrate: 14 gms; Cholesterol: 0; Sodium: 7 mgs; Allowances: 2½ vegetables

Kitty's Steamed Veggies

Topped with balsamic vinegar and freshly ground black pepper, this is one of my favorite meals.

8 new potatoes
2 large onions, peeled and halved
2 large carrots, halved
2 large heads of broccoli, with stems
½ head cauliflower
2 ears of corn, shucked
1 cup chopped red cabbage
8 small mushrooms
1 bunch fresh kale

Place a stainless steel steamer in a large pot or a bamboo steamer in a steel wok, with 1½ inches of water below it. As the water heats, wash and prep the vegetables.

The only trick to steaming a variety of vegetables is timing—so that they will all be ready at the same time. So start to cook the harder vegetables before the faster-cooking ones. With the above mixture, place the potatoes, onion, and carrots in the steamer first. Give them a 10-15-minute head start, depending upon the size of the vegetables. Obviously, the larger a vegetable, the longer it will take to cook. If you would like to expedite the process, you can cut the vegetables in smaller pieces, but remember that the smaller they are cut, the more nutrients are lost.

If you are using a bamboo steamer, place the second group of vegetables in another steamer tray that fits above the first one. The broccoli, cauliflower, corn, and red cabbage need up to 5 minutes more cooking time than the remaining mushrooms and kale. This also will depend upon how large you want to keep the vegetables and how much time you have to cook.

Yield: 4 servings ■ One serving contains approximately: Calories: 211 (5% from fat); Protein: 9 gms; Fat: 1.25 gms; Carbohydrate: 46 gms; Cholesterol: 0; Sodium: 58 mgs; Allowances: 2 starches + 1½ vegetables

Twice-Baked Garlic Sweet Potatoes

1–2 head(s) of garlic (dependent upon love for garlic!)
¼ teaspoon extra virgin olive oil
6 small to medium unpeeled sweet potatoes

½ cup plain nonfat yogurt
¼ teaspoon freshly ground black pepper

Preheat oven to 400 degrees.

Remove the outer covering from garlic, but do not peel or separate the cloves. With a paring knife slice off the smallest end of the garlic cloves. Using the palms of your hands, coat the garlic with olive oil, then wrap in aluminum foil. Bake garlic and sweet potatoes on a baking sheet for 1 hour and 15 minutes. (Leave oven on.) After cooking, separate garlic cloves and squeeze to extract 2 to 4 teaspoons of pulp—dependent upon how garlicky you want it.

Slice the top skin off each sweet potato, and carefully scoop out most of the insides, leaving the shells intact. Mash the sweet potato pulp, stir in garlic pulp, yogurt, and pepper. Spoon this mixture back into the shells, and bake at 400 degrees for 15 minutes or until thoroughly heated.

Yield: 6 servings ■ Each serving contains approximately: Calories: 143 (2% from fat); Protein: 4 gms; Fat: .3 gm; Carbohydrate: 32 gms; Cholesterol: trace; Sodium: 29 mgs; Allowances: 1¼ starches + ½ vegetable + ⅓ dairy

Gingered Peas, Peppers, and Carrots

1 teaspoon extra virgin olive oil
1 teaspoon minced garlic
2 teaspoons minced ginger root
3 tablespoons chopped scallions
½ cup wine, red or white
2 carrots, julienned

½ pound sugar snap peas, de-capped and de-veined
1 red pepper, sliced in strips
1 tablespoon chopped fresh cilantro

Heat olive oil in wok on high and add garlic. Before garlic browns, add ginger root and scallions. Stir occasionally. Add wine before mixture begins to stick, then add carrots. Continue to stir every couple of minutes, giving the carrots approximately 5 minutes of cooking before adding the remaining ingredients. Stir-fry for another few minutes then serve over brown rice, quinoa, or any whole grain.

Yield: 4 servings; serving size 4 cups ■ Each serving contains approximately: Calories: 104 (14% from fat); Protein: 8 gms; Fat: 1.6 gms; Carbohydrate: 17 gms; Cholesterol: 0; Sodium: 16 mgs; Allowances: ¾ starch + 1 vegetable + ¼ fat

Holiday Brussels Sprouts and Chestnuts with Orange Glaze

24 small fresh brussels sprouts
½ teaspoon extra virgin olive oil
12 shelled chestnuts, quartered
4 shallots, thinly sliced crosswise
½ cup unsweetened orange juice
½ cup *Basic Veggie Stock* (see page 249)
2 teaspoons molasses
1 teaspoon fresh lemon juice
¼ teaspoon freshly ground black pepper

Wash brussels sprouts carefully, removing discolored leaves and stem ends. Place in a vegetable steamer over boiling water, cover, and steam for 8 minutes, or until tender. Drain and set aside.

Heat oil in a large skillet over medium-high heat; add chestnuts and shallots. Sauté for 5 minutes or until tender, adding some stock as needed to prevent scorching. Combine orange juice, *Basic Veggie Stock,* molasses, and lemon juice. Stir well and add to the chestnut mixture. Bring the mixture to a boil and cook for about 5 minutes. Stir in the brussels sprouts and cook for another 5 minutes.

Yield: 4 servings; serving size 1 cup ■ Each serving contains approximately: Calories: 160 (11% from fat); Protein: 4 gms; Fat: 2 gms; Carbohydrate: 35 gms; Cholesterol: 0; Sodium: 28 mgs; Allowances: 1 starch + 2 vegetables + $\frac{1}{3}$ fruit + $\frac{1}{10}$ fat

Tsimmes
by Rhoda Harris

4 large sweet potatoes
4 large carrots
1 pound seedless prunes
$\frac{1}{2}$ pound dried apricots
Vegetable cooking spray
2 cups orange juice
2 cups water
1 large lemon, thinly sliced

Preheat oven to 350 degrees.

Precook sweet potatoes and carrots in a microwave for 10 minutes, then turn them and cook another 10 minutes. Slice them into $\frac{1}{8}$- to $\frac{1}{4}$-inch slices. Cut the prunes and apricots in half, then mix them with the sweet potatoes and carrots.

Coat a 4- or 5-quart glass casserole with vegetable cooking spray. Add fruit mixture and cover with orange juice and water. Place lemon slices on top of fruit. Cover and bake for 45 minutes.

Yield: 24 servings; serving size $\frac{3}{4}$ cup ■ Each serving contains approximately: Calories: 102 (2% from fat); Protein: 1 gm; Fat: .2 gm; Carbohydrate: 26 gms; Cholesterol: 0; Sodium: 8 mgs; Allowances: $\frac{1}{4}$ starch + 1 vegetable + 1 fruit

Persimmon and Cranberry Stuffed Squash

2 large acorn squash, split lengthwise and seeded
1 pear, chopped
1 cup raw cranberries
1 persimmon, peeled and cubed
2 tablespoons orange juice concentrate
2 tablespoons honey
$\frac{1}{2}$ teaspoon ground allspice
2 teaspoons ground cinnamon

Preheat oven to 400 degrees.

Pour water 1-inch deep into a 9×12-inch casserole and place squash cut side up. Stir the remaining ingredients together and spoon the mixture into the center of each squash half. Spoon and brush extra liquid onto the cut edges of the squash. Bake for 45 to 60 minutes or until the squash is tender.

Yield: 4 servings ■ Each squash half contains approximately: Calories: 161 (2% from fat); Protein: 1 gm; Fat: .3 gm; Carbohydrate: 28 gms; Cholesterol: 0; Sodium: 4 mgs; Allowances: 1 starch + $1\frac{1}{3}$ fruits

Guvec or Turlu (Or you could say, Vegetable Casserole!)
by Farida Gindi

2 long thin eggplants or 1 medium oval
    eggplant
4 small zucchini
3 small green peppers
½ pound okra
½ cup vinegar
½ pound green beans
5 small ripe tomatoes
1 tablespoon extra virgin olive oil
3 small onions, sliced
2 garlic cloves, minced
¼ cup chopped fresh parsley
Freshly ground black pepper to taste

Preheat oven to 300 degrees.

Wash vegetables. Remove stems from the eggplants, then slice into ½-inch slices. Oval eggplant should be quartered, then sliced. Trim zucchini and cut into ½-inch pieces. Remove stem and seeds from peppers, and slice into ½-inch pieces.

To prepare okra the Middle Eastern way is worth the effort because it really does prevent the okra from becoming slimy. Wash the okra well and handle gently. Trim stem end and around conical stem attached to pod, removing a thin layer. This is the correct way to prepare okra, as it serves to remove the fine brown ring just above the pod and the outer layer of the stem. Middle Eastern cooks prefer to do this as the whole vegetable then becomes edible. If okra is not very young, use a fine nylon scourer to remove the fuzz under running water. After okra is washed and trimmed, spread it out on a cloth or paper towel to dry.

When dry, place in a bowl and cover with ½ cup of vinegar, and toss occasionally for 30 minutes. Drain, rinse, and dry.

Remove ends from string beans and slit in half length-wise (French cut). Slice tomatoes. Heat half the oil in a frying pan and fry eggplant until lightly browned. Remove to a plate. Add remaining oil to pan and sauté onions until transparent, then stir in garlic, and cook for 1 minute.

Place a layer of eggplant in the bottom of a casserole dish, followed by layers of zucchini, peppers, and beans. Spread some onion mixture on top and cover with tomato slices, pepper, and parsley. Repeat until all ingredients are used, reserving some tomato and parsley for the top. Place prepared okra on top, and cover with the last of the tomato, parsley, and pepper. Cover casserole and bake for one hour.

Yield: 6 servings ■ Each serving contains approximately: Calories: 96 (19% from fat); Protein: 3 gms; Fat: 2 gms; Carbohydrate: 17 gms; Cholesterol: 0; Sodium: 18 mgs; Allowances: 3 vegetables + ½ fat

Soulouk Moukala (Fried Mustard Greens)
by Farida Gindi

This is great topped with hot pepper vinegar or lemon juice. Serve with a nice whole grain bread and follow with a fresh fruit salad.

2 pounds fresh or frozen mustard greens
2 onions, chopped
5 garlic cloves, minced
2 16-ounce cans no-salt garbanzo beans

$\frac{1}{2}$ cup chopped fresh oregano, or $\frac{1}{4}$ teaspoon dried oregano
1 tablespoon extra virgin olive oil
$\frac{1}{2}$ teaspoon allspice
2 stalks celery, finely diced

Wash mustard greens, tear into pieces, and boil for 10 minutes. Or, prepare frozen greens according to package directions. Drain, then rinse to reduce bitter compounds from greens, and return to pot. Sauté onions then add to greens. Add remaining ingredients, and simmer for 1 hour.

Yield: 9 servings; serving size 1 cup ■
Each serving contains approximately: Calories 99 (18% from fat); Protein: 6 gms; Fat: 2 gms; Carbohydrate: 13 gms; Cholesterol: 0; Sodium: 26 mgs; Allowances: $\frac{3}{4}$ starch + 1 vegetable + $\frac{1}{3}$ fat

Kim Chee
with Ms. Lan Tan

This Korean version of sauerkraut is wonderful ''straight'' or enjoyed as a chutney on beans, grains, or vegetables needing a kick! Of course, more of the ginger, garlic, or chili powder may be used depending upon your personal tastes.

1$\frac{1}{2}$ pounds Napa cabbage
2–3 garlic cloves, chopped or 1–2 teaspoons garlic powder
1–2 teaspoons grated ginger or 1 teaspoon powdered ginger
2 teaspoons chili powder (or more to taste)
1–2 tablespoons sugar
1$\frac{1}{2}$ tablespoons rice vinegar
$\frac{1}{2}$ cup grated carrots

Blanch cabbage for approximately 1 minute. A quick dip in a wok full of boiling water will do. Then rinse with cold water. Squeeze out the excess water and chop into 1-inch pieces. Mix the remaining ingredients and pour over chopped cabbage, mixing thoroughly. Place in a quart jar and let sit on the counter for 2 days. If the mixture has then soured enough to suit you, refrigerate.

Yield: 6 servings; serving size $\frac{1}{4}$ cup ■
Each serving contains approximately: Calories: 18 (8% from fat); Protein: 1 gm; Fat: .15 gm; Carbohydrate: 8 gms; Cholesterol: 0; Sodium: 38 mgs; Allowances: $\frac{3}{4}$ vegetable

Marinated Roasted Peppers

This is probably my favorite food in the entire world! It is absolutely delicious on bread or pasta.

5 yellow peppers
5 red peppers
8–12 garlic cloves, minced
$\frac{1}{2}$ cup balsamic vinegar
1 tablespoon extra virgin olive oil
$\frac{1}{4}$ cup chopped fresh basil
$\frac{1}{2}$–1 teaspoon freshly ground black pepper

Wash and core the peppers, removing the seeds from the insides. Place peppers on their shoulders (or where their stems were before they were deseeded) on a rack in a large broiler pan, with $\frac{1}{2}$ inch of water below the rack to ensure an easy clean-up. Peppers should be placed so that they are approximately 3 inches from the broiler unit. Broil peppers until the bottoms are blackened, then turn on their sides. Broil until this side is blackened, turn and burn, and turn and burn again until thoroughly roasted. This process can also be done on a gas burner or grill.

Wrap roasted peppers in moistened paper towels and put the wrapped peppers in a paper bag to let them sweat for 10 to 15 minutes. This will facilitate the removal of the peppers' skin. The moistened paper towel can be used to stroke the charred skin from the pepper. (Most recipes suggest that you skin them under running water, but why rinse valuable flavors down the drain?!)

Slice the peppers in $\frac{1}{2}$-inch wide strips and combine with the remaining ingredients. Place in a tightly sealed container in the refrigerator for a few days.

Yield: 14 servings; serving size $\frac{1}{4}$ cup ■ Each serving contains approximately: Calories: 44 (20% from fat); Protein: 1 gm; Fat: 1 gm; Carbohydrate: 9 gms; Cholesterol: 0; Sodium: 6 mgs; Allowances: $1\frac{1}{2}$ vegetables + $\frac{1}{5}$ fat

Lorraine and Maria's Garlicky Greens
by Maria Zagorianos and Lorraine Deieso

3 pounds fresh spinach or other greens
1 teaspoon extra virgin olive oil
$\frac{1}{4}$ teaspoon red pepper flakes or to taste
6–12 garlic cloves, minced (or more if desired)
1 large onion, chopped
Juice of 2 lemons

Carefully clean the spinach of any dirt or imperfections in the leaves. Heat the olive oil, then add the red pepper, garlic,

and onions; saute for 2 to 3 minutes. Add the freshly torn spinach and lemon juice and stew until the spinach leaves are tender, approximately 3 to 4 minutes more.

Yield: 8 servings; serving size $\frac{1}{2}$ cup ■ Each serving contains approximately: Calories: 52 (17% from fat); Protein: 4 gms; Fat: 1 gm; Carbohydrate: 9 gms; Cholesterol: 0; Sodium: 11 mgs; Allowances: $1\frac{2}{3}$ vegetables + $\frac{1}{4}$ fat

Basic Marinated Veggies
by Carol Ericsson

3 heads broccoli, with stems
1 head cauliflower
3 *Marinated Roasted Peppers,* chopped (see page 270)
1 cucumber, peeled, de-seeded and thinly sliced
$\frac{1}{2}$ cup fat-free sour cream
1 cup *Stupendous Cooked Salad Dressing* (see page 264)
$\frac{1}{2}$ teaspoon chopped fresh dill
2 green onions, sliced

Steam the broccoli and cauliflower until crisp but tender. Cut into small bite-size pieces, excluding most of the stems, if desired. Mix with peppers and cucumber. Blend the remaining ingredients, pour over vegetables, and refrigerate overnight.

Yield: approximately 8 servings ■ Each serving contains approximately: Calories: 39 (6% from fat); Protein: 8 gms; Fat: .26 gm; Carbohydrate: 8 gms; Cholesterol: 0; Sodium: 27 mgs; Allowances: $1\frac{1}{4}$ vegetables + $\frac{1}{10}$ dairy

Spring Veggies and Squash
by Carol Ericsson

$\frac{1}{2}$ cup *Basic Veggie Stock* (see page 249)
1 pound baby asparagus
3 yellow squash
1 scallion, julienned
1 small *Marinated Roasted Pepper,* sliced (see page 270)

Wash asparagus and bend near the base, throwing away the tougher end that breaks off. Cut diagonally into thirds and steam asparagus until al dente. Cut squash into halves, then slice into julienne strips. Heat *Basic Veggie Stock* and stir-fry squash for 3 to 4 minutes, then add asparagus, roasted pepper, and scallion for the last minute of stir-frying.

Yield: 4 servings ■ Each serving contains approximately: Calories: 40 (13% from fat); Protein: 3 gms; Fat: .58 gm; Carbohydrate: 8 gms; Cholesterol: 0; Sodium: 6 mgs; Allowances: $1\frac{1}{3}$ vegetables

Broccoli Rabe and Artichoke Stir-Fry

This makes a fabulous meal simply served over pasta, or with added sun-dried tomatoes if you can find them without salt.

1 10-ounce package frozen artichokes
$\frac{1}{4}$ cup *Basic Veggie Stock* (see page 249)
3–4 cloves garlic, minced (more if desired)
1 bunch broccoli rabe (rapini), or 1 bunch each broccoli and arugala or spinach, chopped
Pinch of red pepper flakes, to taste

Cook artichokes according to package instructions. Heat stock in a wok and stir-fry the remaining ingredients until crisp and tender. Drain artichokes and mix with stir-fried vegetables.

Yield: approximately 4 cups or 2 2-cup servings (if you want to make a meal of it!) ■ Each serving contains approximately: Calories: 86 (5% from fat); Protein: 7 gms; Fat: .5 gm; Carbohydrate: 8 gms; Sodium: 103 mgs; Allowances: $3\frac{1}{2}$ vegetables

15-Minute Meals

Pasta Bean Pronto!

Good with no-fat/no-salt crackers, like Cracottes or Health Valley crackers and a fruit or vegetable salad.

1 15-ounce can no-salt beans, drained and rinsed
5 ounces pasta (any no-fat/no-salt variety)
3 large tomatoes, chopped
Pinch or 2 of garlic powder and cumin to taste

1 jalapeño pepper, seeded and minced to taste

Cook pasta for recommended time. While waiting for water to boil, microwave the beans for 3 to 4 minutes. Meanwhile, combine remaining ingredients and toss in beans and pasta when done.

Yield: 4 servings ■ Each serving contains approximately: Calories: 208 (11% from fat); Protein: 10 gms; Fat: 2.5 gms; Carbohydrate: 42 gms; Cholesterol: 0; Sodium: 12 mgs; Allowances: 2⅓ starches + ¾ vegetable

Refried Beans and Salsa with Chips

Many salsa companies now have a no-salt version. Enrico's is presently my favorite. Enjoy with any no-fat/no-salt chips. The Baked Tostitos and Smart Temptations are thinner, thus crispier, than Guiltless Gourmet.

1 16-ounce can no-salt Bearitos refried beans
6 ounces salsa
Juice of 1 lime
2 tablespoons chopped fresh cilantro
Minced fresh jalapeño to taste
60–80 no-fat/no-salt corn chips

Mix refried beans with salsa. Blend in the lime juice, cilantro, and jalapeños to taste! (Beware of pickled jalapeños, which are loaded with sodium.)

Yield: 5 servings ■ Each serving contains approximately: Calories: 188 (14% from fat); Protein: 7gms; Fat: 3 gms; Carbohydrate: 35 gms; Cholesterol: 0; Sodium: 32 mgs; Allowances: 2 starches + 1 vegetable

Spontaneous Spaghetti or Polenta

You could also toss a quick vegetable salad (topped with no-fat salad dressing), within the 15-minute prep time. Enjoy with no-fat/no-salt bread or crackers.

6 ounces pasta or polenta
1 jar any no-salt spaghetti sauce

Boil water, add pasta or polenta, and cook for recommended time. While waiting for water to boil, heat spaghetti sauce. Drain pasta and mix with sauce.

If you like pasta, you'll probably like it topped with just about anything else you like! This quickie recipe can be varied by adding canned no-salt clams or beans, fresh or frozen spinach, etc. Or for a 10-minute meal, simply add a can of no-salt sardines to pasta, vinegar to taste, and toss.

Yield: 4 servings ■ Each serving contains approximately: Calories: 325 (17% from fat); Protein: 12 gms; Fat: 6.2 gms; Carbohydrate: 58 gms; Cholesterol: 0; Sodium: 13 mgs; Allowances: 2 starches + 4⅕ vegetables + 1 fat

Super Swift Pasta or Polenta

¼ cup texturized vegetable protein, optional
¼ cup water or *Basic Veggie Stock* (see page 249)
1 onion, chopped
1 sweet red pepper, chopped
1 yellow pepper, chopped
½ cup chopped mushrooms, preferably shiitake mushrooms
24 ounces no-salt vegetarian spaghetti sauce
8 ounces pasta or 8¾ ounces of polenta

Put a gallon of water to boil for pasta or polenta. In a saucepan, heat vegetable stock; add vegetables and sauté until still slightly crisp. Add spaghetti sauce. Add the TVP to sauce if you would like a chewy, meatlike consistency. As your "new and improved sauce" is warming, add pasta or polenta to boiling water and cook for the amount of time specified on package.

When pasta is al dente (tender but firm), strain off water and top with sauce. If using polenta, simply serve 1½ cups of cooked polenta per plate and top with one fourth of the sauce. Enjoy with a nice vegetable salad.

Yield: 4 servings ■ Each serving (calculated using rice pasta fettuccini) contains approximately: *With TVP:* Calories: 340 (18% from fat); Protein: 11 gms; Fat: 6.9 gms; Carbohydrate: 59 gms; Cholesterol: 0; Sodium: 19 mgs; Allowances: 3 starches + 2 vegetables + 1 fat. *Without TVP:* Calories: 322 (19% from fat); Protein: 9 gms; Fat: 6.7 gms; Carbohydrate: 57 gms; Cholesterol: 0; Sodium: 18 mgs; Allowances: 2¾ starches + 2 vegetables + 1 fat

Vegetarian Chili Immediato!

1 can Health Valley no-salt vegetarian chili
2 tablespoons fresh lime juice or more to taste
2 tablespoons freshly chopped cilantro
Freshly minced jalapeño to taste
24–32 no-fat/so salt corn chips

Mix the vegetarian chili with lime juice, cilantro, and jalapeño to taste. Heat until warm throughout.

Yield: 2 servings ■ Each serving contains approximately: Calories: 354 (15% from fat); Protein: 18 gms; Fat: 6 gms; Carbohydrate: 54 gms; Cholesterol: 0; Sodium: 45 mgs; Allowances: 3 starches + 1⅓ vegetables

Swift Summer Fruit Plate

3 cups ½% dry curd cottage cheese
2 apples, chopped
2 oranges, peeled and chopped
2 bananas, sliced
1 cup seedless grapes
1 cup cubed melon
1 cup cubed pineapple
1 cup berries
4 tablespoons raisins
Cinnamon and vanilla to taste

Wash and prep fruit. Mix cinnamon and vanilla into cottage cheese and place ¾ cup in center of each of 4 plates. Surround with fruit. Or, if you prefer, mix the cottage cheese with the fruit. It's best to do this just before serving.

Good with bagels, Mini-Rice Cakes (Honey Nut and Apple Cinnamon) or Crispy Cakes (Apple Cinnamon).

Yield: 4 servings ■ Each serving contains approximately: Calories: 314 (5% from fat); Protein: 21 gms; Fat: 1.6 gms; Carbohydrate: 57 gms; Cholesterol: 8 mgs; Sodium: 26 mgs; Allowances: 3¾ fruits + 1 dairy

The Best "Burger" Out!

Good served on a slice of no-salt bread (*Pane Paesano,* page 240 or *Basic Whole Wheat Bread,* page 239), topped with no-salt-added mustard, and freshly sliced tomato and lettuce.

2 cubes very-low-sodium chicken or vegetable bouillon
1½ cups plus 3 tablespoons warm water or *Basic Veggie Stock* (see page 249)
12 ounces Better Than Burger? mix
Vegetable cooking spray

Dissolve the bouillon in the warm stock or water. Add the Better Than Burger? mix. Stir until well blended and let stand for 20 to 30 minutes. Mix again and form into ¼-inch-thick patties.

Fry in a nonstick pan or in a pan sprayed with vegetable cooking spray. Turn only once when the "burger" is light brown in color. Then brown the second side.

Yield: 10 to 12 burgers ■ Each serving contains approximately: *If 10 "burgers":*

Calories: 165 (11% from fat); Protein: 20 gms; Fat: 2 gms; Carbohydrate: 25 gms; Cholesterol: 0; Sodium: 53 mgs; Allowances: 2 starches + ⅕ vegetable. *If 12 "burgers":* Calories: 138 (11% from fat); Protein: 17 gms; Fat: 1.6 gms; Carbohydrate: 21 gms; Cholesterol: 0; Sodium: 43 mgs; Allowances: 1¾ starches

Main Dishes

Italian Flag Pasta
by Carol Ericsson

1 pound tricolor fusilli
1½ cups of *Basic Veggie Stock* (see page 249)
1 tablespoon potato starch, dissolved in ¼ cup of the *Basic Veggie Stock,* cold
2 9-ounce packages of frozen artichoke hearts
1 Vidalia onion, chopped
1 tablespoon chopped garlic
⅓ cup chopped sun-dried tomatoes
1 yellow pepper, chopped
¼ cup chopped fresh Italian parsley
¼ cup fresh basil, julienned
Freshly ground black pepper to taste

Boil water for pasta, preferably in a steamer which facilitates the removal of the pasta. Cook until al dente and set aside. Heat the stock and add the potato starch, artichoke hearts, onion, garlic, and tomatoes, stir-frying for approximately 5 minutes. Then add the yellow peppers and seasonings and cook another 2 minutes.

Toss the previously cooked pasta into the seasoned vegetables and cook another minute.

Yield: 12 servings ■ Each serving contains approximately: Calories: 183 (11% from fat); Protein: 7 gms; Fat: 2.3 gms; Carbohydrate: 33 gms; Cholesterol: 0; Sodium: 33 mgs; Allowances: 1⅕ starches + 1½ vegetables

Carol's Lentil Loaf
by Carol Ericsson

1 pound lentils, preferably red
1 quart *Basic Veggie Stock* (see page 249)
1 small onion, finely diced
1 garlic clove, chopped
¼ cup chopped fresh Italian parsley
¼ teaspoon freshly ground black pepper
1 6-ounce can no-salt tomato paste
5 ounces fresh bread crumbs
2 egg whites
Vegetable cooking spray

Preheat oven to 375 degrees.

Reserve 2 tablespoons of the *Basic Veggie Stock.* Cook lentils in the rest of the stock for 35 to 45 minutes, then drain well. Sauté onion and garlic in the 2 tablespoons of stock until limp and fairly dry. Add parsley and pepper and sauté another minute. Add lentils and remaining ingredients, and mix well.

Spray a $8\frac{1}{4} \times 4\frac{1}{2}$-inch loaf pan with vegetable cooking spray; add lentil mixture and bake for 1 hour.

Yield: 8 servings ■ Each serving contains approximately: Calories: 225 (5% from fat); Protein: 14 gms; Fat: 1.2 gms; Cholesterol: 0; Sodium: 30 mgs; Allowances: $2\frac{1}{2}$ starches + 1 vegetable

Maria's Lenten Stuffed Peppers or Tomatoes
by Maria Zagorianos

1 cup brown rice
8 large or 10 small bell peppers or tomatoes
5 zucchini, grated
4 medium onions, chopped
1 tablespoon extra virgin olive oil
1 16-ounce can no-salt tomatoes, drained and chopped
$1\frac{1}{2}$ teaspoons plus $\frac{1}{2}$ teaspoon freshly ground black pepper
2 tablespoons chopped fresh mint
2–3 tablespoons chopped fresh dill
Juice of 1 lemon
$\frac{1}{2}$ cup water
4 ounces no-salt tomato sauce

Boil 1 cup water and add brown rice; parboil for 20 minutes or until it is approximately halfway done.

Mix together the zucchini, onions, oil, canned tomatoes, parboiled rice, $1\frac{1}{2}$ teaspoons pepper, mint, dill, and lemon juice. Place the mixture in a covered container and refrigerate for 2 to 12 hours.

Preheat oven to 350 degrees.

Core and de-seed peppers or tomatoes, saving the tops. If using peppers, roast, parboil, or steam them for 3 to 5 minutes. Stuff the rice mixture in the peppers or tomatoes and cover with the vegetable tops. Place in baking dish with $\frac{1}{2}$ cup water, $\frac{1}{2}$ teaspoon black pepper, and the tomato sauce. Bake for 1 hour.

Yield: 4 servings; serving size 2 stuffed vegetables ■ Each stuffed pepper or tomato contains approximately: Calories: 208 (19% from fat); Protein: 6 gms; Fat: 4.4 gms; Carbohydrate: 40 gms: Cholesterol: 0; Sodium: 42 mgs; Allowances: $\frac{2}{3}$ starch + 6 vegetables + $\frac{2}{3}$ fat

Greek Style Lentils
by Maria Zagorianos

1 pound lentils
1 large onion, chopped
4–5 large garlic cloves, minced
1 tablespoon extra virgin olive oil
1–2 bay leaves
1 16-ounce can no-salt tomatoes
$\frac{1}{2}$ 6-ounce can no-salt tomato paste
Freshly ground black pepper to taste
$\frac{1}{4}$ cup vinegar or to taste
$\frac{1}{4}$–$\frac{1}{2}$ cup red wine, optional

Wash and sort lentils; place in 2 quarts water over medium heat. When lentils begin to simmer, add all the other ingredients. Continue to simmer, uncovered, until the lentils are cooked and sauce is thickened, approximately 30 minutes.

Yield: 10 servings; serving size 1 cup ■ Each serving contains approximately: Calories: 147 (12% from fat); Protein: 9 gms;

Fat: 1.9 gms; Carbohydrate: 25 gms; Cholesterol: 0; Sodium: 11 mgs; Allowances: $1\frac{1}{3}$ starches + $1\frac{1}{5}$ vegetables + $\frac{1}{3}$ fat

Pasta with Escarole and Beans

This is one of our favorite 15- to 20-minute meals. It is great served with *Basic Whole Wheat Bread* topped with *Marinated Peppers.*

1 pound pasta
$\frac{1}{2}$ cup water
10 sundried tomatoes, finely diced
1 large head escarole or any dark green leafy vegetable
9 garlic cloves, minced
2 tablespoons extra virgin olive oil
$\frac{1}{2}$ – 1 teaspoon crushed red pepper flakes (dependent upon desired hotness)
1 can white beans
Juice of 2 limes

Put a gallon of water to boil for pasta.

In a separate pan, heat the $\frac{1}{2}$ cup water, then place the diced sundried tomatoes in the hot water to reconstitute. Thoroughly wash escarole, trim ends, and chop into 1- to 2-inch pieces. Heat olive oil in large pot over medium heat. When oil is hot, add garlic. Within a minute or so (before garlic browns) add escarole, sundried tomatoes with their water, and crushed red pepper. Sauté for 5 to 10 minutes, stirring frequently. When escarole is limp and dark green, add beans with their liquid. Heat for another 5 minutes. Place pasta in boiling water, and cook according to package directions.

When pasta is al dente, drain and combine with the sautéed vegetables and lime juice.

Yield: 12 servings; serving size 1 cup ■
Each serving contains approximately: Calories: 201 (15% from fat); Protein: 8 gms; Fat: 3.4 gms; Carbohydrate: 37 gms; Cholesterol: 0; Sodium: 39 mgs; Allowances: 2 starches + 1 vegetable + $\frac{1}{2}$ fat

Pasta e Fagioli

2 cups dried cannellini or pinto beans
1 cup water or *Basic Veggie Stock* (see page 249)
2 large onions, chopped
4 garlic cloves, minced
1 red or green bell pepper, chopped
2 1-pound cans no-salt whole tomatoes
2 carrots, chopped
1 teaspoon dried basil
1 teaspoon oregano
$\frac{1}{2}$ pound macaroni
$\frac{1}{4}$ cup red wine, optional

Cook beans as described in Chapter 12.

Heat the vegetable stock in a large soup pot. Sauté onions, garlic, and peppers until the onions are translucent. Drain the tomatoes and save the juice, setting it aside. Break the tomatoes up into small pieces with your fingers. Add the tomatoes, carrots, basil, and oregano to the sautéed vegetables. Simmer over low heat, stirring occasionally, for about 20 minutes. Add macaroni, wine, cooked beans, and reserved tomato juice. Simmer another 10 to 15 minutes, or until pasta is cooked al dente.

Yield: 10 servings; serving size 1 cup ■
Each serving contains approximately: Calories: 210 (11% from fat); Protein: 10 gms; Fat: 2.6 gms; Carbohydrate:

38 gms; Cholesterol: 0; Sodium: 21 mgs;
Allowances: $2\frac{1}{3}$ starches + 1 vegetable

Legal Lasagna
with Julie Mozzella

Tomato Sauce:
2 tablespoons olive oil
10 cloves garlic, chopped
2 tablespoons chopped fresh parsley
Freshly ground black pepper to taste
Pinch of cayenne pepper or to taste
2 teaspoons vinegar
2 35-ounce cans no-salt Italian peeled tomatoes
1 carrot, chopped

Lasagna:
$\frac{1}{2}$ cup plain nonfat yogurt
1 tablespoon wheat flour
1 pound $\frac{1}{2}$% dry curd cottage cheese
2 egg whites or equivalent portion of egg
   substitute
Freshly ground black pepper, optional
1 pound uncooked lasagna noodles
1 pound fresh spinach, cooked and
   drained 1 10-ounce package frozen
   spinach, defrosted

Make the sauce: Heat olive oil, then sauté
chopped garlic, parsley, black and red
pepper, and vinegar for 5 minutes. Add
the tomatoes and carrot and cook over
low heat until carrot is soft. Purée in
blender and set aside.

Stir the yogurt and flour together (to prevent yogurt from separating); stir in the
cottage cheese, egg whites, and pepper.
Squeeze excess water from spinach.

Preheat oven to 375 degrees.

Lightly oil two 13 × 8″ casserole dishes
with olive oil. Layer tomato sauce, pasta,
spinach, and cheese mixture in alternating layers. Continue to the top of pan, fin-
ishing with tomato sauce on top. Bake,
covered, for 45 minutes. Uncover for
the last 10 to 15 minutes of baking, if
you like lasagna less moist with top
browned.

Yield: 16 servings; serving size one 4 ×
3-inch square ■ Each serving contains approximately: Calories: 178 (7% from fat);
Protein: 12 gms; Fat: 1.4 gms; Carbohydrate: 28 gms; Cholesterol: 2 mgs; Sodium: 70 mgs; Allowances: $1\frac{1}{3}$ starches +
$1\frac{3}{8}$ vegetables + $\frac{1}{4}$ dairy + $\frac{1}{6}$ fat

Veggie Spaghetti Sauce

This sauce is delicious on pasta, polenta,
brown rice, or any whole grain. For lower
fat option, omit the walnuts.

1 tablespoon extra virgin olive oil
4–5 garlic cloves, minced
2 cups chopped onions
1 carrot, grated
1 cup chopped celery
2 cups chopped green peppers
2 cups cubed eggplant
8 ounces tempeh
2 cups chopped mushrooms
$\frac{1}{2}$ cup chopped fresh parsley
2 teaspoons basil
2 teaspoons oregano
1 bay leaf
2 28-ounce cans no-salt plum tomatoes
$\frac{1}{2}$ cup chopped walnuts
2 18-ounce cans no-salt tomato paste
2 cups water

Heat olive oil in large cast iron skillet. Sauté garlic and the next 7 ingredients (onions through mushrooms) in the order listed. When the vegetables are al dente, or slightly crisp, add spices and walnuts and cook for another 2 to 3 minutes. Stir in tomato paste and water and simmer for an hour or so.

Yield: 20 1-cup servings. ■ Each serving contains approximately: *Sauce:* Calories: 118 (40% from fat); Protein: 7 gms; Fat: 5.3 gms; Carbohydrate: 14 gms; Cholesterol: 0; Sodium: 42 mgs; Allowances: $\frac{1}{4}$ starch + 2 vegetables + 1 fat. *With 1 cup of spaghetti:* Calories: 273 (20% from fat); Protein: 11 gms; Fat: 6.1 gms; Carbohydrate: 48 gms; Cholesterol: 0; Sodium: 42 mgs; Allowances: $2\frac{1}{4}$ starches + 2 vegetables + 1 fat

My Favorite Marinara Sauce

1 teaspoon extra virgin olive oil
5 garlic cloves, minced
1 large onion, chopped (about 1 cup)
1 cup water or *Basic Veggie Stock* (see page 249)
2 teaspoons fresh lime juice
1 cup tomato purée
$\frac{1}{4}$ cup tomato paste
6 canned no-salt plum tomatoes
1 tablespoon minced fresh basil
1 teaspoon minced fresh oregano
1 teaspoon minced fresh parsley
$\frac{1}{4}$ teaspoon dried thyme
$2\frac{1}{4}$ teaspoons honey

Heat olive oil in a large pot (preferably cast iron). Sauté garlic for a few seconds, and then add onion, stirring occasionally until translucent. Add the remaining ingre-

dients and simmer over low heat for 30 minutes to 2 hours, depending upon available time and personal preference. More water may be needed if your preference is for a long, slow simmer.

Yield: 4 servings; serving size 1 cup plus 1 tablespoon ■ Each serving contains approximately: Calories: 96 (16% from fat); Protein: 3 gms; Fat: 1.7 gms; Carbohydrate: 20 gms; Cholesterol: 0; Sodium: 25 mgs; Allowances: $3\frac{1}{3}$ vegetables + $\frac{1}{4}$ fat

Gnocchi via Mangione

This recipe was inspired by a wonderful meal served by Mangione Ignazio at l'Osteria di via Solata in Bergamo, Italy. His enthusiasm for food and life spilled over into some of the best gnocchis I have ever had. This is a modified version that he translated from their chef, Andrea Corrone.

3 pounds boiling potatoes (do not use new, red, or Idaho baking potatoes)
5 cups enriched all-purpose flour
2 egg whites

Boil potatoes for approximately 2 hours, or until skins are cracked. Allow to cool a bit, then peel. Mash well (a potato ricer works best for this). Gradually add all but $\frac{1}{2}$ cup of the flour, which will be needed to keep your board floured. Knead into a dough ball. Place the dough on a floured board. Create a well in the middle of the dough ball and add egg whites; knead them well into the dough.

Cut off approximately one fourth of the dough, placing the remaining portion on a well-floured cookie sheet in the freezer to be rolled out later. Roll the dough into cylinders about the thickness of your thumb. Cut cylinders into 1-inch pieces. Traditionally, these little potato dumplings are indented with your thumb, or imprinted with a fork. The indentations will give the marinara sauce more surface area to adhere to.

Place gnocchis on a floured cookie sheet in the freezer. Retrieve another portion of dough from the freezer to continue gnocchi-making process. Store frozen gnocchis in a large zip-lock freezer bag for future use. Of course, the amount you choose to cook now does not need to be frozen.

To cook, place gnocchis in pot of boiling water. After they float to the top of the water, boil them for 2 minutes more. Drain and enjoy topped with marinara sauce!

Yield: approximately 170 gnocchis, or 13 meals of 13 gnocchis per person ■ Each serving contains approximately: Calories: 284 (2% from fat); Protein: 8 gms; Fat: .6 gm; Carbohydrate: 61 gms; Cholesterol: 0; Sodium: 14 mgs; Allowances: $3\frac{1}{2}$ starches

Bowtie and Bean Bonanza

4 medium carrots
4 stalks broccoli
16 ounces pasta (bowties or shells)
1 tablespoon extra virgin olive oil
2 15-ounce cans no-salt black beans, drained
4 medium tomatoes, diced
6 green onions, chopped
2 tablespoons no-salt prepared mustard

1 tablespoon freshly ground horse-radish
Juice of 3 large lemons
$\frac{1}{2}$ cup finely chopped fresh cilantro
Freshly ground black pepper to taste

Before you begin prepping the other ingredients, put a large pot of water to boil for the pasta. Steam carrots for 7 to 8 minutes, then add broccoli and steam for another 8 minutes or until both are barely tender. Add pasta to boiling water. Stir occasionally and check for doneness as directed on package. When *al dente* (tender but slightly firm) pour into a colander, rinse with cold water, and drain. Toss with olive oil.

Slice the carrots julienne style (thinly sliced lengthwise). Chop the broccoli widthwise, taking care to maintain the flowerets. Mix all ingredients into a large bowl and refrigerate.

Yield: 25 cups ■ Each cup contains: Calories: 108 (10% from fat); Protein: 5 gms; Fat: 1.2 gms; Carbohydrate: 20 gms; Cholesterol: 0; Sodium: 14 mgs; Allowances: 1 starch + 1 vegetable + $\frac{1}{10}$ fat

Mihshi Malfuf Bi Zayt (Meatless Cabbage Rolls)
by Farida Gindi

18 cabbage leaves (1 large head)

Stuffing:
1 cup brown basmati rice (or hulled or pearled barley)
1 teaspoon extra virgin olive oil
$1\frac{1}{2}$ cups chopped scallions
$\frac{1}{2}$ cup finely chopped parsley
1 cup chopped tomatoes

½ teaspoon ground allspice
1 cup cooked chickpeas (cooked from ½ cup dried) or 1 cup canned chickpeas, drained
Freshly ground black pepper to taste

Sauce:
3 garlic cloves, minced
1 teaspoon minced fresh mint
¼ cup fresh lemon juice
1 tablespoon extra virgin olive oil

Preheat oven to 350 degrees. Boil 2 cups water, add rice, and cook for at least 45 minutes. Core the cabbage and steam for 5 to 10 minutes. When slightly cooled, the leaves will more easily pull apart. Heat olive oil and sauté scallions for 2 to 3 minutes. (When minimizing oil, you can always add some water to prevent sticking or scorching.) Put scallions into a bowl and add rice and remaining stuffing ingredients. Season to taste with pepper. Place 2 generous tablespoons of stuffing on the base of each leaf. Roll up once and leave the seam underneath to help maintain the roll. Repeat for the 18 rolls. Place rolls in baking dish.

For the sauce: blend the minced garlic with the mint, lemon juice, and olive oil. Pour mixture over the cabbage rolls. Add enough water to the dish to prevent scorching, approximately ¼ inch. Cover and bake for 20 to 30 minutes.

Yield: 6 servings; serving size 3 cabbage rolls ■ Each serving contains approximately: Calories: 181 (20% from fat); Protein: 6 gms; Fat: 4 gms; Carbohydrate: 31 gms; Cholesterol: 0; Sodium: 101 mgs; Allowances: 1 starch + 2⅘ vegetables + ⅔ fat

Armenian Nivik

Serve with bread, rice, or pasta and/or salad as a light meal. It is great hot or cold.

2⅖ cups dried chickpeas (garbanzo beans) or 6 cups no-salt canned
2 large onions, chopped
1 tablespoon extra virgin olive oil
½ cup no-salt tomato paste
1 teaspoon honey
Freshly ground black pepper to taste
3 pounds fresh spinach

Wash dried chickpeas, then place in a bowl and cover with water, covering the beans by a few inches. Soak overnight in a cool place if weather is hot. Rinse beans the next day. Then cover beans again with fresh water and bring to a boil. Reduce heat, cover, and simmer for 1¼ to 1½ hours or until tender.

Sauté onions in olive oil until transparent. Add tomato paste, honey, and black pepper.

Wash spinach carefully, removing all dirt, stems, and blemished leaves; chop or tear into small pieces. Add spinach and onion mixture to cooked chickpeas; mix well.

Cover and simmer for 20 to 30 minutes, adding enough water to prevent sticking.

Yield: 9 servings; serving size 1 cup ■ Each serving contains approximately: *Without rice:* Calories: 190 (16% from fat); Protein: 13 gms; Fat: 3.3 gms; Carbohydrate: 34 gms; Cholesterol: 0; Sodium: 111 mgs; Allowances: 1½ starches + 2 vegetables + ⅓ fat. *With 1 cup rice:* Calories: 422 (10% from fat); Protein: 18 gms; Fat: 4.5 gms; Carbohydrate: 83 gms; Cholesterol: 0; Sodium: 111 mgs; Allowances: $4\frac{1}{2}$ starches + 2 vegetables + $\frac{1}{3}$ fat

Progressive Persian Rice

2 cups brown basmati rice, uncooked
3 cups water
2 cups orange juice
$\frac{2}{3}$ cup raisins or any diced dried fruit, including sundried tomatoes
$\frac{1}{2}$ teaspoon grated orange rind
2 tablespoons chopped fresh mint
2 tablespoons chopped fresh parsely

Place rice in a skillet and cook over moderate heat. Stir frequently until slightly toasted. Add water, orange juice, and raisins. Cover and simmer over low heat until rice is tender, 45 to 50 minutes. Remove from heat and fluff rice with a fork, mixing in the remaining ingredients.

Yield: 5 servings; serving size 1 cup ■
Each serving contains approximately: Calories: 246 (4% from fat); Protein: 4 gms; Fat: 1 gm; Carbohydrate: 56 gms; Cholesterol: 0; Sodium: 4 mgs; Allowances: $2\frac{2}{5}$ starches + 1 fruit

Indian Subzi

This is excellent served with brown rice. Hot peppers can be added if a spicier flavor is desired.

1 tablespoon extra virgin olive oil
1 tablespoon ground turmeric
2 tablespoons ground cumin
3 tablespoons ground coriander
2 onions, chopped

3 garlic cloves, minced
3 new potatoes, cubed
2 cups green beans, snapped
1 small cauliflower, cut into small flowerets
1 small eggplant, cubed
4 tomatoes, diced
1 cup green peas
1 red pepper, chopped
2 tablespoons chopped fresh cilantro
3 cups plain nonfat yogurt

Heat oil in a wok or cast iron pan; add spices, onion, garlic, and potatoes. Cook potatoes at least 10 minutes before adding other vegetables, adding tablespoons of water as needed to prevent sticking or scorching. Then add green beans, cauliflower, and eggplant. Sauté for approximately 15 minutes. Add tomatoes, peas, peppers, and cilantro, and sauté another 5 to 15 minutes depending upon desired tenderness. Stir in yogurt 2 to 3 minutes before removing from heat.

Yield: 9 servings; serving size 1 cup ■
Each serving contains approximately: Calories: 123 (18% from fat); Protein: 8 gms; Fat: 2.5 gms; Carbohydrate: 17 gms; Cholesterol: 0; Sodium: 71 mgs; Allowances: $\frac{1}{3}$ starch + $2\frac{2}{5}$ vegetables + $\frac{2}{5}$ dairy + $\frac{1}{3}$ fat

Hoppin' John Vinaigrette

Hoppin' John without bacon fat will definitely enhance your New Year's blessings. It is beyond luck!

Dressing:
2 tablespoons no-fat/no-salt Dijon mustard
$\frac{1}{2}$ cup red wine vinegar

4 chipotle peppers, reconstituted and minced
1 tablespoon extra virgin olive oil, optional

$1\frac{1}{4}$ pounds dried black-eyed peas
4 garlic cloves, minced
Pinch of dried thyme
1 bay leaf
1 cup uncooked brown basmati rice
3 small carrots, halved lengthwise and thinly sliced
4 scallions, thinly sliced
1 medium red or yellow bell pepper, cored and diced
4 ripe plum tomatoes
4 tablespoons chopped fresh parsley
Freshly ground black pepper to taste

Prepare dressing ingredients, whisking in the oil last, and set aside.

Rinse and sort black-eyed peas. Cover with 2 inches of water and boil with garlic, thyme, and bay leaf for 30 to 40 minutes or until tender. Drain well and place in a large bowl. While the beans are cooking, cook rice for approximately 45 minutes. Add the carrots during the last 5 minutes of cooking. Drain if necessary and add to the black-eyed peas, along with the remaining salad ingredients.

Pour the dressing over the salad while it is still warm and toss gently. Try to let it stand at room temperature for at least one hour before serving to allow the flavors to mingle. It is best served at room temperature.

Yield: 8 servings ■ Each serving contains approximately: *Without dressing:* Calories: 225 (4% from fat); Protein: 11 gms; Fat: 1.1 gms; Carbohydrate: 43 gms; Cholesterol: 0; Sodium: 15 mgs; Allowances: $2\frac{1}{2}$ starches + $\frac{1}{2}$ vegetable + $\frac{1}{2}$ fat. *With dressing:* Calories: 246 (11% from fat); Protein: 11 gms; Fat: 3 gms; Carbohydrate: 44 gms; Cholesterol: 0; Sodium: 15 mgs; Allowances: $2\frac{1}{2}$ starches + $\frac{1}{2}$ vegetable + $\frac{1}{3}$ fat

Kashi Bean Burgers

Freeze extras for future use so that *Kashi Bean Burgers* will be more convenient than meat. Enjoy with *Carolina Cukes,* no-salt mustard, lettuce, and tomato on *Basic Whole Wheat Bread.* Delicious!

$2\frac{1}{2}$ cups uncooked Kashi cereal or try your own mixture of whole oats, barley, brown rice, rye, buckwheat groats, and sesame seeds
$3\frac{1}{2}$ cups uncooked black beans
$\frac{1}{4}$ cup wine (any dry wine will do)
6 garlic cloves, minced
2 large onions, chopped
1 green pepper, chopped
3 cups sliced mushrooms
$\frac{1}{4}$ cup chopped fresh parsley
1 teaspoon freshly ground black pepper
28 ounces no-salt tomato purée
$1\frac{1}{8}$ cups whole wheat flour
Vegetable cooking spray

Cook beans as described in Chapter 12. Bring 5 cups of water to a boil, add Kashi or grain mixture and lower heat to medium. Cook, covered, for 25 minutes, or until water has been absorbed. Remove from heat and let the cereal rest, covered, for 5 minutes.

Heat wine and add garlic, onions, green pepper, mushrooms, parsley, and black pepper. Sauté for 10 to 15 minutes, or until vegetables are tender. Add vegetable mixture and tomato purée to cooked cereal. Add cooked beans and mix thoroughly. Put mixture in food processor and process until approximately $\frac{1}{4}$ of original volume. The mixture should not be puréed into a paste, but left chunky enough to hold together in a patty.

Preheat oven to 400 degrees.

Coat a large baking pan with vegetable cooking spray. Place $\frac{1}{4}$ cup whole wheat flour on a plate or piece of waxed paper. Measure out $\frac{1}{2}$ cup of bean/cereal mixture into the palm of your hand and form into a burger-shaped patty. Lightly dip patties in flour, then place on oiled baking pan. Bake for 20 minutes.

Yield: 18 cups or 36$\frac{1}{2}$-cup burgers. ■
Each burger contains approximately: Calories: 103 (9% from fat); Protein: 4.5 gms; Fat: 1 gm; Carbohydrate: 20 gms; Cholesterol: 0; Sodium: 10 mgs; Allowances: $\frac{3}{4}$ starch + 1$\frac{3}{4}$ vegetables

Prudent Potato Latkes

2 cups freshly mashed potatoes
2 egg whites
1 small onion, grated
1 small green pepper, chopped
1 tablespoon chopped fresh parsley
$\frac{1}{2}$ teaspoon minced fresh basil
$\frac{1}{4}$ cup whole wheat flour
1 teaspoon extra virgin olive oil
Plain nonfat yogurt, optional

In a mixing bowl combine the mashed potatoes, egg whites, onion, pepper, parsley, and basil; mix well. Divide into eight

cakes, and coat with whole wheat flour. Coat skillet or grill with olive oil and pan fry latkes on each side until golden brown. Serve hot, topped with a dollop of plain nonfat yogurt.

Yield: 4 servings; serving size 2 latkes ■
Each contains approximately: Calories: 124 (9% from fat); Protein: 6 gms; Fat: 1.2 gms; Carbohydrate: 24 gms; Cholesterol: 0; Sodium: 30 mgs; Allowances: 1$\frac{3}{5}$ starches + $\frac{2}{3}$ vegetable + $\frac{1}{4}$ fat

Grilled Gourmet Vegetables

Making plenty of vegetables for a meal for four, this would be delicious over quinoa, rice, or pasta.

Marinade:
2 tablespoons extra virgin olive oil
Juice of 5 large limes
5 garlic cloves, minced
1 tablespoon chopped fresh basil
Freshly ground black pepper to taste

20 cherry tomatoes
2 large Vidalia onions or 16 pearl onions
1 large red pepper
1 large yellow pepper
1 large orange or green pepper
12 mushrooms
1 medium eggplant, sliced widthwise into
  $\frac{1}{2}$-inch slices

Combine marinade ingredients and set aside. Wash all vegetables. Cut Vidalia onions and each pepper into 8 pieces. Thread the vegetables pieces (except eggplant) on wooden skewers, putting all of the same type vegetable on the same skewers (for example, all the onions together). This is because the vegetables will cook at different times. Place the sliced eggplant in a shallow, flat casserole, and place skewers of vegetables over them. Pour marinade over vegetables. Cover with plastic wrap and refrigerate for at least an hour. Occasionally spoon marinade over vegetables.

Grill vegetables, preferably over a gas grill. These could be done under a carefully watched oven on broil, turning the skewers over when one side is slightly burnt.

Yield: 4 servings ■ Each serving contains approximately: Calories: 131 (31% from fat); Protein: 5 gms; Fat: 4.1 gms; Carbohydrate: 24 gms; Cholesterol: 0; Sodium: 17 mgs; Allowances: $3\frac{3}{4}$ vegetables + $\frac{3}{4}$ fat. *With 1 cup cooked pasta:* Calories: 290 (14% from fat); Protein: 10 gms; Fat: 4.8 gms; Carbohydrate: 58 gms; Cholesterol: 0; Sodium: 18 mgs; Allowances: 2 starches + $3\frac{3}{4}$ vegetables + $\frac{3}{4}$ fat

Veggie-Stuffed Potatoes

Even people who are confirmed veggie haters are pleasantly surprised by this dish.

4 baking potatoes
1 large head lettuce of choice, chopped
$\frac{1}{4}$ head red cabbage, grated
2 carrots, julienned
2 bell peppers, chopped
1 cucumber, sliced
3 large tomatoes, diced, or carton of cherry tomatoes
$\frac{1}{2}$ head cauliflower, chopped
$\frac{1}{2}$ pound mushrooms, sliced
2 cups plain nonfat yogurt
4 tablespoons no-fat/no-salt salad dressing

Wash potatoes, then microwave for about 10 to 13 minutes or bake at 400 degrees for 1 hour until done. While potatoes are cooking, wash, prep, and mix together the other vegetables. To serve, place one potato on each plate, cut in half, and spread open wide to prepare for toppings. First top each with $\frac{1}{2}$ cup nonfat yogurt, then with mixed vegetables, and finally with 1 tablespoon of salad dressing.

Yield: 4 servings ■ Each serving contains approximately: Calories: 349 (3% from fat); Protein: 15 gms; Fat: 1.2 gms; Carbohydrate: 74 gms; Cholesterol: 2 mgs; Sodium: 137 mgs; Allowances: 3 starches + $\frac{2}{3}$ dairy + 2 vegetables

Seasoned Pinto Beans

These beans freeze beautifully, which makes next week's and next month's suppers a breeze! Great served over any grain or pasta.

6 cups dried pinto beans
1 tablespoon extra virgin olive oil
4 garlic cloves, minced
2 large onions, minced
2 bell peppers, chopped
4 teaspoons cumin
2 teaspoons chili powder
2 teaspoons oregano
1 teaspoon basil
1 16-ounce can no-salt tomatoes
Freshly ground black or red pepper to taste

Cook pinto beans as described in Chapter 12.

Heat olive oil, add garlic, onion, and bell peppers, and sauté until vegetables are still slightly crisp. Add spices and tomatoes, and cook for another 2 to 3 minutes.

Add spiced vegetables to cooked beans and simmer for 15 to 20 minutes. Add pepper to taste.

Yield: approximately 32 servings; serving size ½ cup ■ Each serving contains approximately: Calories: 103 (8% from fat); Protein: 5 gms; Fat: .86 gm; Carbohydrate: 29 gms; Cholesterol: 0; Sodium: 5 mgs; Allowances: 1 starch + 1 vegetable

Basic Black-Eyed Peas
by Dr. Robert Rosati

1 pound dried black-eyed peas
1 onion, chopped
1 tablespoon extra virgin olive oil
12 fresh sage leaves, crushed, or 1 teaspoon dried sage
3 tomatoes, chopped
Freshly ground black pepper to taste

Soak the black-eyed peas overnight, rinsing occasionally to reduce gaseous compounds. Cover with 2 inches of water and simmer with the onion until tender, approximately 40 minutes. Heat the oil with the sage leaves in a large, heavy pot over medium heat until the oil is almost smoking. Then add the cooked beans and stir for 3 minutes. Water may be added to prevent scorching the beans. Add the tomatoes and black pepper, stirring until the tomatoes are warm and a desired consistency is achieved. Serve as your main course or add to *Rosati's Insalata alla Contadina,* page 260.

Yield: 5 servings; serving size a bit more than 1 cup ■ Each serving contains approximately: Calories: 202 (16% from fat); Protein: 11 gms; Fat: 3.7 gms; Carbohydrate: 33 gms; Cholesterol: 0; Sodium: 11 mgs; Allowances: 2¼ starches + vegetables

Bayou Baked Bourbon Beans

5 cups dried navy beans
1 large yellow onion, chopped
¾ cup molasses
2 teaspoons dry mustard or 2 tablespoons no-salt prepared mustard
½ cup brown sugar (brown sugar substitute is available for diabetics)
10 whole cloves
½ teaspoon freshly ground black pepper
1 tablespoon minced ginger root, optional
1 cup bourbon

Preheat oven to 300 degrees.

Wash and sort the beans in cold water. Place chopped onion in the bottom of a 1-gallon bean pot. Pour the drained beans on top of the onions.

Combine remaining ingredients in a bowl except for the bourbon. Pour mixture over the beans and add enough water to cover. Bake, covered, for 5 hours, stirring hourly and adding water to keep the beans covered. Then stir in the bourbon and bake, uncovered, for 1 hour more.

Yield: 14 servings; serving size 1 cup ■ Each serving contains approximately: Calories: 264 (4% from fat); Protein: 12 gms; Fat: 1.2 gms; Carbohydrate:

52 gms; Cholesterol: 0; Sodium: 10 mgs; Allowances: $2\frac{1}{3}$ starches + 1 fruit + 1 vegetable

"Boss" Black Beans

Enjoy on *Salmon and Bean Burritos with Cucumber Salsa,* on page 294. Beans will easily keep for a week if covered with a tight-fitting lid. Freeze what you do not eat this week in pint containers to make "convenience food" for the upcoming months.

5 cups dried black beans
1 large onion, chopped
1 yellow pepper, chopped
1 red pepper, chopped
4 jalapeño peppers, de-seeded and chopped
1 teaspoon ground cumin
1 bay leaf
1–3 chipotle peppers (dependent upon desired hotness)
3 quarts *Basic Veggie Stock* (see page 249)
Juice of 1 lemon

Sort and wash beans, removing any debris. Cook beans as described in Chapter 12. Combine all ingredients except the lemon juice in a stockpot and bring to a boil. Reduce heat to low and simmer, uncovered, until the beans are soft, about $1\frac{1}{2}$ hours. Add more stock as needed to keep the beans immersed during the cooking process. Add lemon juice to taste.

Yield: 17 servings; serving size $\frac{2}{3}$ cup ■ Each serving contains approximately: Calories: 144 (4% from fat); Protein: 10 gms; Fat: .6 gm; Carbohydrate: 26 gms; Cholesterol: 0; Sodium: 2 mgs; Allowances: $1\frac{1}{5}$ starches + 2 vegetables

Southern Succotash

This is almost as good frozen as fresh picked! It's the simplest of summer meals but served with freshly cut tomatoes, it is impossible to beat!

$\frac{1}{2}$ cup *Basic Veggie Stock* (see page 249)
$4\frac{1}{2}$ cups fresh or frozen lima beans
4 cups fresh corn kernels (9 ears) or frozen corn
1 cup chopped Vidalia onion
1 bell pepper, chopped

Mix all ingredients together and simmer for about 20 minutes, or until desired tenderness is obtained.

Yield: 8 servings; serving size a bit more than 1 cup ■ Each serving contains approximately: Calories: 216 (6% from fat); Protein: 10 gms; Fat: 1.4 gms; Carbohydrate: 46 gms; Cholesterol: 0; Sodium: 8 mgs; Allowances: $2\frac{1}{2}$ starches + $\frac{1}{2}$ vegetable

Cornbread and Mushroom Stuffing

This is a great stuffing for turkey, if you still eat turkey. Or, serve it as a base for your favorite beans.

$\frac{1}{4}$ cup white wine
11 cups chopped mushrooms (mixture of portobello, shiitake, chanterelle, or any edible wild mushrooms)
3 cups sliced shallots
1 fennel bulb, thinly sliced
3 cups corn
$\frac{3}{4}$ cup Italian parsley, chopped
1 teaspoon freshly ground black pepper
1 cup *Basic Veggie Stock* (see page 249)

6 cups cubed *D'Liteful Cornbread* (see page 240)

1½ cups homemade mashed potatoes (preferably made with Yukon Gold potatoes)

Vegetable cooking spray

Heat wine in a wok. Add the mushrooms, shallots, and fennel and cook 5 to 10 minutes or until tender. Stir in the corn, parsley, and pepper and sauté for another 1 or 2 minutes. Add a little stock, if needed, to prevent scorching. Add cubed cornbread, mashed potatoes, and remaining stock; stir well.

Preheat oven to 450 degrees. Spray a 13½ × 8¾ × 1¾-inch casserole and an 8-inch round baking dish with vegetable cooking spray.

Place mixture in prepared baking dishes and bake for 30 minutes or until browned.

Yield: 15 servings ■ Each serving contains approximately: Calories: 156 (4% from fat); Protein: 6 gms; Fat: .75 gm; Carbohydrate: 35 gms; Cholesterol: 0; Sodium: 35 mgs; Allowances: 1⅔ starches + ¾ vegetable

Seafood

Fresh Pasta with Smoked Bluefish

½ cup no-salt/no-fat sundried tomatoes

8 ounces fresh fettuccine or 12 ounces dried pasta, preferably tomato fettuccine

2 teaspoons extra virgin olive oil

1 garlic clove, minced

2 tablespoons fresh lime juice

2 tablespoons orange juice

1 pound low-sodium smoked bluefish, diced

1½ cups snow peas, cut into thirds

½ cup plain nonfat yogurt

2 tablespoons white wine

1 tablespoon chopped fresh cilantro

Freshly ground black pepper to taste

Reconstitute dried tomatoes by covering them with warm water for 10 minutes, then drain and coarsely chop. Cook fettuccine in boiling water until *al dente,* or tender to the bite. Heat oil, add garlic, and sauté 30 seconds. Stir in lime juice, orange juice, and tomatoes, and sauté for another minute. Then add fish and snow peas and simmer for about 3 minutes. Stir in yogurt, white wine, and cilantro. Continue cooking over low heat until hot throughout.

Drain fettuccine and rinse with warm water. Add to fish mixture and toss to coat pasta. Serve immediately, topped with freshly ground black pepper.

Yield: 6 servings; serving size 1 cup ■ Each serving contains approximately: Calories: 323 (19% from fat); Protein: 28 gms; Fat: 7 gms; Carbohydrate: 35 gms; Cholesterol: trace; Sodium: 86 mgs; Allowances: 2 starches + ½ vegetable + 2⅖ meats + ⅑ dairy + ⅓ fat

Salmon Cakes

1 $15\frac{1}{2}$-ounce can no-fat/no-salt red sockeye salmon
3 scallions, chopped
2 teaspoons fresh lemon juice
1 tablespoon chopped fresh parsley
$\frac{1}{4}$–$\frac{1}{2}$ small green pepper, chopped
$\frac{1}{4}$–$\frac{1}{2}$ stalk celery, minced
2 teaspoons dry mustard
1 teaspoon ground fresh horseradish
$\frac{1}{4}$ teaspoon dill weed
Dash of garlic powder
1 cup no-fat/no-salt flake cereal
1 egg white, beaten
Extra virgin olive oil

Preheat oven to 350 degrees.

Mix together all ingredients except the cereal, the egg white, and the olive oil. Pat into portions of $\frac{1}{3}$ cup each. Crush cereal into bread crumb consistency by placing it in a small plastic bag and rolling it with a rolling pin. Dip each salmon cake into the beaten egg white then roll in cereal crumbs until coated.

Lightly oil a casserole dish with olive oil. Place salmon cakes in dish and bake for approximately 25 minutes.

Yield: 6 salmon cakes ■ Each salmon cake contains approximately: Calories: 153 (33% from fat); Protein: 17 gms; Fat: 5.7 gms; Carbohydrate: 8 gms; Cholesterol: 32 mgs; Sodium: 69 mgs; Allowances: $\frac{1}{4}$ starch + $\frac{1}{4}$ vegetable + $2\frac{1}{2}$ meats. *With 1 cup brown rice:* Calories: 385 (16% from fat); Protein: 22 gms; Fat: 6.9 gms; Carbohydrate: 58 gms; Cholesterol: 32 mgs; Sodium: 69 mgs; Allowances: $3\frac{1}{4}$ starches + $\frac{1}{4}$ vegetable + $2\frac{1}{2}$ meats

Hot 'n' Sweet Salmon

For an interesting presentation, place a serving of *Corn and Black Bean Salsa* (page 296) on each plate, and top with the salmon. Served with a green vegetable, such as steamed broccoli, this is almost as much fun to view as to eat! Almost!

The combination of honey and chili powder is called Red Chili Honey in the Taos area of northern New Mexico. Natives would suggest that you make it by combining wildflower honey, Chimayo chili powder, and a little crushed, roasted garlic, then let it sit (unrefrigerated) for a few weeks.

4 tablespoons honey
2 tablespoons chili powder
4 6-ounce salmon fillets

Place a well-seasoned cast iron skillet in a preheated 450-degree oven. Combine honey and chili powder and stir well. Thoroughly clean salmon and remove any bones. Pat salmon dry with a paper towel before placing it in the heated skillet in the oven. Sear the fillets for 2 minutes on one side. Before turning them over, brush the top side of each fillet with $1\frac{1}{2}$ teaspoons of the honey-chili mixture. This may be done with a brush, spatula, or knife. Then turn them and cook the other side for 5 minutes, brushing the tops of the salmon with the remaining mixture for the last minute of cooking.

Yield: 4 servings ■ Each serving contains approximately: Calories: 382 (42% from fat); Protein: 35 gms; Fat: 18 gms; Carbohydrate: 19 gms; Cholesterol: 112 mgs; Sodium: 83 mgs; Allowances: 1 fruit + 5 meats. *With 1 cup brown rice:* Calories: 614 (28% from fat); Protein: 40 gms; Fat:

19.2 gms; Carbohydrate: 69 gms; Cholesterol: 112 mgs; Sodium: 83 mgs; Allowances: 3 starches + 1 fruit + 5 meats

Salmon Steaks Topped with Cranberry Sauce

This beautiful and succulent dish proves that cranberries go with more than turkey!

1 cup coarsely chopped fresh cranberries
$\frac{3}{4}$ cup unsweetened orange juice
2 tablespoons finely chopped celery
1 large tomato, chopped
1 tablespoon finely chopped red onion
1 large orange, peeled and coarsely
   chopped
1 tablespoon finely sliced scallion tops
4 4-ounce salmon steaks
Vegetable cooking spray
Orange slices
Sprigs of watercress
Freshly ground black pepper

Combine cranberries and $\frac{1}{2}$ cup of the orange juice in a large skillet. Bring to a boil, reduce heat, and simmer, uncovered, for 8 to 10 minutes or until mixture reduces to the consistency of chunky applesauce. Stir occasionally to prevent sticking. Add celery, tomato, and onion, and cook for another minute. Spoon into a serving bowl; add chopped orange and scallion tops.

While the sauce is cooking, place the fish on a rack coated with cooking spray. If the rack is placed in a roasting pan with a $\frac{1}{2}$ inch of water in the bottom, you dramatically reduce your clean-up hassle! Brush fish with 2 tablespoons orange juice, and broil approximately 4 inches from the heat for 5 minutes. Turn the fish, brush with the remaining 2 tablespoons orange juice, and broil an additional 3 minutes or until fish flakes easily and is starting to brown. Place on a serving plate, spoon sauce over fish, and garnish with orange slices and watercress sprigs, and pepper to taste.

Yield: 4 servings ■ Each serving contains approximately: Calories: 219 (72% from fat); Protein: 24 gms; Fat: 9.5 gms; Carbohydrate: 9 gms; Cholesterol: 74 mgs; Sodium: 61 mgs; Allowances: $\frac{1}{3}$ vegetable + $\frac{3}{4}$ fruit + 3 meats

Foolproof Fish

20 ounces fresh red snapper or grouper fillets (although just about any fish will do)
1 large bell pepper, chopped
1 small red onion, chopped or $\frac{1}{2}$ cup
   chopped scallions
1 large tomato, chopped
Juice of 2 limes
2 tablespoons chopped fresh parsley
2 garlic cloves, minced
Freshly ground black pepper to taste
Dash of white wine or sherry, optional

Preheat oven to 450 degrees.

Place freshly washed and dried fish on a sheet of aluminum foil, $2\frac{1}{2}$ times its size. Combine remaining ingredients, top fish with the mixture, and wrap aluminum foil around your creation. Make sure the seam where the foil meets is on top, so that it will be easier to check for doneness. Place in a pan and bake for 15 to 25 minutes, depending upon the thickness of the fish.

This recipe is fool proof unless you over-cook it! Fish should flake easily with a fork when it is done.

Yield: 4 servings ■ Each serving contains approximately: Calories: 178 (8% from fat); Protein: 30 gms; Fat: 1.5 gms; Carbo-hydrate: 10 gms; Cholesterol: 0; Sodium: 105 mgs; Allowances: 1 vegetable + $3\frac{3}{4}$ meats

"Outta Banks" Seafood Gumbo

$4\frac{1}{2}$ cups cooked brown rice ($1\frac{1}{2}$ cups raw brown rice)
2 cups cooked lentils (1 cup dried lentils)
2 tablespoons extra virgin olive oil
3 tablespoons wheat flour
3 large garlic cloves, minced
3 cups chopped onion (2 large)
6 cups water
2 14-ounce cans no-salt tomatoes or 7 fresh tomatoes, chopped
$\frac{1}{4}$ teaspoon freshly ground black pepper
$\frac{1}{2}$–1 teaspoon crushed red pepper or to taste
1 cup chopped celery
$\frac{3}{4}$ pound okra, trimmed and chopped
1 large red, orange, yellow, or green pepper, chopped
1 pound shrimp, shelled and de-veined
$\frac{1}{2}$ pound fresh fish fillet, cut into bite-size pieces
3 tablespoons chopped fresh parsley
2 teaspoons very-low-sodium Worcester-shire sauce
$\frac{1}{2}$ pound crab meat
$3\frac{1}{2}$ teaspoons filé powder

Start rice and lentils cooking in separate pans while you prepare the other ingredi-ents. Heat oil in Dutch oven, or any large heavy kettle or soup pot over medium heat. Add flour and stir constantly until flour has turned a warm golden brown. (This brown roux is a flour base common to all true gumbos.) Add garlic and onion and sauté for 4 or 5 minutes. Add water and all the remaining ingredients except for crab and the filé powder. Simmer for another 10 minutes. Then add the crab and simmer for another 10 minutes.

If you are not sure that you will finish the gumbo in one meal, it is best to add filé powder only to the amount of gumbo you are going to serve—approximately $\frac{1}{2}$ tea-spoon per $2\frac{1}{2}$ cups. Stir thoroughly as mix-ture thickens. If filé is added initially to the gumbo batch, it will become stringy when reheated.

Yield: 18 servings; serving size 1 cup ■ Each serving contains approximately: Calories: 164 (16% from fat); Protein: 13 gms; Fat: 2.9 gms; Carbohydrate: 22 gms; Cholesterol: 43 mgs; Sodium: 84 mgs; Allowances: $\frac{4}{5}$ starch + 1 vegeta-ble + $1\frac{1}{3}$ meats + $\frac{1}{3}$ fat

Mock Fried Fish

1 pound fresh fish fillets (catfish, floun-der, or red snapper are good)
$\frac{1}{8}$ cup skim milk
1 cup no-fat/no-salt/no-sugar cereal
$\frac{1}{2}$ teaspoon paprika
$\frac{1}{4}$ teaspoon garlic powder
$\frac{1}{8}$ teaspoon dry mustard
$\frac{1}{2}$–1 teaspoon salt-free Spike, Mrs. Dash, or Italian seasonings
1 teaspoon extra virgin olive oil
Lemon slices
Fresh parsley sprigs

Preheat oven to 350 degrees.

Rinse fish, pat day, and place in dish with milk. Put the cereal, paprika, garlic powder, mustard, and seasoning in a zip-lock plastic bag, close it, and crush with a rolling pin. Empty dry mixture onto a plate and dip fillets into it, coating fish on both sides.

Place coated fish on baking sheet that has been lightly greased with the olive oil. Bake 15 to 20 minutes, or until fish is browned and flakes easily with a fork. Garnish with lemon slices and parsley sprig.

Yield: 4 servings ■ Each serving contains approximately: Calories: 157 (8% from fat); Protein: 24 gms; Fat: 1.5 gms; Carbohydrate: 10 gms; Cholesterol: 40 mgs; Sodium: 57 mgs; Allowances: $\frac{1}{3}$ starch + 3 meats

Carolina Country Pickled Shrimp

These shrimp will keep for a week, but they never last that long at our house!

1$\frac{1}{4}$ cups tarragon vinegar
$\frac{3}{4}$ cup water
6 nickel-size slices fresh gingerroot
1 teaspoon honey
$\frac{1}{4}$ cup coriander seeds
1 tablespoon fennel seeds
1 tablespoon mustard seeds
1 teaspoon whole allspice berries
2 pounds medium-large shrimp
1 large red or Vidalia onion, thinly sliced
2 large lemons, thinly sliced and seeded
8 garlic cloves
3 dried chipotle peppers, reconstituted in $\frac{1}{4}$ cup hot water, drained and finely chopped

5 bay leaves
1 tablespoon freshly grated horseradish, optional
$\frac{1}{2}$ cup extra virgin olive oil
1 tablespoon no-salt prepared mustard

In a stainless steel saucepan, combine the vinegar, water, gingerroot, honey, coriander, fennel, mustard seed, and allspice berries. Bring to a boil over moderately high heat, then lower heat and simmer for approximately 10 minutes. Let the pickling mixture cool. Add the shrimp to a large pot of boiling water. Remove from the heat and let stand for 3 minutes or until the shrimp turn pink. Drain, cool, then shell and de-vein the shrimp.

In a large-mouth half-gallon glass jar, alternate layers of the shrimp, onions, lemon, garlic, peppers, bay leaves, and horseradish. Whisk the olive oil and mustard into the pickling mixture, then pour over the shrimp. Cover the jar tightly and refrigerate for at least two days.

Yield: 10 servings; serving size about thirteen shrimp ■ Each serving contains approximately (As olive oil solidifies with refrigeration and many of the spices are not eaten, calculation was estimated for actual consumption of $\frac{1}{4}$ the oil and $\frac{1}{2}$ the spices.): Calories: 145 (20% from fat); Protein: 19 gms; Fat: 3 gms; Carbohydrate: 6 gms; Cholesterol: 138 mgs; Sodium: 137 mgs; Allowances: 3 meats + $\frac{3}{5}$ fat

Tuna Salad

4–8 radicchio and Bibb lettuce leaves
16$\frac{1}{8}$-ounce can tuna or 6$\frac{1}{8}$ ounces fresh grilled tuna

5 teaspoons mustard
1 teaspoon honey
½ tomato, chopped
Freshly ground black pepper to taste

Place radicchio and lettuce leaves on a plate, alternating the red and green leaves. Blend the remaining ingredients and place on radicchio and lettuce leaves. This is also great served between two slices of *Basic Whole Wheat Bread*, page 239.

Yield: 2 servings ■ Each serving contains approximately: Calories: 117 (15% from fat); Protein: 29 gms; Fat: 2 gms; Carbohydrate: 4.5 gms; Cholesterol: 30 mgs; Sodium: 48 mgs: Allowances: ¼ vegetable + 3 meats

Blastin' Blackened Red Snapper

1½ teaspoons garlic powder
2 teaspoons onion powder
1½ teaspoons dry mustard
1 teaspoon ground thyme
⅛ teaspoon freshly ground black pepper
¼–½ teaspoon crushed red pepper
4 4-ounce red snapper fillets or any fish
¼ teaspoon extra virgin olive oil
1 lemon, quartered

Combine the garlic and onion powders, mustard, thyme, and peppers. Sprinkle approximately ⅛ of the seasoning mixture on each side of the fillets.

Coat a cast iron skillet (or any fry pan) with the olive oil. Place the skillet on a medium-high burner and when hot, add the fillets. Cook 4 minutes. Turn and cook for 3 or 4 minutes more or until fish flakes easily. Squeeze a quarter of a

lemon on each fillet, as needed, to prevent sticking.

Yield: 4 servings ■ Each fillet contains approximately: Calories: 122 (10% from fat); Protein: 23 gms; Fat: 1.4 gms; Carbohydrate: 3 gms; Cholesterol: 42 mgs; Sodium: 78 mgs; Allowances: 3 meats

Asparagus and Salmon Surprise

1 teaspoon olive oil
1 large garlic clove, minced
6 scallions, chopped
½ teaspoon minced fresh gingerroot
½ cup *Basic Veggie Stock* (see page 249) or water with no-sodium bouillon cube)
2 tablespoons plus 1 tablespoon freshly squeezed lemon juice
2 cups fresh asparagus cut into 1-inch pieces, (if using frozen asparagus, thaw first)
8 ounces thin spaghetti (vermicelli)
1 9-ounce package of frozen artichoke hearts, chopped
1 7½-ounce can red sockeye salmon, drained, rinsed, and broken into large chunks
Freshly ground black pepper to taste

Start heating a large pot of water for the pasta. Heat olive oil in a large saucepan or cast iron skillet. When oil is hot, add the garlic, scallions, and ginger. Sauté for approximately one minute, stirring as needed. Add the stock, 1 tablespoon of the lemon juice, and the asparagus, and simmer for 1 or 2 minutes. (If using frozen asparagus, cook for only 1 minute.) Put vermicelli in boiling water (it should be ready in about 5 minutes when your topping will be). Microwave artichokes as directed on package, then coarsely chop. Add the artichokes to the stock and sauté for another couple of minutes, then add the salmon and pepper. Sauté 1 or 2 minutes more to ensure a consistent temperature.

When pasta is *al dente* (tender but still firm), drain it in a colander, then toss with the remaining 2 tablespoons of lemon juice. Divide the pasta among four plates and top with the asparagus-salmon mixture.

Yield: 4 servings ■ Each serving contains: Calories: 352 (18% from fat); Protein: 21 gms; Fat: 7 gms; Carbohydrate: 53 gms; Cholesterol: 18 mgs; Sodium: 54 mgs; Allowances: $2\frac{3}{4}$ starches + 1 vegetable + $1\frac{4}{5}$ meats + $\frac{1}{4}$ fat

International Flavors

Mexican/Southwestern

New Mexican Green Chili Sauce

This sauce is splendid with eggs, potatoes, bean burritos, or fish. The sauce can be refrigerated for up to 4 days or frozen for up to 2 months. Re-heat slowly as you do not want to scorch this precious stuff!

$2\frac{1}{2}$ pounds fresh green chilis, roasted, peeled, seeded, de-veined, and chopped to measure 3 cups (see note)
4 cups water
$\frac{1}{2}$ medium white onion, diced
4 teaspoons roasted Mexican oregano
1 teaspoon roasted ground cumin
8 garlic cloves, finely minced

Note: You can substitute Anaheim and jalapeño or serrano chilis for the New Mexican green chilis if you must.

Buy green chilis already roasted (see Appendix A) or prepare as instructed in About Ingredients. Place all the ingredients in a large saucepan over medium heat. Simmer 20 to 30 minutes or until the liquid has thickened. Stir occasionally to ensure that the chilis are not sticking to the bottom of the pan. If you prefer a less chunky sauce, you can put one half of the sauce into a food processor and pulse lightly until desired consistency is achieved.

Yield: 14 servings; serving size $\frac{1}{4}$ cup ■ Each serving contains approximately: Calories: 12 (16% from fat); Protein: .5 gm; Fat: .2 gm; Carbohydrate: 3 gms; Cholesterol: 0; Sodium: 2 mgs; Allowances: $\frac{1}{2}$ vegetable

Salmon–Black Bean Burrito with Cucumber Salsa

Cucumber Salsa:
2 cucumbers, peeled in alternating strips and thinly sliced
$\frac{1}{2}$ yellow bell pepper, seeded and finely chopped
$\frac{1}{2}$ red bell pepper, seeded and finely chopped
$\frac{1}{4}$ cup finely diced red onion

2 teaspoons finely chopped fresh dill
  leaves
3 tablespoons coarsely chopped fresh
  cilantro
1 serrano chili, stemmed, seeded, and
  finely minced (any hot pepper will do)
2 tablespoons red wine vinegar

Burrito:
$\frac{1}{2}$ cup *Yogurt Cheese* (see page 247)
4 teaspoons finely minced fresh thyme
  leaves
4 teaspoons finely minced fresh basil
  leaves
4 teaspoons finely minced fresh Italian
  parsley
1 tablespoon fresh lime juice
2 teaspoons olive oil
2 tablespoons chili powder (Chimayo chili
  powder if available)
4 6-ounce salmon fillets
$1\frac{1}{3}$ cups *"Boss" Black Beans* (see page
  287)
4 flour tortillas

Combine the salsa ingredients in a large bowl and mix thoroughly. This may be prepared an hour before serving.

Blend the yogurt cheese, thyme, basil, and parsley in another bowl with a spatula. Cover and refrigerate until you are ready to assemble the burrito.

Prepare a charcoal or gas grill. Wash and dry the salmon fillets, checking carefully for any hidden bones. Mix the lime juice, olive oil, and chili powder together, then paint this on each side of the salmon fillets. When the fire is hot, place the salmon fillets on the grill rack and cook 2 to 3 minutes per side, depending upon the thickness of the fillets and personal preference for doneness.

While the salmon is grilling, heat the beans. Next, warm the tortillas in a cast iron skillet on medium heat, approximately 15 seconds per side. (The tortillas can also be wrapped in foil, sprinkled with water, and heated in the oven or on the grill.) Take care not to overcook them, as they lose their pliability. They can be kept warm wrapped in a dry cloth towel.

To assemble: Place a tortilla on a warmed serving plate. Spread 2 tablespoons of the seasoned yogurt cheese on the tortilla, then $\frac{1}{4}$ cup of the beans in the center, and top with a grilled salmon fillet. Wrap the tortilla around these ingredients, then roll the seam or end underneath to hold the burrito closed. Top each burrito with one fourth of the cucumber salsa.

Yield: 4 servings ■ Each serving contains approximately: Calories: 464 (20% from fat); Protein: 49 gms; Fat: 10.5 gms; Carbohydrate: 45 gms; Cholesterol: 88 mgs; Sodium: 216 mgs; Allowances: $1\frac{4}{5}$ starches + $\frac{3}{4}$ vegetable + $4\frac{1}{2}$ proteins + $\frac{1}{3}$ dairy + $\frac{1}{2}$ fat

Kitty's Sassy Salsa

$\frac{1}{2}$ bell pepper, finely chopped
3 fresh tomatoes, diced
5 scallions, chopped (use both green and
  white parts)
2 garlic cloves, minced
$1\frac{1}{2}$ tablespoons chopped fresh cilantro
Juice of 1 lemon
$\frac{1}{2}$–1 jalapeño pepper, seeded and minced
  to taste

This is so simple—just combine all ingredients and prepare yourself for the best salsa you have ever had!

Yield: 2½ cups ∎ Each 2-ounce serving contains approximately: Calories: 10 (8% from fat); Protein: .4 gm; Fat: .09 gm; Carbohydrate: 2 gms; Cholesterol: 0; Sodium: 4 mgs; Allowances: ⅖ vegetable

Latin Bean Dip

2 cups *Seasoned Pinto Beans* (see page 285)
½ cup plain nonfat yogurt
1 fresh jalapeño pepper, seeded (or more if you like it hot)
1 cup *Kitty's Sassy Salsa* (see page 295)

Combine pinto beans, yogurt, and jalapeño pepper in a food processor and purée. Then add the salsa, and blend to desired consistency. The less you blend it after the salsa addition, the better the color and texture.

Yield: 3½ cups ∎ Each 2-ounce serving contains approximately: Calories: 37 (7% from fat); Protein: 2 gms; Fat: .3 gm; Carbohydrate: 7 gms; Cholesterol: 0; Sodium: 24 mgs; Allowances: ⅓ starch + ⅛ vegetable

Fat-Free Tortilla Chips

Although no-fat/no-salt corn chips are now on the market, this recipe is supplied in case they are not available in your area.

24 no-fat/no-salt corn tortillas
Garlic powder, cumin, chili powder, or any salt-free spice that you would like to try
Vegetable cooking spray

Preheat oven to 350 degrees.

Line a baking sheet with parchment or mist with vegetable cooking spray. Cut each tortilla into 8 equal pieces and spread them over the baking sheet. Bake for 10 minutes or until the chips curl and are slightly browned.

Remove from the oven and spray lightly with the vegetable cooking spray. Sprinkle with the spice or herb of your choice.

Yield: 24 servings; serving size 8 chips ∎ Each serving contains approximately: Calories: 67 (15% from fat); Protein: 2 gms; Fat: 1.1 gms; Carbohydrate: 13 gms; Cholesterol: 0; Sodium: 53 mgs; Allowances: ⅘ starch

Corn and Black Bean Salsa

Delicious as a colorful base for *Hot 'n' Sweet Salmon* (page 289). Or, double the portion for a main dish.

1½ cups fresh corn kernels
½ cup chopped red pepper
2 teaspoons chopped jalapeño
½ teaspoon honey
½ cup water
1½ cups *"Boss" Black Beans* (see page 287), or canned no-salt black beans
½ cup chopped tomatoes
3 tablespoons vinegar
1 teaspoon extra virgin olive oil
Juice and grated zest of 1 lime
½ cup chopped fresh cilantro or basil

Cook corn, peppers, and honey in water over medium heat, covered, for 2 to 3 minutes. Add beans and their juice, tomatoes, vinegar, and oil; cook for 2 to 3 minutes more. Remove from heat and toss in lime juice and zest and basil or cilantro.

Yield: 4 cups, or 8 servings; serving size $\frac{1}{2}$ cup ■ Each serving contains approximately: Calories: 71 (17% from fat); Protein: 4 gms; Fat: 1.3 gms; Carbohydrate: 16 gms; Cholesterol: 0; Sodium: 12 mgs; Allowances: $\frac{3}{4}$ starch + $\frac{1}{2}$ vegetable

Green Chili Salsa

Enjoy this as a dip with your no-fat/no-salt corn chips or as a spicy topping for fish or eggs.

5 large tomatoes
$1\frac{1}{4}$ pounds green chilis, roasted and peeled (approximately $1\frac{1}{2}$ cups, chopped) (see note)
6 garlic cloves, minced
2 tablespoons chopped fresh cilantro

Note: Buy green chilis already roasted (see mail order source in Appendix A), or roast your own as directed in the About Ingredients section.

Remove stems, seeds, and veins from the inside of the chilis, and chop coarsely. Roast tomatoes by placing them in a broiler pan a few inches from the broiling unit. Scorch skin completely by turning the tomatoes until they are blackened evenly. Remove stems, skins, and seeds and chop. Mix all of the ingredients together.

Yield: 4 cups, or 16 servings; serving size $\frac{1}{4}$ cup ■ Each serving contains approximately: Calories: 14 (12% from fat); Protein: .6 gm; Fat: .2 gm; Carbohydrate: 3 gms; Cholesterol: 0; Sodium: 6 mgs; Allowances: $\frac{1}{2}$ vegetable

Mexican Bean Salad

10 ounces frozen corn kernels
1 teaspoon olive oil
2 garlic cloves, minced
1 small onion, chopped
2 tablespoons apple cider vinegar
3 Anaheim peppers, chopped
1 small sweet red pepper, chopped
1 15-ounce can no-salt black beans
2 tablespoons chopped fresh cilantro
$\frac{1}{2}$ teaspoon oregano
$\frac{1}{2}$ teaspoon cumin
$\frac{1}{2}$ teaspoon chili powder

Cook the frozen corn and set aside. In a wok, heat olive oil over high heat. Add garlic, onion, vinegar, and peppers. Stir-fry until more liquid is needed.

Drain beans, reserving $\frac{1}{2}$ cup of the bean juice. Add the bean juice and the remaining spices to the wok. Add beans, corn, cilantro, and spices to the vegetable mixture, mix well, and heat for 10 minutes to blend flavors.

Refrigerate and enjoy later on top of a mixed tossed salad.

Yield: $4\frac{1}{2}$ cups, or 4 servings just over 1 cup each ■ Each serving contains approximately: Calories: 130 (10% from fat); Protein: 8 gms; Fat: 1.5 gms; Carbohydrate: 32 gms; Cholesterol: 0; Sodium: 13 mgs; Allowances: $1\frac{2}{5}$ starches + $\frac{1}{3}$ vegetable + $\frac{1}{4}$ fat

Chipotle and Rosemary Barbecue Sauce

This is great to use on *Barbecued Tempeh on Quinoa* (see below).

¾ cup double strength Postum
1 cup no-salt ketchup
¼ cup molasses
4 tablespoons apple cider or balsamic
   vinegar
2 teaspoons orange juice concentrate
2 teaspoons no-fat/no-salt Dijon mustard
3 sprigs fresh rosemary
2 chipotle peppers, pierced with fork

Combine all ingredients in a small saucepan and simmer over low heat for 15 minutes. Cook uncovered, stirring occasionally. Remove the rosemary sprigs and chipotle peppers.

Yield: approximately 2 cups, or 8 servings; serving size ¼ cup ■ Each serving contains approximately: Calories: 29 (1% from fat); Protein: trace; Fat: 0.5 gm; Carbohydrate: 6 gms; Cholesterol: 0; Sodium: 12 mgs; Allowances: 1 vegetable

Barbecued Tempeh on Quinoa

This is delicious accompanied by *Grilled Gourmet Vegetables,* page 284.

16 ounces no-salt tempeh
1½ cups quinoa
½ cup *Chipotle and Rosemary Barbecue Sauce* (on this page)

Put four cups of water to boil in a medium saucepan. Cut tempeh into finger-sized strips, coat with the barbeque sauce, then grill (for approximately 4 minutes per side). While tempeh is grill-ing, cook quinoa. Rinse quinoa until the water runs clear, then add to boiling water and cook, covered, 15 minutes. Remove from heat and set aside for 5 minutes, then fluff with a fork.

When tempeh has been grilled until slightly browned, remove and serve atop quinoa.

Yield: 4 servings ■ Each serving contains approximately: Calories: 421 (19% from fat); Protein: 32 gms; Fat: 9 gms; Carbohydrate: 53 gms; Cholesterol: 0; Sodium: 23 mgs; Allowances: 5 starches + ½ vegetable

Chilis Rellenos Sin Aceite o Sal (Stuffed Chilis Without Oil or Salt)

This vegetable stuffing can also be served wrapped in a warm flour or corn tortilla. It's also a great side dish with salmon or as a luncheon dish.

3 cups cooked brown rice
1 cup *Boss Black Beans* (see page 287) or
   canned no-salt black beans
3 tomatoes
1 ear of corn
3 tablespoons red wine or *Basic Veggie Stock* (see page 249)
4 garlic cloves, minced
1 medium onion, chopped
6 okra pods, chopped
2 tablespoons chopped fresh cilantro
8 New Mexico roasted green chilis (see note)

Note: Order green chilis roasted from Appendix A source or roast as directed in About Ingredients.

Roast tomatoes in a broiler pan 4 inches below broiler unit. Turn tomatoes until all surfaces are blackened evenly. Remove peels, cores, and seeds, then chop tomatoes. Remove corn kernels from the cob. Heat wine or stock to sauté the corn, tomatoes, garlic, onion, okra, and cilantro. Sauté until tender, then add the beans and rice. Peel chilis, slit them lengthwise and remove the seeds and veins within. Fill the chilis with the vegetable stuffing mixture and microwave for 2 minutes, or heat in a 350-degree oven until warm.

Yield: 4 servings; serving size 2 chilis
■ Each serving contains approximately:
Calories: 324 (6% from fat); Protein: 11 gms; Fat: 2 gms; Carbohydrate: 69 gms; Cholesterol: 0; Sodium: 23 mgs; Allowances: $2\frac{4}{5}$ starches $+$ $3\frac{1}{2}$ vegetables

Green Chili Cream Sauce
by Joy Nelson

Enjoy this sauce on bean burritos, vegetables, or seafood dishes. Add some jalapeños if you prefer it a little hotter.

5 fresh green chilis (such as Anaheim peppers), finely chopped
$\frac{1}{4}$ cup chopped onion
2 teaspoons canola or olive oil
2$\frac{1}{2}$ cups skim milk
3 tablespoons wheat flour
1$\frac{1}{2}$ teaspoons finely chopped fresh cilantro
$\frac{1}{8}$ teaspoon white pepper
1 tablespoon white wine

Heat the oil and sauté the chopped chilis and onion over low heat for 8 to 10 minutes. While the chili mixture is sautéing, bring the milk to the boiling point, taking care not to scorch it (use a microwave, if available). Put the chili mixture, flour, and cilantro in the container of a food processor and process until smooth. Add the purée to the heated milk and stir with a wire whisk until thickened, about 5 minutes. Stir in pepper and wine; cover and let stand for a minute or two before serving to allow wine to blend with the sauce.

Yield: 16 servings; serving size $\frac{1}{4}$ cup
■ Each serving contains approximately:
Calories: 30 (19% from fat); Protein: 2 gms; Fat: .7 gms; Carbohydrate: 4 gms; Cholesterol: 0; Sodium: 21 mgs; Allowances: $\frac{2}{5}$ vegetable $+$ $\frac{1}{7}$ dairy $+$ $\frac{1}{7}$ fat

Poblano and Tomatillo Chili

6 poblano peppers
1$\frac{1}{2}$ pounds tomatillos (25 medium)
1$\frac{1}{2}$ cups chopped onion
5 garlic cloves, minced
1 cup texturized vegetable protein (TVP)
1 tablespoon cumin
1 tablespoon minced fresh oregano or 1 teaspoon dried
$\frac{1}{2}$ cup chopped fresh cilantro
2 tablespoons fresh lemon or lime juice
5 no-fat/no-salt corn tortillas
5 tablespoons plain nonfat yogurt
Freshly grated lemon rind, optional

Place peppers within 3 inches of the broiler in the oven. Broil, turning them approximately three times, until they are evenly scorched. When peppers are thoroughly blackened, wrap in moist paper towels and place in a paper bag to "sweat" for 5 to 10 minutes. Remove from bag and peel scorched skin from peppers with the paper towel. Slice peppers lengthwise into $\frac{1}{4}$-inch strips; set aside.

Remove the papery husks from tomatillos, rinse, place in saucepan, and cover with water. Bring to a boil and cook 8 minutes or until tender. Drain tomatillos, reserving $1\frac{1}{2}$ cups cooking liquid. Set aside.

Sauté peppers, onion, and garlic in 1 cup of reserved tomatillo liquid for 5 minutes, stirring frequently. Add TVP, cumin, and oregano, stirring well. Bring to a boil, reduce heat, and simmer for $1\frac{1}{2}$ hours, stirring occasionally. Add more tomatillo liquid, if needed. Stir in cilantro and lemon juice, and cook for an additional 5 minutes.

Wrap tortillas in damp paper towels, then in aluminum foil and heat in a 350-degree oven for 10 minutes. They can also be warmed in a cast iron skillet on the stove top (medium-high). Ladle chili into colorful soup bowls, top with yogurt, and garnish with lemon rind, if desired. Serve with warm tortillas.

Yield: 5 servings; serving size 1 cup
■ Each serving contains approximately: Calories: 149 (20% from fat); Protein: 9 gms; Fat: 3.5 gms; Carbohydrate: 32 gms; Cholesterol: 0; Sodium: 38 mgs; Allowances: $1\frac{2}{5}$ starches + $1\frac{1}{3}$ vegetables + $\frac{1}{10}$ dairy

Tremendous Chili with TVP

This great fall or winter dish freezes beautifully. A guaranteed hit for vegetarians and meat lovers!

8 cups cooked pinto beans (4 cups uncooked)
6 garlic cloves, minced
2 cups chopped onions
$\frac{1}{4}$ cup red wine
1 green pepper, chopped
1 yellow pepper, chopped
4 tablespoons fresh lime juice
2 tablespoons chili powder
2 teaspoons cumin
1 teaspoon oregano
1 teaspoon sage
2 teaspoons paprika
$\frac{1}{4}$ teaspoon ground bay leaf
28 ounces no-salt tomato purée
2 16-ounce cans no-salt tomatoes
3 cups texturized vegetable protein (TVP)
2 dried chipotle peppers (3 to 5 if you like it really hot)
$\frac{1}{4}$ cup grits
Fresh lime juice and chopped fresh cilantro to taste

Cook pinto beans as outlined in *Tips on Cooking Beans* in Chapter 12. In a large saucepan (preferably cast iron) sauté garlic and onions in wine for 3 or 4 minutes. Add the green and yellow peppers and cook for 3 more minutes, then add the lime juice, spices and herbs, tomato purée, and tomatoes.

Add the TVP and cooked beans to the tomato mixture. Add the dried chipotle peppers, then the grits, and simmer for 20 minutes or more. Remove chipotle peppers, and top with fresh lime juice and cilantro as desired before serving.

Yield: 17 servings; serving size 1 cup ■ Each 1 cup serving contains approximately: Calories: 196 (11% from fat); Protein: 11 gms; Fat: 2.4 gms; Carbohydrate: 35 gms; Cholesterol: 0; Sodium: 32 mgs; Allowances: $1\frac{4}{5}$ starches + 2 vegetables

Rancheros Frittata

This wonderful dish can be breakfast, lunch, or dinner! Serve with flour or corn tortillas.

Vegetable cooking spray
12 egg whites
1 teaspoon turmeric
3 tablespoons skim milk or soy milk, optional
1½ cups *Green Chili Salsa* (see page 297)
1 cup *Boss Black Beans* (see page 287), or canned no-salt black beans
1 cup *New Mexican Green Chili Sauce* (see page 294)

Coat a large cast iron skillet with vegetable cooking spray and warm it over medium heat. Combine the egg whites, turmeric, and milk (if using) in a bowl and beat together with a whisk. Add to skillet when oil is warm and cook, covered, until frittata is almost done. Heat the *Green Chili Salsa* and the black beans. Mix them together and use to coat the top of the frittata. Put the skillet under a broiler to cook the top for a few minutes or until the surface has tightened.

Yield: 4 servings ■ Each serving contains approximately: Calories: 161 (6% from fat); Protein: 16 gms; Fat: 1 gm; Carbohydrate: 23 gms; Cholesterol: trace; Sodium: 172 mgs; Allowances: ¾ starch + 1½ vegetables + 1 protein

Huevos con Frijoles y Chipotles (*Eggs with Beans and Smoked Jalapeños*)

This is great served with no-fat/no-salt corn tortillas which can be just slightly browned in a well-seasoned iron skillet.

Viva con salud, y sin cholesterol! (Live with health, and without cholesterol!)

¼ cup wine
1 chipotle pepper
Juice of 1 lime
3 garlic cloves, minced
1 large onion, chopped
½ green pepper, chopped
½ yellow pepper, chopped
6 mushrooms, sliced
1 large tomato, chopped
¼ cup chopped fresh cilantro
12 egg whites
¼ cup skim milk
½ teaspoon olive oil
8 ounces canned no-salt refried beans

Heat wine and add chipotle pepper to reconstitute. Mince chipotle and save wine to use for sautéing. Prep the vegetables. Heat the wine and lime juice and sauté vegetables, adding them in the order listed above. Beat egg whites with a whisk and add the skim milk while whisking them. When vegetables are just slightly done, set aside.

In an iron skillet or omelet pan, heat olive oil on medium-high. When warm, add beaten egg whites and milk. Cover and cook for a few minutes or until egg mixture is ¾ cooked or semi-solid. Then place skillet under broiler and broil, which will tighten the top of the egg mixture and reduce the odds of scorching the bottom. When omelet is almost firm, remove from broiler and coat it with the refried beans, then top with the spicy vegetable mixture. Serve immediately or return to oven for a last-minute warmup.

Yield: 4 servings ■ Each serving contains approximately: Calories: 153 (16% from fat); Protein: 16 gms; Fat: 2.7 gms; Cholesterol: 0; Sodium: 186 mgs; Allowances: $\frac{3}{5}$ starch + 1½ vegetables + 1 protein + $\frac{1}{16}$ dairy + $\frac{1}{8}$ fat

Guaca-Asparagus

A great alternative to traditional fat-loaded avocado guacamole. Serve with no-fat/no-salt corn chips.

1 pound fresh asparagus
2 tablespoons minced onion
1 large garlic clove, minced
$\frac{1}{8}$ teaspoon white pepper
$\frac{1}{4}$ teaspoon cumin
2 tablespoons no-salt tomato paste
1 tablespoon minced fresh cilantro
1 tablespoon fresh lime juice
Minced fresh chili peppers to taste
1 medium tomato, diced

Wash asparagus. Remove and discard the tough ends by bending the stems at the base until they break. Steam for 10 minutes, or until very soft. Purée in blender. Add remaining ingredients, mix well, and chill.

Yield: 4 servings; serving size ½ cup ■ Each serving contains approximately: Calories: 47 (11% from fat); Protein: 3 gms; Fat: .6 gm; Carbohydrate: 9 gms; Cholesterol: 0; Sodium: 13 mgs; Allowances: 2 vegetables

Tortilla Soup
by Carol Ericsson

1 whole lime
4 cups *Basic Veggie Stock* (see page 249)
6 ounces canned no-salt tomatoes, or 1 large fresh tomato, quartered

1 sprig fresh cilantro
1 jalapeno, chopped
2 corn no-fat/no-salt tortillas

Garnish:
2 no-fat/no-salt corn tortillas
Vegetable cooking spray
2 Roma tomatoes, peeled and de-seeded (any tomato will do if Romas are not available)
Fresh corn from 1 ear or ½ cup frozen corn kernels, thawed
1 scallion, julienned
1 teaspoon diced jalapeño

Simmer all ingredients (except those for garnish) until disintegrated, then strain through cheesecloth or fine strainer.

Fold or cut corn tortillas in half and then julienne into fine strips. Spray lightly with the vegetable cooking spray and bake in a 350-degree oven until golden brown. Garnish soup with browned tortilla strips and remaining garnish ingredients.

Yield: 4 servings ■ Each serving contains approximately: Calories: 111 (11% from fat); Protein: 4 gms; Fat: 1.4 gms; Carbohydrate: 24 gms; Cholesterol: 0; Sodium: 25 mgs; Allowances: 1¼ starches + ½ vegetable

Potato Enchiladas with Chili Sauce
by Carol Ericsson

Superb "straight," and beyond description if topped with *Tomatillo Glaze,* page 303.

4 cups cooked potatoes (use a mixture of New, Yukon Gold, white and sweet potatoes)

2 scallions, chopped
Freshly ground black pepper
12 ounces no-salt salsa
2 tablespoons chili powder
Vegetable cooking spray
8 no-fat/no-salt corn tortillas

Preheat oven to 325 degrees.

Dice and steam potatoes. Fold scallions, black pepper, and 2 tablespoons of salsa into cooked potatoes. Bring remaining salsa and chili powder to a simmer and immerse tortillas for 20 to 30 seconds or until soft and pliable. Roll approximately ½ cup of potato mixture into the softened tortilla; then lay, seam down, in a baking dish that has been lightly coated with a vegetable cooking spray. Spoon 1 tablespoon of the salsa on each enchilada and cover the baking dish with aluminum foil that has been sprayed with vegetable cooking spray—sprayed side toward food. Bake for 20 minutes.

Yield: 4 servings; serving size 2 enchiladas ■ Each serving contains approximately: Calories: 287 (9% from fat); Protein: 8 gms; Fat: 3 gms; Carbohydrate: 60 gms; Cholesterol: 0; Sodium: 136 mgs; Allowances: 3¼ starches + 1 vegetable

Tomatillo Glaze
by Carol Ericsson

Perfect over *Potato Enchiladas with Chili Sauce* (see page 302), this glaze would be delicious topping any bean or grain dish.

1 cup *Basic Veggie Stock* (see page 249)
6 tomatillos
1 small white onion
1 garlic clove
Few sprigs fresh cilantro

Remove papery husks and quarter the tomatillos. Place all ingredients in saucepan and simmer 15 minutes, or until soft. Purée.

Yield: 4 servings; serving size ¼ cup
■ Each serving contains approximately: Calories: 26 (1% from fat); Protein: 1 gm; Fat: 3 gms; Carbohydrate: 6 gms; Cholesterol: 0; Sodium: 8 mgs; Allowances: 1 vegetable

Chinese

Sweet and Sour Cabbage—Peking Style
with Ms. Lan Tan

Seasoning Sauce:
1 tablespoon sugar
3 tablespoons white rice vinegar
2 teaspoons tapioca starch
1 pound Chinese cabbage

1 tablespoon rice wine
¼ cup shredded carrots
1 teaspoon shredded fresh gingerroot
1 teaspoon toasted sesame oil, optional
1 scallion, chopped

Mix the seasoning sauce and set aside.

Clean the cabbage, discarding the discolored and tough parts. Rinse, drain, and cut cabbage into $\frac{1}{2}$ × 2-inch pieces, keeping tougher stem sections separate from the more tender leaves.

Heat the rice wine in a wok on medium-high heat. Add ginger and cabbage stems. Stir-fry for about 2 minutes. Add carrots and the remaining cabbage and stir-fry for another minute. Add the seasoning sauce to the wok, stirring it in thoroughly. Serve hot or cold, garnished with sesame oil and chopped scallion.

Yield: 4 servings ■ Each serving contains approximately: Calories: 52 (26% from fat with oil; 2% without oil); Protein: 2 gms; Fat: 1.5 gms; Carbohydrate: 10 gms; Cholesterol: 0; Sodium: 77 mgs; Allowances: $1\frac{2}{3}$ vegetables + $\frac{1}{4}$ fat

Eggplant Szechuan Style
with Ms. Lan Tan

Seasoning Sauce:
1 tablespoon rice wine
2 teaspoons sugar
1 teaspoon rice wine vinegar
6 tablespoons fat-free, very-low-sodium vegetable or chicken bouillon

1 medium eggplant (1 pound)
1 teaspoon extra virgin olive oil
1 teaspoon shredded fresh gingerroot
1 garlic clove, chopped
2 teaspoons chili powder
1 teaspoon *No-Salt Hoisin Sauce* (see page 307)
1 teaspoon tapioca starch mixed with 1 tablespoon water

1 scallion, chopped
1 teaspoon freshly ground black pepper

Combine ingredients for seasoning sauce and set aside.

Wash eggplant, remove stem, and cut the eggplant into $\frac{1}{2}$-inch slices. Steam over boiling water for 15 to 20 minutes, or until soft. Remove and set aside.

Heat the olive oil in a wok, add ginger, garlic, chili powder, and *No-Salt Hoisin Sauce*. Stir a few seconds and add cooked eggplant and seasoning sauce. Mix well and bring to a boil. Thicken with dissolved tapioca starch. Serve hot, garnished with chopped scallion and freshly ground black pepper.

Yield: 3 servings ■ Each serving contains approximately: Calories: 70 (28% from fat); Protein: 2 gms; Fat: 2 gms; Carbohydrate: 13 gms; Cholesterol: 0; Sodium: 21 mgs; Allowances: $1\frac{1}{2}$ vegetables + $\frac{1}{3}$ fruit + $\frac{1}{3}$ fat. *With 1 cup white rice:* Calories: 293 (7% from fat); Protein: 6 gms; Fat: 2.2 gms; Carbohydrate: 62 gms; Cholesterol: 0; Sodium: 21 mgs; Allowances: 3 starches + $1\frac{1}{2}$ vegetables + $\frac{1}{3}$ fruit + $\frac{1}{3}$ fat

Stir-Fried Fish with Black Bean Sauce
with Ms. Lan Tan

Seasoning Sauce:
2 tablespoons fat-free, very-low-sodium vegetable or chicken bouillon
2 tablespoons rice wine
$\frac{1}{4}$ teaspoon sugar
Pinch white pepper

½ pound fresh grouper (or any medium to firm-fleshed fish, such as snapper)
1 tablespoon tapioca starch
1 tablespoon cooked black beans
2 garlic cloves
2 quarter-sized slices of fresh ginger
1 teaspoon extra virgin olive oil
1 scallion, chopped

Mix the seasoning sauce and set aside.

Clean and dry the fish. Cut into small cubes and sprinkle with the tapioca starch. Chop black beans, garlic, and ginger together.

Heat the oil in a wok, add fish, and stir-fry for about 2 minutes per side. Add the seasoning sauce at any time to prevent scorching. Stir in the black bean mixture, and stir gently for a few moments. Serve hot, garnished with chopped scallion.

Yield: 3 servings ■ Each serving contains approximately: Calories: 97 (23% from fat); Protein: 15 gms; Fat: 2.4 gms; Carbohydrate: 4 gms; Cholesterol: 52 mgs; Sodium: 46 mgs; Allowances: ¼ vegetable + 2 proteins + ⅓ fat. *With 1 cup brown rice:* Calories: 329 (10% from fat); Protein: 20 gms; Fat: 3.6 gms; Carbohydrate: 54 gms; Cholesterol: 52 mgs; Sodium: 46 mgs; Allowances: 3 starches + ¼ vegetable + 2 proteins + ⅓ fat

Chinese Cabbage with Bean Curd
with Ms. Lan Tan

Seasoning Sauce:
2 tablespoons Chinese rice wine
⅛ teaspoon white pepper

¾ cup fat-free, very-low-sodium vegetable or chicken bouillon

4 dried mushrooms
11 tablespoons tree ears
¼ cup golden needles
½ pound Chinese cabbage
8 ounces firm tofu (bean curd)
¼ cup sliced carrots
1 scallion, chopped
1 teaspoon chopped shallots
1 teaspoon freshly grated ginger
1 teaspoon chopped garlic
1 teaspoon extra virgin olive oil
1½ tablespoons tapioca starch mixed with 2 tablespoons water

Combine the seasoning sauce and set aside. Soak the mushrooms, tree ears, and golden needles in hot water for about 15 minutes or until soft. Cut into small pieces. Cut the cabbage into 1 × 2-inch pieces. Cut the bean curd into 1½″ square pieces. Keep the scallion and shallots separate from the ginger and garlic when chopping these.

Heat olive oil in wok until hot. Add ginger and garlic. Stir for a few seconds, then add the seasoning sauce. Next add cabbage, carrots, mushrooms, tree ears, and golden needles. Stir for about 2 minutes, mixing well. Add the bean curd. Cover and cook over medium heat for 2 more minutes or until cabbage is tender. Add the starch mixture. Garnish with chopped scallion and shallots.

Yield: 3 servings ■ Each serving contains approximately: Calories: 135 (35% from fat); Protein: 8 gms; Fat: 5.2 gms; Carbohydrate: 13 gms; Cholesterol: 0; Sodium: 66 mgs; Allowances: ¾ starch + 2½ vege-

tables + $\frac{1}{3}$ fat. *With 1 cup of brown rice:*
Calories: 367 (15% from fat); Protein:
13.2 gms; Fat: 6.4 gms; Carbohydrate:
62.7 gms; Cholesterol: 0; Sodium:
66 mgs; Allowances: $3\frac{3}{4}$ starches +
$2\frac{1}{2}$ vegetables + $\frac{1}{3}$ fat

Rice Noodles with Shrimp and Vegetables
by Ms. Lan Tan

Seasoning Sauce:
Pinch of white pepper
$\frac{2}{3}$ cup no-fat, very-low-sodium vegetable
   or chicken bouillon

Marinade:
1 tablespoon no-fat, very-low-sodium vegetable or chicken bouillon
1 tablespoon rice wine
1 teaspoon tapioca starch

$\frac{1}{2}$ pound shrimp, peeled and de-veined
8 ounces rice noodles
$\frac{1}{2}$ pound cabbage
2 scallions
3 teaspoons extra virgin olive oil,
   divided
1 tablespoon chopped shallots
$\frac{1}{2}$ pound bean sprouts
1 tablespoon curry powder

Combine ingredients for seasoning sauce
and set aside. In another bowl, combine
ingredients for marinade. Rinse shrimp
with cold water, drain, and place in marinade for about 30 minutes.

Soak the rice noodles in warm water
for about 10 minutes. Drain. Shred
the cabbage and scallions into thin strips
and keep shredded vegetables separate.

Heat 1 teaspoon of the olive oil in a
wok until hot. Add shrimp and stir-fry
until the shrimp change color. Remove
and set aside. Heat another teaspoon of
oil in the wok and add the shallots and
cabbage. Stir until soft, then add the
bean sprouts. Mix well. Remove. Heat
the last teaspoon of oil in the wok and
add scallions, curry powder, and rice
noodles. Fry for about 1 minute. Stir in
the seasoning sauce and stir-fry over
medium-high heat until the liquid is almost absorbed. Add the cooked shallots,
cabbage, bean sprouts, and shrimp. Mix
thoroughly.

Yield: 8 servings ■ Each serving contains
approximately: Calories: 177 (19% from
fat); Protein: 11 gms; Fat: 3.8 gms; Carbohydrate: 24 gms; Cholesterol: 43 mgs; Sodium: 57 mgs; Allowances: $1\frac{1}{3}$ starches +
1 vegetable + $\frac{3}{4}$ protein + $\frac{1}{3}$ fat

Steamed Fish, Cantonese Style
by Ms. Lan Tan

Seasoning Sauce:
4 teaspoons no-fat, very-low-sodium vegetable or chicken bouillon
1 tablespoon rice wine
2 teaspoons extra virgin olive oil
Pinch of white pepper

1 pound fresh fish (red snapper, sea bass,
   or sole)
3 scallions
3 quarter-sized slices of fresh ginger

Mix the seasoning sauce and set aside.
Clean fish and pat dry with a paper
towel. Score fish crosswise on both sides
at 1-inch intervals. If the fish is more

than 6 inches long, cut it in half to steam. Place the fish in a shallow bowl.

Slice the scallions in half lengthwise and slice into julienne-shaped pieces 3 inches long. Shred the gingerroot into small matchstick-sized pieces. Pour the seasoning sauce over the fish, and sprinkle on the scallions and ginger.

Steam fish over boiling water. This is best done by placing the bowl containing the fish and toppings into a bamboo steamer, which is then placed over a wok containing a few inches of water. Medium-high heat will be needed for the fish, steaming for about 12 minutes or until the fish flakes with a fork. Remove the fish bowl and transfer the fish and sauce to a larger platter. Serve immediately.

Yield: 4 servings ■ Each serving contains approximately: Calories: 105 (34% from fat); Protein: 16 gms; Fat: 4 gms; Carbohydrate: 0; Cholesterol: 35 mgs; Sodium: 219 mgs; Allowances: 3 proteins + $\frac{1}{2}$ fat. *With 1 cup white rice:* Calories: 328 (12% from fat); Protein: 20 gms; Fat: 4.2 gms; Carbohydrate: 50 gms; Cholesterol: 35 mgs; Sodium: 219 mgs; Allowances: 3 starches + 3 proteins + $\frac{1}{2}$ fat

No-Salt Hoisin Sauce
with Ms. Lan Tan

Traditionally Hoisin Sauce is used on Mu Shu dishes, but it would be good anywhere you want a sweet touch. Use sparingly though, as calories could quickly add up!

1 teaspoon tapioca starch
1 tablespoon water

1 tablespoon no-salt catsup
1 tablespoon no-fat, very-low-sodium vegetable or chicken bouillon
4 tablespoons sugar
2 tablespoons rice vinegar
Pinch of white pepper
2 garlic cloves, minced
$\frac{1}{4}$ teaspoon chili powder
$\frac{1}{2}$ teaspoon fresh lemon juice
$\frac{1}{2}$ teaspoon toasted sesame oil

In a saucepan, dissolve tapioca starch in water. Add all but the sesame oil and stir over low heat. Heat until fairly thick. Remove from heat and stir in sesame oil.

Yield: 5 servings; serving size 1$\frac{1}{2}$ teaspoons ■ Each serving contains approximately: Calories: 41 (11% from fat); Protein: .2 gm; Fat: .5 gm; Carbohydrate: 9 gms; Cholesterol: 0; Sodium: 2 mgs; Allowances: $\frac{1}{8}$ vegetable + $\frac{3}{5}$ fruit + $\frac{1}{10}$ fat

Mu Shu Vegetables with Rice
by Ms. Lan Tan

2 tablespoons tree ears, soaked
4–6 dried mushrooms, soaked
$\frac{1}{4}$ cup dried lily flowers, soaked
$\frac{1}{2}$ cup bamboo shoots
$\frac{1}{2}$ pound Chinese cabbage, stems only
3 teaspoons extra virgin olive oil, divided
1 egg white, slightly beaten
2 scallions, shredded
1 tablespoon *No-Salt Hoisin Sauce* (see this page)
1 tablespoon no-fat, very-low-sodium vegetable or chicken bouillon

Wash the soaked tree ears carefully. Shred the tree ears, mushrooms, lily flowers, bamboo shoots, and cabbage and set aside. Heat 1 teaspoon oil in a wok; scramble the beaten egg white until firm chopping into small pieces with spatula as you stir-fry. Remove. Heat another 1 teaspoon oil in wok. Add half the scallions, stirring over high heat. Add the *No-Salt Hoisin Sauce,* mixing well. Remove and set aside. Heat the last 1 teaspoon oil in wok. Add tree ears, mushrooms, lily flowers, bamboo shoots and cabbage, and stir-fry until the cabbage turns soft. Add the cooked egg white, scallions, and the bouillon.

Serve on rice or wrapped with *Chinese Pancakes,* see this page.

Yield: 4 servings ■ Each serving contains approximately: Calories: 102 (35% from fat); Protein: 3 gms; Fat: 4 gms; Carbohydrate: 16 gms; Cholesterol: 0; Sodium: 51 mgs; Allowances: 2 vegetables + $\frac{1}{3}$ fruit + $\frac{3}{4}$ fat. *With 1 cup brown rice:* Calories: 334 (13% from fat); Protein: 8 gms; Fat: 5 gms; Carbohydrate: 66 gms; Cholesterol: 0; Sodium: 51 mgs; Allowances: 3 starches + 2 vegetables + $\frac{1}{3}$ fruit + $\frac{3}{4}$ fat

Chinese Pancakes
with Ms. Lan Tan

2 cups all-purpose flour
$\frac{3}{4}$ cup boiling water
1 tablespoon toasted sesame oil

Place flour in a large bowl. Gradually add boiling water and mix until smooth. Place on a lightly floured board and knead until the dough is smooth, about 3 to 5 minutes. Cover and let rest for about

15 minutes. Knead the dough again lightly.

Roll the dough into a long sausagelike roll, about 1 inch in diameter. Divide the dough into 16 pieces. Gently roll each piece into a small ball. Flatten each ball with the palm of your hand, and brush sesame oil on one side of the pancake. Place another pancake on top of oiled pancake. Press together and roll again, rotating to keep the circle as uniform as possible. The pancake should be 6 to 7 inches in diameter.

Heat wok until hot, then turn to medium-low. Cook one pair of pancakes over low heat for about 2 minutes or until small bubbles form. Turn over and cook the other side. Remove and separate into two very thin pancakes. Cover with a damp cloth. Continue until all pancakes are cooked.

Serve the pancake with *Mu Shu Vegetables,* page 307, and *No-Salt Hoisin Sauce,* page 307.

Yield: 16 pancakes ■ Each pancake contains approximately: Calories: 70 (13% from fat); Protein: 2 gms; Fat: 1 gm; Carbohydrate: 13 gms; Cholesterol: 0; Sodium: trace; Allowances: $\frac{3}{4}$ starch + $\frac{1}{5}$ fat

Stir-Fried Grouper with Asparagus
with Ms. Lan Tan

Seasoning Sauce:
1 tablespoon no-fat, very-low-sodium vegetable or chicken bouillon
1 tablespoon rice wine

¼ teaspoon sugar
Pinch of cayenne pepper

½ pound fresh fish, preferably grouper
2 teaspoons plus 1 teaspoon tapioca
  starch
3 garlic cloves, chopped
1 tablespoon freshly chopped ginger
1 scallion, chopped
1 pound fresh asparagus
1 tablespoon extra virgin olive oil
3 tablespoons water

Combine ingredients for seasoning sauce and set aside.

Clean and dry the fish. Cut into small cubes and sprinkle with 2 teaspoons of the tapioca starch. Remove the tough ends of the asparagus by bending the stems at the base until they break. Break the asparagus into 1-inch pieces.

Heat the olive oil in a wok, add fish, and stir-fry for about 2 minutes per side. Remove. In the same wok, add the chopped ginger, garlic, and asparagus. Stir for 2 to 3 minutes, then add the cooked fish and the seasoning sauce. Stir and mix gently. Mix 1 teaspoon tapioca starch in 3 tablespoons water, then mix thoroughly into the stir-fry. Serve hot, garnished with chopped scallion.

Yield: 3 servings ■ Each serving contains approximately: Calories: 165 (33% from fat); Protein: 18 gms; Fat: 6 gms; Carbohydrate: 10 gms; Cholesterol: 27 mgs; Sodium: 47 mgs; Allowances: ½ vegetable + 2 proteins + 1 fat. *With 1 cup white rice:* Calories: 388 (14% from fat); Protein: 22 gms; Fat: 6.2 gms; Carbohydrate: 60 gms; Cholesterol: 27 mgs; Sodium: 47 mgs; Allowances: 3 starches + ½ vegetable + 2 proteins + 1 fat

Vegetable Lo Mein
with Ms. Lan Tan

4 dried black mushrooms
½ pound fresh or dried noodles
1 teaspoon toasted sesame oil
3 tablespoons rice wine
1 scallion, cut into 1-inch pieces
¼ cup shredded carrot
½ cup shedded snow peas
½ pound Chinese cabbage, shredded
2 teaspoons chopped shallots
½ cup shredded bamboo shoots
Fresh ginger to taste, optional
1 cup bean sprouts
⅛ teaspoon white pepper
Five spice powder to taste, optional

Soak the mushrooms in hot water for about 20 minutes, then drain and shred into long, thin strips.

Drop the noodles into boiling water for about 3 minutes. Drain and rinse under cold water. Drain well and mix with the sesame oil. Set aside.

Heat the rice wine in a wok until hot. Stir-fry scallions and carrots for about 1 minute, then add the snow peas and stir-fry for another minute. Add the cabbage, black mushrooms, shallots, bamboo shoots and ginger. Stir-fry another 2 minutes and mix well. Then spread the cooked noodles on top of the vegetable mixture and toss over high heat for a few minutes. Add the bean sprouts and spices to taste, mixing thoroughly.

Yield: 5 servings ■ Each serving contains approximately: Calories: 226 (14% from fat); Protein: 9 gms; Fat: 3.5 gms; Carbohydrate: 39 gms; Cholesterol: 0; Sodium: 41 mgs; Allowances: $2\frac{1}{5}$ starches + $1\frac{2}{3}$ vegetables + $\frac{1}{5}$ fat

Carbohydrate: 22 gms; Cholesterol: 24 mgs; Sodium: 45 mgs; Allowances: $2\frac{1}{2}$ vegetables + $1\frac{1}{2}$ proteins + $\frac{1}{4}$ fat

Kung Pao Fish
with Ms. Lan Tan

Seasoning Sauce:
2 teaspoons sugar
1 teaspoon black vinegar
1 teaspoon tapioca starch
1 teaspoon toasted sesame oil

6 tablespoons rice wine, divided
1 teaspoon tapioca starch
$\frac{1}{2}$ pound fresh cod
$\frac{1}{2}$ cup diced green pepper
$\frac{1}{2}$ cup diced red pepper
$\frac{1}{2}$ cup diced bamboo shoots
$\frac{1}{4}$ cup diced water chestnuts
1 teaspoon finely chopped fresh ginger
2 scallions, chopped
8 dried red peppers
3 garlic cloves, minced

Mix seasoning sauce and set aside.

Mix 2 tablespoons of the rice wine and 1 teaspoon tapioca starch. Cut fish into $\frac{1}{2}$-inch cubes and marinate in the tapioca/wine mixture for about 30 minutes.

Heat 2 tablespoons of the rice wine in a wok, and stir in the diced fish until the fish turns white. Remove and set aside. Heat the remaining 2 tablespoons rice wine in wok and add all of the remaining ingredients. Stir and mix well. Cook until tender. Add seasoning sauce to the stir-fry. Finally add the cooked fish. Serve immediately.

Yield: 4 servings ■ Each serving contains approximately: Calories: 156 (11% from fat); Protein: 13 gms; Fat: 1.9 gms;

Shrimp with Tofu and Snow Peas
with Ms. Lan Tan

Seasoning Sauce:
1 teaspoon toasted sesame oil
$\frac{1}{8}$ teaspoon white pepper
1 tablespoon tapioca starch mixed with 1 cup *Basic Veggie Stock* (see page 249)

Marinade:
1 tablespoon rice wine
1 teaspoon tapioca starch

$\frac{1}{2}$ pound shrimp, shelled and de-veined
6 dried mushrooms, soaked in warm water
$\frac{1}{4}$ pound snow peas
3 tablespoons rice wine
1 scallion, cut into 1-inch pieces
1 teaspoon finely chopped fresh ginger
1 garlic clove, crushed
1 teaspoon chopped shallots
10 ounces tofu, crumbled

Combine seasoning sauce ingredients and set aside.

Prepare marinade and marinate the shrimp for about 30 minutes.

Cut the soaked mushrooms into quarters. Steam the snow peas and shrimp for 4 minutes.

Heat the rice wine in a wok until hot, then stir-fry the chopped vegetables and tofu on high, for 2 or 3 minutes. Add the seasoning sauce, mixing well. Add the cooked shrimp and snow peas, and stir-fry another minute. Serve hot.

Yield: 6 servings ■ Each serving contains approximately: Calories: 145 (34% from fat); Protein: 16 gms; Fat: 5.5 gms; Carbohydrate: 8 gms; Cholesterol: 58 mgs; Sodium: 59 mgs; Allowances: 1 vegetable + $1\frac{2}{3}$ proteins + $\frac{1}{6}$ fat. *With 1 cup cooked brown rice:* Calories: 377 (16% from fat); Protein: 21 gms; Fat: 6.7 gms; Carbohydrate: 58 gms; Cholesterol: 58 mgs; Sodium: 59 mgs; Allowances: 3 starches + 1 vegetable + $1\frac{2}{3}$ proteins + $\frac{1}{6}$ fat

Jasmine Tea and Ginger Rice Salad

Dressing:
1 tablespoon canola oil
4 tablespoons rice vinegar
$1\frac{1}{2}$ teaspoons grated fresh gingerroot

2 teaspoons loose jasmine tea or 1 jasmine tea bag
$1\frac{3}{4}$ cups water
1 cup uncooked jasmine rice
4 ounces fresh snow peas
$\frac{1}{4}$ cup minced carrot
$\frac{1}{4}$ cup thinly sliced scallions
1 teaspoon sesame seeds, toasted

Blend the dressing ingredients and set aside. Steep the jasmine tea in boiling water for 5 minutes. Discard the tea bag or tea leaves, and transfer tea to a medium saucepan or rice steamer. Add rice to the jasmine-flavored water and cook until the rice is tender (see Chapter 12 for rice cooking times).

Prepare snow peas by snapping off the stem and gently pulling the attached vein down the shorter side of the pea. Steam the snow peas in a vegetable steamer un-til crisp-tender, about 3 to 4 minutes. Remove from steamer and rinse with cold water to refresh. Set aside to cool. Cut snow peas into $\frac{1}{4}$-inch diagonal slices.

Just before serving, combine the cooled rice, snow peas, carrot, and all but 2 tablespoons of scallion tops. Add dressing and toss into salad. Spoon into serving dish and garnish with the sesame seeds and remaining green scallion tops.

Yield: 4 servings ■ Each serving contains approximately: *With dressing:* Calories: 201 (20% from fat); Protein: 5 gms; Fat: 4.4 gms; Carbohydrate: 35 gms; Cholesterol: 0; Sodium: 3 mgs; Allowances: $1\frac{3}{4}$ starches + 1 vegetable + $\frac{3}{4}$ fat. *Without dressing:* Calories: 169 (5% from fat); Protein: 5 gms; Fat: 1 gm; Carbohydrate: 34 gms; Cholesterol: 0; Sodium: 3 mgs; Allowances: $1\frac{3}{4}$ starches + 1 vegetable

Sweet and Sour Fish
with Ms. Lan Tan

Seasoning Sauce:
1 tablespoon rice wine vinegar
1 teaspoon tapioca starch
2 tablespoons no-salt catsup
1 tablespoon sugar
1 tablespoon rice vinegar
$\frac{1}{3}$ cup pineapple juice

Marinade:
2 tablespoons rice wine
1 teaspoon tapioca starch

$\frac{1}{2}$ pound fresh fish, such as grouper
1 teaspoon extra virgin olive oil
1 tablespoon chopped fresh gingerroot
3 garlic cloves, crushed and chopped
1 tablespoon rice wine

½ cup diced green pepper
½ cup diced tomato
½ cup diced onion
½ cup pineapple chunks

Make seasoning sauce and set aside.

Mix marinade ingredients together. Cut the fish into small cubes and marinate for 1 hour.

Heat the olive oil in a wok. When hot, add chopped ginger and garlic, and stir-fry for about 15 seconds. Add the marinated fish. Stir gently for about 2 minutes or until the fish turns white. Remove and set aside. Heat the rice wine in wok, and stir in the green pepper, tomatoes, onions, and pineapple chunks. Stir over high heat for about 2 minutes. Add the seasoning sauce. Stir until it thickens, then add the cooked fish. Serve hot.

Yield: 3 servings ■ Each serving contains approximately: Calories: 173 (13% from fat); Protein: 16 gms; Fat: 2.6 gms; Carbohydrate: 19 gms; Cholesterol: 27 mgs; Sodium: 45 mgs; Allowances: 1¼ vegetables + ¼ fruit + 2 proteins + ⅓ fat

Hot and Sour Soup
with Ms. Lan Tan

4 dried black mushrooms
2 tablespoons dried tree ears
¼ cup dried lily flowers
¼ cup bamboo shoots
1 pound tofu
3 tablespoons tapioca starch
2 scallions
6 cups *Basic Veggie Stock* (see page 249)
2 tablespoons rice wine

1 tablespoon freshly grated gingerroot
2 tablespoons no-fat, very-low-sodium vegetable or chicken bouillon
Pinch of sugar
4 tablespoons rice wine vinegar
¼ teaspoon white pepper
2 egg whites, slightly beaten
1 teaspoon toasted sesame oil
1 teaspoon chili oil, optional
1 tablespoon chopped fresh cilantro

In separate bowls soak the mushrooms, tree ears, and lily flowers for about 20 minutes until softened. Wash the tree ears carefully and then shred them. Shred the bamboo shoots and tofu. Dissolve starch in a little water. Chop the scallions.

Bring the vegetable broth to a boil. Add the rice wine, ginger, bouillon, sugar, mushrooms, tree ears, lily flowers, and bamboo shoots. Let boil for about 1 minute, then add tofu. Bring the soup to a boil again. Stir in the tapioca starch until soup thickens. Add the rice vinegar and white pepper, and stir well. Finally, add the beaten egg whites. Immediately turn off heat. Garnish with sesame oil, chili oil, cilantro, and scallions.

Yield: 10 servings ■ Each serving contains approximately: Calories: 67 (40% from fat, 32% from fat if no oil is added); Protein: 5 gms; Fat: 3 gms; Carbohydrate: 5 gms; Cholesterol: 0; Sodium: 15 mgs; Allowances: 1 vegetable + ⅔ protein + ⅕ fat

Bean Sheet Salad
with Ms. Lan Tan

Seasoning Sauce:
1 teaspoon sesame seed paste
  (tahini)
2 teaspoons sugar
3 tablespoons rice vinegar
1 teaspoon chili oil, optional
1 teaspoon peppercorns

5 dried bean sheets
3 baby cucumbers or 3 cups bean
  sprouts
1 carrot
2 scallions, finely chopped
1 teaspoon finely chopped fresh ginger
1 garlic clove, finely chopped

Prepare seasoning sauce, stirring gently until smooth, and set aside.

Cook the bean sheets in boiling water for about 10 minutes. Drain and leave in cold water until cool, then cut into 3-inch-long strips. Put on a plate. Rinse and shred the cucumber (or bean sprouts) and carrot into long thin strips. Lay on top of bean sheet strips. Sprinkle the chopped scallions, ginger, and garlic over this.

Just before serving, pour the sauce over the salad and mix thoroughly. Serve cold.

Yield: 4 servings ■ Each serving contains approximately: Calories: 100 (20% from fat); Protein: 5 gms; Fat: 2.2 gms; Carbohydrate: 17 gms; Cholesterol: 0; Sodium: 12 mgs; Allowances: $\frac{2}{3}$ starch + $\frac{1}{2}$ vegetable + $\frac{2}{5}$ fat

Spicy String Beans
with Ms. Lan Tan

2 ounces cellophane noodles (mung bean
  threads)
1 tablespoon rice wine
1 teaspoon minced garlic
1 tablespoon freshly minced ginger
$\frac{1}{4}$ teaspoon red pepper
1 pound fresh string beans, snapped
$\frac{3}{4}$ cup *Basic Veggie Stock* (see page
  249)
1 teaspoon toasted sesame oil
1 scallion, chopped

Soak the cellophane noodles in warm water for about five minutes. Drain and cut into 3-inch-long sections.

Heat the rice wine in a wok until hot, then stir in the garlic, ginger, red pepper, and string beans, mixing well. Add the vegetable stock. Cover and simmer over medium heat for about 10 minutes, stirring twice. Remove from heat and add the cellophane noodles, mixing thoroughly. Return to heat and cook, covered, 2 or 3 minutes more or until the liquid is absorbed. Garnish with sesame oil and scallions. Serve hot or cold.

Yield: 4 servings ■ Each serving contains approximately: Calories: 98 (28% from fat); Protein: 3 gms; Fat; 3 gms; Carbohydrate: 15 gms; Cholesterol: 0; Sodium: 3 mgs; Allowances: $\frac{1}{2}$ starch + $1\frac{3}{4}$ vegetables + $\frac{1}{4}$ fat. *With 1 cup white rice:* Calories: 321 (9% from fat); Protein: 7 gms; Fat: 3.2 gms; Carbohydrate: 65 gms; Cholesterol: 0; Sodium: 3 mgs; Allowances: $3\frac{1}{2}$ starches + $1\frac{3}{4}$ vegetables + $\frac{1}{4}$ fat

Vegetable Fried Rice
with Ms. Lan Tan

2 egg whites
3 tablespoons rice wine
1 teaspoon minced fresh gingerroot
½ cup diced carrots
½ cup diced onion
½ cup snow peas, stemmed and stringed
1 tablespoon extra virgin olive oil, divided
1 teaspoon freshly minced garlic
2 scallions, chopped
3½ cups cooked brown rice
1 cup mung bean sprouts
Pinch of white pepper

Beat the egg whites. Heat rice wine in a wok and add ginger, carrots, and onions. Stir-fry for 1 or 2 minutes, then add snow peas and cook for another 1 or 2 minutes. Set aside.

Heat 1 teaspoon of the oil in wok. Stir in the beaten egg whites. Scramble and break into small pieces. Remove and set aside. Heat the remaining 2 teaspoons of oil in wok. Stir-fry garlic and half of the scallions, until light brown.

Add the cooked rice and stir until the rice is separated and thoroughly heated. Finally add the scrambled egg, bean sprouts, and white pepper. Stir until well blended. Garnish with the remaining scallions. Serve hot.

Yield: 8 servings ■ Each serving contains approximately: Calories: 143 (14% from fat); Protein: 4 gms; Fat: 2.3 gms; Carbohydrate: 25 gms; Cholesterol: 0; Sodium: 16 mgs; Allowances: 1⅖ starches + ½ vegetable + ⅓ fat

My Favorite Stir-Fry

1 teaspoon extra virgin olive oil
4 garlic cloves, minced
½ cup chopped onion
¼ cup wine
1 teaspoon grated fresh ginger
2 cups julienned carrots
2 cups chopped broccoli
2 cups chopped red cabbage
2 cups chopped snow peas
Juice of ½ lime or to taste
1 tablespoon toasted slivered almonds, optional

Heat olive oil in a wok, add garlic, onion, wine, and ginger. Stir well, then add the carrots and sauté for about 5 minutes.

Add the broccoli, cabbage, snow peas, and lime juice, and sauté for another 5 to 10 minutes until tender but slightly crisp. Keeping the mixture covered except to stir will hasten the cooling process. While this is cooling you can toast some slivered almonds in the oven, if this topping is desired.

Yield: 4 servings ■ Each serving contains approximately: *Without almonds:* Calories: 147 (9% from fat); Protein: 5 gms; Fat: 1.5 gms; Carbohydrate: 17 gms; Cholesterol: 0; Sodium: 46 mgs; Allowances: 1 starch + 2 vegetables + ¼ fat. *With almonds:* Calories: 167 (17% from fat); Protein: 6 gms; Fat: 3.2 gms; Carbohydrate: 18 gms; Cholesterol: 0; Sodium: 47 mgs; Allowances: 1 starch + 2 vegetables + ½ fat

Curried Fish with Peppers and Onions
with Ms. Lan Tan

Seasoning Sauce:
2 tablespoons rice wine
Pinch of white pepper
Pinch of sugar

Marinade:
1 tablespoon rice wine
1 teaspoon tapioca starch

$\frac{1}{2}$ pound fresh fish, such as grouper
1 teaspoon extra virgin olive oil
2 tablespoons rice wine
2 teaspoons curry powder
2 medium onions, sliced
3 garlic cloves, minced
1 green pepper, chopped
1 teaspoon freshly minced ginger
1 tablespoon tapioca starch mixed with 2 tablespoons *Basic Veggie Stock* (see page 249), or water

Prepare seasoning sauce and set aside.

Combine marinade ingredients. Rinse the fish, cut into thin slices, and put in marinade for 30 minutes.

Heat the olive oil in a wok. Add fish and stir-fry until the fish turns white. Remove and set aside. Heat the wine and add curry powder first, then onion, garlic, green pepper, and ginger. Stir-fry for about 1 minute, then add the seasoning sauce. When the onion turns soft, add the tapioca starch mixture. Stir until liquid thickens, and add the cooked fish. Mix thoroughly. Serve hot.

Yield: 4 servings ■ Each serving contains approximately: Calories: 106 (17% from fat); Protein: 12 gms; Fat: 2 gms; Carbohydrate: 10 gms; Cholesterol: 21 mgs; Sodium: 33 mgs; Allowances: $\frac{1}{2}$ vegetable + $1\frac{1}{2}$ proteins + $\frac{1}{4}$ fat

No-Salt Soy Sauce Substitute
by Judy Ladner

$1\frac{1}{2}$ cups boiling water
2 tablespoons no-fat, very-low-sodium vegetable or chicken bouillon
$\frac{1}{8}$ teaspoon freshly ground black pepper
1 tablespoon dark molasses
4 tablespoons apple cider vinegar
1 teaspoon toasted sesame oil
$1\frac{1}{2}$ tablespoons cornstarch

Boil water and add all the ingredients except the cornstarch. Dissolve the cornstarch in a few tablespoons of cold water before adding to the mixture. Simmer for a minute or two, until slightly thickened.

Yield: almost 2 cups, or 32 1-tablespoon servings ■ Each serving contains approximately: Calories: 11 (40% from fat); Protein: 0; Fat: .5 gm; Carbohydrate: 1 gm; Cholesterol: 0; Sodium: 4 mgs; Allowances: trace amounts of starch, fruit, and fat. *With My Favorite Stir-Fry:* Calories: 158 (11% from fat); Protein: 5 gms; Fat: 2 gms; Carbohydrates: 18 gms; Cholesterol: 0; Sodium: 50 mgs

Desserts and Beverages

Healthy Oatmeal Cookies

3 bananas
$\frac{1}{4}$ cup WonderSlim (if not available, use 2
    tablespoons applesauce and 2 addi-
    tional egg whites)
2 egg whites, beaten
1 teaspoon vanilla extract
$\frac{1}{4}$ cup molasses
$1\frac{1}{4}$ cups whole wheat pastry flour
1 teaspoon low-sodium baking powder
$3\frac{1}{2}$ cups rolled oats
$\frac{1}{2}$ cup reconstituted coffee substitute
1 cup plain nonfat yogurt (or more if bat-
    ter needs moisture)
1 cup raisins
1 teaspoon cinnamon
1 teaspoon extra virgin olive oil

Preheat oven to 350 degrees.

Purée bananas in food processor or
blender. Add WonderSlim (or the substitute) and mix with the bananas. Beat the
egg whites and stir in the vanilla and the
molasses and set aside. Sift together flour
and baking powder.

If you are using thick-cut rolled oats (the
kind that is sold in bulk at health food
stores), grind the oats slightly in a
blender or food processor, with a few
quick spurts. This step is not necessary if
you are using a more refined product,
such as Quaker Oats.

Blend flour mixture into the banana mixture, then add all the remaining ingredients except olive oil. Mix thoroughly.

Grease cookie sheet with the olive oil.
Drop rounded teaspoons of batter onto
cookie sheet and flatten with a fork to desired width. Bake 13 to 15 minutes or until slightly browned. Remove from cookie
sheet while still hot, and cool on a rack.

Yield: 4 dozen ■ Each cookie contains approximately: Calories: 59 (13% from fat);
Protein: 2 gms; Fat: less than .5 gm; Carbohydrate: 12 gms; Cholesterol: trace; So-
dium: 7 mgs; Allowances: $\frac{1}{2}$ starch + $\frac{1}{3}$
fruit

Oat Bran Brownies
with May Segal

1 teaspoon extra virgin olive oil
1 cup oat bran
$\frac{1}{2}$ teaspoon low-sodium baking powder
3 tablespoons cocoa
2 tablespoons powdered coffee substitute
3 ripe bananas
$\frac{1}{4}$ cup Wonderslim
4 egg whites
1 teaspoon almond or vanilla extract
2 tablespoons chopped walnuts

Preheat oven to 300 degrees.

Coat a 9-inch square pan with olive oil.
Combine the oat bran, baking powder, cocoa, and coffee substitute in a bowl. In
another bowl, combine all other ingredients except the nuts. Fold the moist mixture into the dry, mix well, then fold in
the nuts.

Pour mixture into pan and bake 35 to 40
minutes. Test to see that the center is
done. Cut into $1\frac{1}{2} \times 2\frac{1}{4}$-inch bars.

Yield: 2 dozen brownies ■ Each brownie contains approximately: Calories: 37 (19% from fat); Protein: 2 gms; Fat: .8 gm; Carbohydrate: 7 gms; Cholesterol: 0; Sodium: 9 mgs; Allowances: $\frac{1}{5}$ starch + $\frac{1}{4}$ fruit + $\frac{1}{12}$ fat

Apple-Oatmeal Delights

4 large apples
5 teaspoons cinnamon
$\frac{3}{4}$ cup oatmeal
$\frac{3}{4}$ cup oat bran
3 egg whites
1 tablespoon fresh lemon juice
1 tablespoon honey
$\frac{1}{2}$ cup powdered nonfat milk
$\frac{1}{2}$ cup raisins
$\frac{1}{4}$ teaspoon canola oil

Wash, core, and chop the apples. Put them in a steamer, sprinkle with cinnamon, and steam until tender, about 10 minutes. If you do not have a steamer, put about 2 inches of water in a pot, place apples in a colander set in the pot, and boil, covered, for approximately 10 minutes.

Preheat oven to 350 degrees.

Combine all the other ingredients and set aside. When apples are tender liquify them in a blender. Mix the liquified apples with the other ingredients. Brush a cookie sheet with canola oil and drop rounded teaspoons of batter onto tray, flattening to form desired cookie shape. Bake for about 20 minutes.

Yield: 2 to 3 dozen cookies, depending upon how large you make them ■ Each cookie contains approximately: *If 2 dozen:*

Calories: 60 (8% from fat); Protein: 3 gms; Fat: .5 gm; Carbohydrate: 13 gms; Cholesterol: trace; Sodium: 21 mgs; Allowances: $\frac{1}{2}$ starch + $\frac{1}{3}$ fruit. *If 3 dozen,* Calories: 40 (8% from fat); Protein: 2 gms; Fat: .3 gm; Carbohydrate: 9 gms; Cholesterol: trace; Sodium: 14 mgs; Allowances: $\frac{1}{3}$ starch + $\frac{1}{4}$ fruit

Healthy Holiday Pumpkin Pie

Touch of extra virgin olive oil to grease pie pan.

Crust:
1 cup Health Valley granola
1 cup whole wheat flour
$\frac{1}{2}$ cup oat bran
$\frac{1}{2}$ teaspoon cinnamon
$\frac{3}{4}$ cup applesauce
$\frac{1}{2}$ cup plain nonfat yogurt

Filling:
3 egg whites, lightly beaten
1 16-ounce can pumpkin
$\frac{1}{2}$ cup maple syrup or honey
1 12-ounce can evaporated skim milk
Dash nutmeg
$\frac{1}{4}$ teaspoon ginger
$\frac{1}{4}$ teaspoon cloves
$1\frac{1}{2}$ teaspoons cinnamon
4 teaspoons arrowroot

Preheat oven to 425 degrees. With a paper towel moistened with olive oil, lightly grease a 10-inch pie pan.

Make the crust: Place granola, flour, oat bran, and $\frac{1}{2}$ teaspoon cinnamon in a food processor and pulverize until everything is well mixed, about 10 to 12 seconds. In a bowl thoroughly mix these dry ingredients with the applesauce and yogurt. Spoon crust mixture into the greased pie pan, smooth out evenly, then bake for 10 minutes.

Beat egg whites and set aside. Combine and mix other filling ingredients, then fold in beaten egg whites. After 10 minutes of baking, remove pie crust from oven, and add filling mixture. Return to oven and bake another 40 to 50 minutes or until a knife inserted in the center comes out clean.

Yield: 8 servings ■ Each serving contains approximately: Calories: 232 (4% from fat); Protein: 10 gms; Fat: 1 gm; Carbohydrate: 47 gms; Cholesterol: 2 mgs; Sodium: 101 mgs; Allowances: $1\frac{1}{4}$ starches + $\frac{1}{2}$ vegetable + $1\frac{1}{6}$ fruits + $\frac{1}{8}$ protein + $\frac{1}{2}$ dairy

Oat Bran Carrot Cake

$\frac{1}{2}$ cup apple juice
3 cups finely shredded carrots
$\frac{1}{4}$ cup honey
1 cup raisins
1 cup applesauce
1 teaspoon canola oil
3 cups oat bran
2 teaspoons low-sodium baking powder
$1\frac{1}{2}$ teaspoons ground cinnamon
6 egg whites

Preheat oven to 350 degrees.

Mix together the apple juice, carrots, honey, raisins, and applesauce in a bowl and set aside. Coat a 13 × 9 × 2-inch baking pan with oil. In another bowl, combine oat bran, baking powder, and cinnamon, mixing well. Stir carrot mix-

ture into dry ingredients. Beat egg whites and then fold into cake mixture. Pour into prepared pan.

Bake for 50 to 60 minutes, or until a toothpick inserted into the center of the cake comes out clean. Cut into 24 portions each approximately $2\frac{1}{4}$ × $2\frac{1}{8}$ inches. This is great topped or "iced" with 2 tablespoons of plain nonfat yogurt flavored with cinnamon, maple syrup, and vanilla to taste.

Yield: 24 servings ■ Each piece of cake contains approximately: Calories: 88 (10% from fat); Protein: 3 gms; Fat: 1 gm; Carbohydrate: 17 gms; Cholesterol: 0; Sodium: 18 mgs; Allowances: $\frac{1}{2}$ starch + $\frac{3}{5}$ fruit + $\frac{1}{8}$ protein

Quinoa Banana Pudding

Enjoy this versatile pudding for breakfast, brunch, snack, or dessert.

1 cup quinoa
2 cups boiling water
$\frac{1}{3}$ cup raisins
$\frac{1}{2}$ cup unsweetened apple juice
2 bananas
$\frac{1}{4}$ teaspoon grated lemon rind
$\frac{3}{4}$ teaspoon fresh lemon juice
1 teaspoon vanilla
$\frac{1}{2}$ teaspoon cinnamon

Rinse quinoa in cold water and drain while waiting for water to boil. Add quinoa to boiling water, then reduce heat to medium-low. Boil quinoa for 10 minutes, then add raisins and boil for another 5 minutes. While quinoa is cooking, put remaining ingredients in a blender or food processor and blend until smooth.

Add the blended ingredients into the quinoa and simmer for 5 more minutes, or until desired consistency is achieved.

Yield: 4 servings; serving size ¾ cup ■ Each serving contains approximately: Calories: 230 (11% from fat); Protein: 6 gms; Fat: 2.9 gms; Carbohydrate: 51 gms; Cholesterol: 0; Sodium: 20 mgs; Allowances: 1⅓ starches + 2 fruits

Banana Cream Kahlua

Whenever your bananas are ripening faster than you can eat them, simply peel them, wrap in plastic wrap or aluminum foil, and place them in the freezer. Then whenever you get that urge for something very cold and sweet, here is an easy and healthful remedy!

4 large bananas, frozen
2 tablespoons Kahlua or other liqueur
⅛ teaspoon cinnamon, optional

Place the frozen bananas in a food processor with the liqueur and cinnamon and purée. If the processor starts to "struggle" a bit, let the bananas soften for a few minutes and then try again.

Yield: 4 servings; serving size ½ cup
■ Each serving contains approximately: Calories: 132 (4% from fat); Protein: 1 gm; Fat: .6 gm; Carbohydrate: 30 gms; Cholesterol: 0; Sodium: less than 1 mg; Allowances: 2⅕ fruits

Angelic Ambrosia

2 cups plain nonfat yogurt
2 small bananas
¼ cup golden raisins
¼ teaspoon cinnamon
½ teaspoon vanilla extract
1½ cups berries
1 cup seedless grapes
2 firm ripe pears, chopped into ½-inch dice
2 oranges, chopped into ½-inch dice
2 apples, chopped into ½-inch dice
4 tablespoons chopped walnuts
1 tablespoon toasted sesame seeds

Blend the yogurt, bananas, raisins, cinnamon, and vanilla in a blender or food processor. Prepare the fresh fruit and mix with the yogurt blend. Top with walnuts and sesame seeds.

Yield: 16 servings; serving size ½ cup
■ Each serving contains approximately: Calories: 79 (20% from fat); Protein: 3 gms; Fat: 1.7 gms; Carbohydrate: 17 gms; Cholesterol: 0; Sodium: 27 mgs; Allowances: ⅘ fruit + ⅙ dairy + ⅓ fat

Poached Pears with Pomegranate Sauce

4 Bosc or Red Bartlett pears
¾ cup pomegranate juice (or any juice, such as cranberry or grape, with color that will contrast with the pears)
1 tablespoon arrowroot powder
3 tablespoons cold water
Sprigs of fresh spearmint

Wash pears and place in a saucepan, stem end up. Add juice and bring to a boil. Reduce heat and simmer for 20 minutes. Remove pears from pan and place on attractive plates. Dissolve arrowroot powder in cold water before adding to juice. Simmer juice for another 3 to 5 minutes or until desired thickness is achieved.

Spoon thickened juice over pears and garnish with mint.

Yield: 4 servings ■ Each serving contains approximately: Calories: 126 (5% from fat); Protein: 1 gm; Fat: .75 gm; Carbohydrate: 31 gms; Cholesterol: 0; Sodium: 2 mgs; Allowances: $\frac{1}{3}$ starch + $1\frac{3}{5}$ fruits

Oat Bran and Fruit Smoothie

$\frac{1}{2}$ cup blueberry nectar
4 tablespoons plain nonfat yogurt
1 tablespoon oat bran
$\frac{1}{2}$ cup ice cubes
$\frac{3}{4}$ cup strawberries
$\frac{1}{2}$ tablespoon wheat germ
$\frac{1}{2}$ banana

Place all ingredients in a blender and whip until smooth. In place of the blueberry nectar, you may use $\frac{1}{2}$ cup unsweetened fruit juice of your choice.

Yield: 1 serving ■ Calories: 209 (6% from fat); Protein: 7 gms; Fat: 1.4 gms; Carbohydrate: 46 gms; Cholesterol: trace; Sodium: 50 mgs; Allowances: $\frac{3}{5}$ starch + $2\frac{1}{8}$ fruits + $\frac{1}{3}$ dairy

Icy Melon Delight

$\frac{1}{2}$ cup chopped cantaloupe
$\frac{1}{2}$ cup chopped pineapple
2 tablespoons plain nonfat yogurt
$\frac{1}{4}$ cup ice cubes
$\frac{1}{4}$ teaspoon vanilla extract
Dash freshly grated nutmeg
Sprigs of fresh mint

Place all ingredients except mint in blender and process on high speed until smooth. Serve over ice in a tall, frosted glass, and garnish with mint.

Yield: 1 serving ■ Calories: 83 (6% from fat); Protein: 3 gms; Fat: .6 gm; Carbohydrate: 19 gms; Cholesterol: trace; Sodium: 29 mgs; Allowances: $1\frac{1}{10}$ fruits + $\frac{1}{15}$ dairy

Mock Mocha Shake

1 cup skim milk
$\frac{1}{2}$ banana
1 tablespoon carob powder
1 teaspoon powdered coffee substitute
$\frac{1}{2}$ teaspoon wheat germ, optional
$\frac{1}{2}$ cup ice cubes

Put all ingredients in a blender and blend on high until smooth.

Yield: 1 serving ■ Calories: 167 (4% from fat); Protein: 10 gms; Fat: .8 gm; Carbohydrate: 34 gms; Cholesterol: 4 mgs; Sodium: 132 mgs; Allowances: $\frac{1}{4}$ starch + 1 fruit + 1 dairy

Appendix A

MAIL ORDER SOURCES FOR HEALTH FOODS

Some of the products mentioned in this book may be difficult or impossible for you to obtain in your community, but are delicious and healthy. Call or write the companies to request information on their products, which will include ordering procedures and costs. Always remember to request only low-fat, no-salt added products.

BAKING PRODUCTS OR BAKED GOODS

King Arthur Flour
P.O. Box 876
Norwich, VT 05055
(800) 827-6836

This company offers superb quality baking ingredients and products. Everything from WonderSlim (a fat and egg substitute) and WonderSlim Cocoa (a caffeine-free, low-fat unsweetened cocoa powder for baking and drinking) to baking stones and Tomato Tapenade (a salt-free paste of finely minced sun-dried tomatoes, garlic, and olive oil). This paste is great on pizzas and in soups, salad dressings, and marinades. For more specific information regarding WonderSlim call (800) 497-6595.

Toufayan Bakeries, Inc.   or   Toufayan Bakeries, Inc.
9255 Kennedy Blvd.   3826 Bryn Mawr Street
N. Bergen, NJ 07047   Orlando, FL 32808
(800) 328-7482   (800) 233-7482

This company makes 8-ounce salt-free white and whole wheat pitas. Their pita bread products, called Pitettes, measure $3\frac{1}{2}$ by 4 inches in diameter and freeze beautifully. Call them to find out the distributor of Pitettes near you. If there is no distributor near you, they will gladly ship via UPS.

CHINESE INGREDIENTS

Lan's Gourmet Food & Chinese Cooking School
4215 University Drive
Durham, NC 27707
(919) 493-1341

Ms. Lan offers an extensive variety of Chinese ingredients and cooking utensils. She will ship by UPS to anywhere in the United States. She also runs a delightful cooking school for local residents.

China Bowl Trading Company
169 Lackawanna Avenue
Parsippany, NJ 07054
(201) 335-1000

This company can provide a wide selection of Chinese ingredients.

DRIED BEANS AND PEAS

Baer's Best
154 Green Street
Reading, MA 01867
(617) 944-8719

The Baers grow fifteen or more different varieties of beans on their farm in St. Albans, Maine. From commonplace to exotic, a wide selection can be ordered in bulk or 1-pound packages.

DRIED MUSHROOMS

Gourmet Treasure Hunters
10044 Adams Avenue, Suite 305
Huntington Beach, CA 92646
(714) 964-3355

This company sells a wide variety of dried mushrooms, from Chinese to American. It is also a good source of specialty rices (basmati and arborio) and Japanese and Vietnamese ingredients.

FRESH FRUIT

Cushman Fruit Company
3325 Forest Hill Blvd.
West Palm Beach, FL 33406
(800) 776-7575

Mack's Groves
1180 N. Federal Hwy.
Pompano Beach, FL 33062
(800) 327-3525

FRUITS AND NATURAL SWEETS

Wax Orchards
22744 Wax Orchard Road SW
Vashon, WA 98070
(800) 634-6132

They sell the best fat-free chocolate sauce you can imagine. Naturally sweetened with fruits, it is a guilt-free treat!

ORGANIC FOODS

Bearitos
Little Bear Organic Foods
Carson, CA 90746

Bearitos Vegetarian Refried Beans, low-fat, no-salt added, are the best. Try jazzing them up with the 15-Minute Meal recipe *Refried Beans and Salsa with Chips.* Be forewarned that many of their other products contain significant amounts of sodium.

Eden Foods Inc.
Clinton, MI 49236

One of the most well-distributed organic food suppliers, Eden has a variety of no-fat/no-salt canned beans. They season them with an edible seaweed, kombu, which offers some flavor and, reportedly, reduces the gaseous compounds in the beans.

Walnut Acres
Penns Creek, PA 17862
(800) 433-3998 (24 hours a day)

This company probably has more wonderful products than any I have ever known. They offer a large selection of practically everything organic and of the best quality imaginable. Really the only products to stay clear of are the sodium-rich cheeses and soups and the fat-rich peanut butter, nuts, and seeds. Otherwise they have a tremendous selection of luscious fruits (fresh, dried, jams, and juices), grains, beans, vegetables, and spices.

SEEDS FOR GROWING HERBS AND VEGETABLES

Burpee
300 Park Avenue
Warminster, PA 18991
(800) 888-1447

This is the seed company that enabled me to first start growing cilantro and arugula. The cilantro plant has a long root and does not like to be transplanted. When you buy it as a plant and transplant it into your garden, it rarely is good for more than a few cuttings before it bolts. Thus, if you really enjoy cilantro, you need to grow it from seed. A small packet of cilantro seeds will provide you with plenty for two years or for life if you let some plants go to seed, and then replant them! Arugula also grows as easily as do weeds, and is easier to grow than to find in most grocery stores.

Shepherd's Garden Seeds
30 Irene Street
Torrington, CT 06790
(203) 482-3638 (Connecticut)
(408) 335-5311 (California)

Shepherd's offers an extraordinary selection of seeds for herbs and vegetables, from common to exotic. They are accompanied by detailed growing instructions for the novice gardener.

Vermont Bean Seed Company
Garden Lane
Fair Haven, VT 05743
(802) 265-4212

Obviously if you are searching for the hard-to-find bean seed, you look for someone who specializes in beans. If it grows in the United States, they will have it.

SPICES AND SOUTHWEST DELIGHTS

The Spice House
P.O. Box 1633
Milwaukee, WI 53203
(414) 272-0977

Fresh herbs, spices, seeds, and no-salt seasoning mixes are sold in amounts ranging from 1 ounce to 1 pound. Orders can be sent UPS COD within 48 hours.

Santa Fe School of Cooking
Upper Level, Plaza Mercado
116 West San Francisco Street
Santa Fe, NM 87501
Phone: (505) 983-4511
FAX: (505) 983-7540

In addition to selling a large variety of herbs, chiles, and seeds to grow them, they also offer an extensive selection of other Southwestern cooking ingredients, such as posole (lime-treated corn) and hard-to-find beans.

Coyote Cocina
1364 Rufina Circle #1
Santa Fe, NM 87501
Phone: (800) 866-4695
FAX: (505) 473-3100

This is a food store associated with Santa Fe's fun-filled restaurant Coyote Cafe (which is now also in Las Vegas, Nevada, and Washington, DC). This store offers an incredible selection of foods, from blue corn meal to epazote, a spice that reduces gaseousness of beans. Many other interesting items are offered as well, from New Mexico red chile wreaths, or *ristras,* to tortilla presses.

Rancho Mesilla Inc.
P.O. Box 39
Mesilla, NM 88046
(505) 525-2266

Stewart, the justifiably proud owner, will send you fresh-picked, roasted, and frozen New Mexican green chiles. Believe it or not, they are actually worth the rather steep price. For those in pursuit of the unusual, he also sells buffalo meat, which is lower in saturated fat than chicken, and llamas—for petting not eating!

VEGETARIAN FOODS

Boca Burger Co.
Ft. Lauderdale, FL 33305
(954) 524-1977

Boca Burger has been on grocery shelves for approximately three years, and has proven to be the best ready-made vegetarian burger on the market. Most meat analogs still contain a lot of fat and sodium, whereas Boca Burger's Vegan Original has no added fat or sodium. Be sure to get the Vegan Original Boca Burger, as there are a few with added cheese, thus higher fat and sodium. Look for this product in health food stores; you may call them to find out the nearest distributor to you, but they do not mail retail.

Dacopa Foods
California Natural Products
Manteca, CA 95336
(209) 858-2525, Ext. 223

The best coffee substitute I have ever tasted! Dacopa is different from the many bitter grain and cereal coffee substitutes; it is slightly sweet from the natural fructose found in its only ingredient: dahlia tuber juice. Although Dacopa is not available in most chain grocery stores, it is worth the extra effort to special order. It's available in individual packets, 2-ounce jars, and 7-ounce canisters. Call for prices and shipping costs, which must be prepaid (no credit cards accepted). Try it with a teaspoon of honey and some Health Valley Soy Moo.

Enrico's
Ventre Packing Co., Inc.
Syracuse, NY 13204
(315) 463-2384

Enrico's makes the best no-salt salsa and pasta sauce on the market. If you cannot find a no-salt salsa or marinara sauce in your area, it would be worth ordering a case of theirs.

Harvest Direct, Inc.
P.O. Box 4514
Decatur, IL 62525
(800) 835-2867

This company sells all-natural vegetarian products that may be difficult for you to find unless you have a health food store nearby. For instance, they sell texturized vegetable protein (TVP) made without added fat or sodium. Be sure that you order their unflavored varieties, which contain only 15 milligrams of sodium per 100 grams. They also sell a nice selection of interesting items, from yogurt cheese funnels, to cookbooks, to egg replacer. Harvest Direct also carries Beano, a food enzyme that breaks down the sugars that can cause gaseousness. Since this product is not recommended for diabetics, or for those with certain other medical conditions, you may wish to call the Beano Company with your questions, (800) 257-8650, before ordering.

Health Valley Foods, Inc.
16100 Foothill Blvd.
Irwindale, CA 91706
Nature Mart (800) 668-9363 (a retail store that will mail direct bulk orders)

Health Valley has one of the largest varieties of no-fat/no-sugar vegetarian processed foods. Many of them are no-salt as well. They have approximately 30 different no-fat, no-salt or no-sugar cold cereals, and make the best vegetarian chili on the market. They have some no-salt soups, but most of their soups generally have 200–300 milligrams of sodium. Their product called Soy Moo contains less fat and sodium than any nondairy "milk" product. Although they do not ship to individuals, the Nature Mart store (noted above with 800 number) will be glad to do so.

Mr. Spice Sauces
Lang Naturals
850 Aquidneck Avenue
Newport, RI 02842-7201
(800) SAUCE4U = (800) 728-2348
(888) MRSPICE

This is one of the better companies producing no-salt/no-fat condiments. They presently sell eight different condiments that are salt- and fat-free, including a popular hot sauce called Tangy Bangy. Their Thai Peanut Sauce is the only one with significant fat; its atherogenic peanut oil should be avoided by those with high cholesterol. With the exception of the Thai Peanut Sauce, their sauces are no-fat. They also are free of added sodium, sugar, cholesterol, gluten, wheat, dairy, soy, MSG, preservatives, and sulfites. All sauces are vegetarian and kosher. Their other sauces include garlic steak sauce, honey barbecue sauce, ginger stir-fry sauce, hot wing sauce, honey mustard sauce, sweet and sour sauce, and Indian curry sauce. They are stocked in many health food stores nationally. Mail orders carry discounts for volume orders.

Pritikin/Direct to You
P.O. Box 9940
Maple Plain, MN 55592
(800) 458-5711

They will send you free catalogs and recipe ideas upon request. Some of their products are salt-free but some now have added sodium, so read the nutritional analysis provided carefully.

R.W. Knudsen and Sons, Inc.
Chico, CA 95928
(916) 899-5000

Their Very Veggie low-sodium Natural Vegetable Cocktail is better than salty tomato juice ever thought of being. They also make delicious canned fruit juice and seltzer water beverages.

Robbie's
1920 North Lake Avenue
Altadena, CA 91001
(818) 798-9944

By far the best no-salt, no-sugar, no-fat condiments on the market. From the best garlic sauce you can imagine, to wonderful Worcestershire, barbecue and sweet and sour sauce, to pancake syrup! Robbie's new Italian-style spaghetti sauce is also superb. The only product that he currently makes that has any added salt is his salsa.

Sovex Natural Foods, Inc.
Collegedale, TN 37315
Vege Way Distributors, Chattanooga, Tenn.
(800) 717-0080

Their product called Better than Burger? is the only no-fat/no-sodium-added vegetable burger mix I have seen on the market. See *The Best Burger Out!* for my modification to the recipe suggestion found on their box. Although Sovex is not able to ship this product to individuals, their distributor (listed above) will do so.

VIDALIA ONIONS

Bland Farms
P.O. Box 506-G2-S89
Glennville, GA 30427
(800) 843-2542

These unbelievably sweet onions are available only in May and June, but this company also sells other Southern items. Each order of onions (minimum 10 pounds) comes with a free recipe booklet, and a call will get you a free catalog.

VINEGARS AND OILS

Community Kitchens
P.O. Box 2311
Baton Rouge, LA 70821
(800) 535-9901

In addition to an impressive selection of vinegars and oils, they also offer a wide variety of kitchen equipment.

COOKBOOKS

The Cookbook Cottage
1279 Bardstown Road
Louisville, KY 40204
(502) 458-5227

They specialize in used and out-of-print cookbooks, and they can and will find *anything* for you!

Jessica's Biscuit Cookbook Catalog
Box 301
Newtonville, MA 02160
(800) 225-4264 from outside Massachusetts
(800) 322-4027 from within Massachusetts
(617) 965-0530 from metropolitan Boston

Kitchen Arts and Letters
1435 Lexington Avenue
New York, NY 10128
(212) 876-5550

Owner Nahum Waxman knows cookbooks. His store is a dream come true for those who love reading about food!

Appendix B

SOURCES FOR MORE INFORMATION

Best Newsletters Available to Support Less Than 20%
Fat Nutritional Approaches or Vegetarian Lifestyles

Center for Science in the Public Interest
1875 Connecticut Avenue, N.W., Suite 300
Washington, DC 20009
(202) 332-9110

Although this nutrition newsletter is not as ambitious with their sodium and fat recommendations as this book, it is the only newsletter that reports information consistently more progressive than the others on limiting fat and sodium. In addition to highlighting a practical comparative survey of some type of food each month, they also guide those interested in making a difference. Their Nutrition Activist Hotline number is (202) 332-9110. As soon as the recorded message begins, press "5" on your touch-tone phone to hear a brief message explaining a current political issue, and *what* you can tell *whom* to be part of the solution.

Vegetarian Dietetics
c/o The American Dietetic Association
216 West Jackson Boulevard
Chicago, IL 60606
WATS Line: 800-877-1600

Vegetarian Dietetics is a newsletter published by the Vegetarian Nutrition practice group of the American Dietetic Association. Although the publication is more interested in vegetarian diets, without particular concern for fat and salt intakes, their "Review of Recent Literature" section is the best I read.

Best Vegetarian Books:

Beware of the lack of sodium concern in the following books.

Ballentine, R. *Transition to Vegetarianism: An Evolutionary Step.* Honesdale, Pa.: The Himalayan International Institute, 1987.

Ballentine, R. *Diet and Nutrition: A Holistic Approach.* Honesdale, Pa.: The Himalayan International Institute, 1978.

Craig, W. *Nutrition for the Nineties.* Eau Claire, Mich.: Golden Harvest Books, 1992.

Any of Dr. John McDougall's books are highly recommended. The recipes are basic and simple, as well as being very low in fat and sodium.

Any of Dr. Dean Ornish's books are also highly recommended. For those seeking prevention and reversal of heart disease, his *Dr. Dean Ornish's Program for Reversing Heart Disease* (New York, N.Y.: Random House, 1990) is a must. Again, be mindful of sodium levels that may excede your goals in some of the recipes.

Robbins, J. *Diet for a New America.* Walpole, N.H.: Stillpoint Publishing. 1987. This is a tender, yet informative book on the health, humane, and political reasons for vegetarianism. Contains no recipes.

Thrash, A. *Nutrition for Vegetarians.* Santa Cruz, Ca.: New Life Books, 1982.

The Following Books Contain Recipes with Very Low Amounts of Sodium and Fat:

Williams, J.B., and G. Silverman. *No Salt, No Sugar, No Fat Cookbook.* San Leandro, Ca.: Bristol Publishing Enterprises, Inc., 1982.

Schell, M. *Chinese Salt-Free Diet Cookbook.* New York, N.Y.: New American Library, 1985.

For Information to Help Quit Smoking:

Smoke Stoppers
The National Center for Health Promotion
3920 Varsity Drive
Ann Arbor, MI 28108
(313) 971-6077

U.S. Office on Smoking and Health
Centers for Chronic Disease Prevention
Centers for Disease Control and Prevention
1600 Clifton Road, N.E.
Atlanta, GA 30333
(404) 488-5703

Smokenders
(800) 323-1126

Smokers Anonymous: See *To Find Anonymous Groups.*

Diabetes:

American Diabetes Association
Communications Department
1660 Duke St.
Alexandria, VA 22314
(800) 232-3472 Ext. 290

Heart Information:

American Heart Association
National Center 7272 Greenville Ave.
Dallas, TX 75231
(214) 373-6300
(800) 242-8721

Cardiac Rehabilitation groups can offer valuable physical, emotional, and spiritual support to the heart patient. These programs can be found throughout the world; the U.S. organization to contact is:

American Association of Cardiovascular and Pulmonary Rehabilitation
7611 Elmwood Avenue, Suite 201
Middleton, WI 53562
(608) 831-6989
FAX: (608) 831-5122

To Find Anonymous Groups:

The following book offers information on a variety of self help groups: *Self Help Source Book: Finding and Forming Mutual Aid Self Help Groups,* 4th Ed., American Self Help Clearing House, 25 Pocono Road, Denville, N.J. 07834; Phone: (201) 625-7101.

Hazelden Education Materials publishes much of the twelve step Anonymous groups' literature. Call (800) 328-9000 [in Minnesota (800) 257-0070].

Adult Children of Alcoholics (ACOA) groups do not require that you are literally a biological child of an alcoholic, but that you are interested in examining your addictive behaviors, such as *controlling or enabling others.* ACOA and information on the other anonymous groups may be found via a phone call to Alcoholics Anonymous (AA), since many of the smaller groups do not have a separate listing. As all the groups are different to some extent, try each group a few times before deciding which is best for you.

Overeaters Anonymous groups are in most cities in the United States and in many throughout the world. If you do not find a listing in your local phonebook, also check under Alcoholics Anonymous. Adult Children of Alcoholics groups and many of the other anonymous groups may be found by calling AA. As all the groups are different to some extent, try each group a few times before deciding which is best for you. To find locales near you, call or write:

Overreaters Anonymous, Inc.
6075 Zenith Ct. N.E.
Rio Rancho, NM 87124
(505) 891-2664

Network for Attitudinal Healing International
1301 Capital of Texas Highway South, Suite B 122
Austin, Texas 78746
(512) 327-4568
FAX: 327-8835

The Attitudinal Healing groups provide support for people who want to explore their abilities to perceive things differently, to choose peace rather than conflict and love rather than fear. The groups are now in fourteen countries and seven continents, and are offered free, with trained peer facilitators. Call or write to obtain the closest Attitudinal Healing group to you.

Christian Retreat Centers:

Aqueduct
716 Mount Carmel Church Road
Chapel Hill, NC 27514
(919) 933-5557

An exceptional retreat center for emotional and spiritual healing, nestled on a hill just south of Chapel Hill, N.C. Their retreats are conducted by priests, preachers, or therapists who are especially gifted in healing. They offer $3\frac{1}{2}$-day retreats approximately monthly, complete with beautiful accomodations and a food service receptive to vegetarian requests.

Benedictine Monastery
Pecos, NM 87552
(505) 757-6415

Snail's Pace
Attn: Melissa Lang
P.O. Box 593
Saluda, NC 28773
(704) 749-4791

Appendix C

FOOD JOURNAL WITH ALLOWANCES

DATE & TIME	FOODS EATEN/PORTIONS PER CUP, TBS., OZ.	FOOD ALLOWANCES	AEROBIC EXERCISE (IN $\frac{1}{2}$, $\frac{3}{4}$, 1 HR)	STRESS LEVEL 1–10 (LEAST–MOST)

	STARCH	PROTEIN	VEGGIE	FRUIT	DAIRY	FAT
Daily Food Allowances						
Allowances Eaten						
Difference						

Appendix D

FOOD JOURNAL WITH FEELINGS

DATE & TIME	PRECEDING EVENTS/FEELINGS 30 MIN. PRIOR	HUNGER LEVEL (1–5) (LEAST– MOST)	FOODS EATEN/PORTIONS PER CUP, TBS., OZ., ETC.	FULLNESS (1–5), & FEELINGS AFTERWARDS	WHERE/WITH WHOM FOOD WAS EATEN

Plan of Abstinence _____

Water (oz.) _____ Aerobic Exercise (type & number of minutes) _____

SELECTED REFERENCES

Chapter 1: Reversing the Risks of Heart Disease

American College of Sports Medicine. *American College of Sports Medicine Fitness Book.* (Champaign, Illinois: Leisure Press, 1992).

American Heart Association. "Heart and Stroke Facts: 1995 Statistical Supplement."

Blankenhorn, D.H., S.A. Nessim, R.L. Johnson, et al. "Beneficial Effects of Combined Colestipol-Niacin Therapy on Coronary Atherosclerosis and Coronary Venous Bypass Grafts." *Journal of the American Medical Association* 257 (1987): 3233–40.

Brensike, J.F., R.I. Levy, S.F. Kelsey, et al. "Effects of Therapy with Cholestyramine on Progression of Coronary Arteriosclerosis: Results of the NHLBI Type II Coronary Intervention Study." *Circulation* 69 (1984): 313–24.

Brown, G., J.J. Albers, L.D. Fisher, et al. "Regression of Coronary Artery Disease as a Result of Intensive Lipid-Lowering Therapy in Men with High Levels of Apolipoprotein B." *New England Journal of Medicine* 323 (1990): 1289–98.

Buchwald, H., J.P. Matts, L.L. Fitch, et al. "Program on the Surgical Control of the Hyperlipidemias (Posch): Design and Methodology." *Journal of Clinical Epidemiology* 42 (1980): 1111–27.

Frick, M.M., O. Elo, K. Haapa, et al. "Helsinki Heart Study: Primary-Prevention Trial with Gemfibrozil in Middle-Aged Men with Dyslipidemia." *New England Journal of Medicine* 317 (1987): 1237–45.

Kane, J.P., M.J. Malloy, T.A. Ports, et al. "Regression of Coronary Atherosclerosis During Treatment of Familial Hypercholesterolemia with Combined Drug Regimens." *Journal of the American Medical Association* 264 (1990): 3007–12.

Kempner, W. "Radical Dietary Treatment of Hypertensive and Arteriosclerotic Vascular Disease, Heart, and Kidney Disease, and Vascular Retinopathy." *General Practitioner* 9 (1954): 71–93.

Ornish, D., S.E. Brown, L.W. Scherwitz, et al. "Can Lifestyle Changes Reverse Coronary Heart Disease?" *Lancet* 336 (1990): 129–33.

Rosati, K.G., and M. Spencer. "Implementing Progressive 'Reversal' Cardiac Diets in a Hospital Setting: A Success Story at Mother Frances Hospital, Tyler, Texas." *Journal of Cardiopulmonary Rehabilitation* 14 (1994): 13–20.

Roussouw, J.E., B. Lewis, and B.M. Rifkind. "The Value of Lowering Cholesterol After Myocardial Infarction." *New England Journal of Medicine* 323 (1990): 1112–19.

Schuler, G., R. Hambreecht, G. Schlierf, et al. "Myocardial Perfusion and Regression of Coronary Artery Disease in Patients on a Regimen of Intensive Physical Exercise and Low Fat Diet." *Journal of the American College of Cardiology* 19 (1992): 34–42.

Watts, G.F., B. Lewis, J.N.H. Brunt, et al. "Effects on Coronary Artery Disease of Lipid-Lowering Diet, or Diet Plus Cholestyramine, in the St. Thomas's Atherosclerosis Regression Study (STARS)." *Lancet* 339 (1992): 563–69.

Chapter 2: Lowering Your Risk of High Cholesterol

Allen, L.H., E.A. Oddoye, and S. Margen. "Protein-Induced Hypercalciuria: A Longer Term Study." *American Journal of Clinical Nutrition* 34 (1979): 741–749.

Altschuler, S.I. "Dietary Protein and Calcium Loss; A Review." *Nutr. Res.* 2: 193–200.

Anderson, J.W., and J. Tietyen-Clark. "Dietary Fiber: Hyperlipidemia, Hypertension and Coronary Heart Disease." *American Journal of Gastroenterology* 81, no. 10 (1986): 907–919.

Anderson, J.W., Johnstone, B.M., and M.E. Cook-Newell. "Meta-analysis of the Effects of Soy Protein Intake on Serum Lipids." *New England Journal of Medicine* 333 (1995): 276–282.

Anderson, J.W., et al. "Hypocholesterolemic Effects of Oat-Bran or Bean Intake for Hypercholesterolemic Men." *American Journal of Clinical Nutrition* 40 (1984): 1146–1155.

Anderson, J.W., et al. "Serum Lipid Response of Hypercholesterolemic Men to Single and Divided Doses of Canned Beans." *American Journal of Clinical Nutrition* 51 (1990): 1013–9.

Anderson, J.W., et al. "Lipid Responses of Hypercholesterolemic Men to Oat-Bran and Wheat-Bran Intake." *American Journal of Clinical Nutrition* 54 (1991): 678–83.

Anderson, J.W., et al. "Prospective, Randomized, Controlled Comparison of the Effects of Low-Fat and Low-Fat Plus High-Fiber Diets on Serum Lipid Concentrations." *American Journal of Clinical Nutrition* 56 (1992): 887–94.

Anderson, K.M., W.P. Castelli, and D. Levy. "Cholesterol and Mortality: 30 Years of Follow-up from the Framingham Study." *Journal of the American Medical Association* 257 (1987): 2176–2180.

Barrett-Connor, E., and T.L. Bush. "Estrogen and Coronary Heart Disease in Women." *Journal of the American Medical Association* 265 (1991): 1861–1867.

Beilin, L.J. "Dietary Fats, Fish, and Blood Pressure." *Annals of the New York Academy of Sciences* 683 (1993): 34–45.

Benson, Herbert. *The Relaxation Response.* (New York: Avon Books, 1975).

Benson, Herbert. *Beyond the Relaxation Response.* (New York: Berkley Publishing Corp., 1984).

Berkman, L.F., L. Leo-Summers, and R.I. Horwitz. "Emotional Support and Survival after Myocardial Infarction: A Prospective, Population-based Study of the Elderly." *Annals of Internal Medicine* 117 (1992): 1003–1009.

Boffetta, P., and L. Garfinkel. "Alcohol Drinking and Mortality among Men Enrolled in an American Cancer Society Prospective Study." *Epidemiology* 1 (1990): 342–348.

Burger, W.C., et al. "Suppression of Cholesterol Biosynthesis by Constituents of Barley Kernel." *Atherosclerosis* 51 (1984): 75–87.

Burr, M.L., J.F. Gilbert, R.M. Holliday, et al. "Effects of Changes in Fat, Fish, and Fibre Intakes on Death and Myocardial Reinfarction: Diet and Reinfarction Trial (DART)." *The Lancet,* September 30 (1989): 757–761.

Byrd, R.C. "Positive Therapeutic Effects of Intercessory Prayer in a Coronary Care Unit Population." *Southern Medical Journal* 81 (1988): 826–829.

Calvo, Mona S. "Dietary Phosphorus, Calcium Metabolism and Bone." *Journal of Nutrition* 123 (1993): 1627–33.

Campbell, T.C., and C. Junshi. "Diet and Chronic Degenerative Diseases: Perspectives from China." *American Journal of Clinical Nutrition* 59(supp) (1994): 1153S–61S.

Cara, L., C. Dubois, P. Borel, et al. "Effects of Oat Bran, Rice Bran, Wheat Fiber, and Wheat Germ on Postprandial Lipemia in Healthy Adults." *American Journal of Clinical Nutrition* 55 (1992): 81–88.

Case, R.B., A.J. Moss, N. Case, et al. "Living Alone After Myocardial Infarction: Impact on Prognosis." *Journal of American Medical Association* 267 (1992): 515–519.

Center for Science in the Public Interest. "Nutrition and Aging." *Nutrition Action* 19, no. 4 (1992): 5–7.

Cerda, J.J., et al. "The Effects of Grapefruit Pectin on Patients at Risk for Coronary Heart Disease Without Altering Diet or Lifestyle." *Clinical Cardiology* 11 (1988): 589–94.

Comstock, G.W., and K.B. Partridge. "Church Attendance and Health." *Journal of Chronic Diseases* 25 (1972): 665–72.

Cooper, M.J., and M.M. Aygen. "A Relaxation Technique in the Management of Hypercholesterolemia." *Journal of Human Stress* 5 (1979): 24–27.

Craig, W.J. *Nutrition for the Nineties.* (Eau Claire, Michigan: Golden Harvest Books, 1992).

de Lorgeril, M., S. Renaud, N. Mamelle, et al. "Mediterranean Alpha-Linolenic Acid-Rich Diet in Secondary Prevention of Coronary Heart Disease." *The Lancet* 343 (1994): 1454–59.

DeVine, A., et al. "A Longitudinal Study of the Effect of Sodium and Calcium Intakes on Regional Bone Density in Postmenopausal Women." *American Journal of Clinical Nutrition* 62 (1995): 740–745.

Diplock, A.T. "Antioxidants Nutrients and Disease Prevention: An Overview." *American Journal Clinical Nutrition* 53 (1991): 189S–193S.

Dossey, Larry. *Healing Words: The Power of Prayer and the Practice of Medicine.* (San Francisco: Harper, 1993).

Duthie, G.G., K.W.J. Wahle, and W.P. James. "Oxidants, Antioxidants, and Cardiovascular Disease." *Nutrition Research Review* 2 (1989): 51–62.

Dwyer, J.T. "Health Aspects of Vegetarian Diets." *American Journal of Clinical Nutrition* 48 (1988): 712–738.

Ellis, F.R., S. Holesh, J.W. Ellis. "Incidence of Osteoporosis in Vegetarians and Omnivores." *American Journal of Clinical Nutrition* 25 (1972): 555–558.

Ellison, R.C. "Cheers!" (Editorial). *Epidemiology* 1 (1990): 337–339.

Esterbauer, H., G. Striegl, H. Puhl, S. Oberreither, M. Rotheneder, M. el-Saadani, and G. Jurgens. "The Role of Vitamin E and Carotinoids in Preventing Oxidation of Low Density Lipoproteins." *Annals of the New York Academy of Sciences* 570 (1989): 254–67.

Expert Panel on Detection, Evaluation, and Treatment of High Blood Cholesterol in Adults. "Summary of the Second Report of the National Cholesterol Education Program (NCEP) Expert Panel on Detection, Evaluation, and Treatment of High Blood Cholesterol in Adults (Adult Treatment Panel II.)" *Journal of the American Medical Association* 269 (1993): 3015–3023.

Ferguson, Tom. *The No-Nag, No-Guilt, Do-It-Your-Own-Way Guide to Quitting Smoking.* (New York: Ballantine Books, 1989).

Fogarty, M. "Garlic's Potential Role in Reducing Heart Disease." *British Journal of Clinical Practice* 47 (1993): 64–65.

Forrow, L., D.R. Calkins, K. Allshouse, et al. "Evaluating Cholesterol Screening." *Archives of Internal Medicine* 155 (1995): 2177–2184.

Freeland-Graves, J. "Mineral Adequacy of Vegetarian Diets." *American Journal of Clinical Nutrition* 48 (1988): 859–862.

Friedlander, Y., J.D. Kark, and Y. Stein. "Religious Orthodoxy and Myocardial Infarction in Jerusalem–A Case Control Study." *International Journal of Cardiology* 10 (1986): 33–41.

Friedlander, Y., J.D. Kark, and Y. Stein. "Religious Observance and Plasma Lipids and Lipoproteins among 17-Year-Old Jewish Residents of Jerusalem." *Preventive Medicine* 16 (1987): 70–79.

Fuhrman, B., A. Lavy, and Michael Aviram. "Consumption of Red Wine with Meals Reduces the Susceptibility of Human Plasma and Low-Density Lipoprotein to Lipid Peroxidation." *American Journal of Clinical Nutrition* 61 (1995): 549–54.

Goulding, A., H.E. Everitt, J.M. Cooney, and G.F.S. Spears. "Sodium and Osteoporosis." In *Recent Advances in Clinical Nutrition,* edited by A.S. Truswell, and M.L. Walqvist, Vol. 2 (London: John Libbey, 1986), 99–108.

Grundy, S.M. "Monounsaturated Fatty Acids, Plasma Cholesterol, and Coronary Heart Disease." *American Journal of Clinical Nutrition* 45 (1987): 1168–1175.

Grundy, S.M., L. Florentin, D. Nix, et al. "Comparison of Monounsaturated Fatty Acids and Carbohydrates for Reducing Raised Levels of Plasma Cholesterol in Man." *American Journal of Clinical Nutrition* 47 (1988): 965–969.

Harvard Heart Letter. "Walking: The Ideal Exercise?" Nov. 1992: 5–7.

Haskell, W.L., et al. "Role of Water-Soluble Dietary Fiber in the Management of Elevated Plasma Cholesterol in Healthy Subjects." *American Journal of Cardiology* 69, no. 5 (1992): 433–39.

Hegsted, D.M. "Calcium and Osteoporosis." *Journal of Nutrition* 17 (1986): 2316–2319.

Helsing, E. "Traditional Diets and Disease Patterns of the Mediterranean, circa 1960." *American Journal of Clinical Nutrition* 61 (suppl) (1995): 1329A–37S.

Herbert, V. "Vitamin B12: Plant Sources, Requirements, and Assay." *American Journal of Clinical Nutrition* 48 (1988): 852–858.

Hernandez-Avila, M., G. Colditz, et al. "Caffeine, Moderate Alcohol Intake, and Risk of Fractures of the Hip and Forearm in Middle-Aged Women." *American Journal of Clinical Nutrition* 54 (1991): 157–63.

Jha, P., M. Flather, E. Lonn, et al. "The Antioxidant Vitamins and Cardiovascular Disease: A Critical Review of Epidemiologic and Clinical Trial Data." *Annals of Internal Medicine* 123 (1994): 860–872.

Judelson, D.R. "Coronary Heart Disease in Women: Risk Factors and Prevention." *Journal of the American Medical Womens Association* 49 (1994): 186–191.

Kannel, W.B. "Lipids, Diabetes, and Coronary Heart Disease: Insights from the Framingham Study." *American Heart Journal* 110 (1985): 1100–7.

Kempner, W. "Radical Dietary Treatment of Hypertensive and Arteriosclerotic Vascular Disease, Heart, and Kidney Disease, and Vascular Retinopathy." *General Practitioner* 9 (1954): 71–93.

Kestin, M., R. Moss, P.M. Clifton, et al. "Comparative Effects of Three Cereal Brans on Plasma Lipids, Blood Pressure, and Glucose Metabolism in Mildly Hypercholesterolemic Men." *American Journal of Clinical Nutrition* 52 (1990): 661–666.

Keys, A. "Coronary Heart Disease in Seven Countries." *Circulation* 41 (suppl 1) (1970): 1–211.

Keys, A., A. Menotti, C. Aravanis, et al. "The Seven Countries Study: 2289 deaths in 15 years." *Journal of Preventative Medicine* 13 (1984): 141–54.

Kiel, D.P., et al. "Caffeine and the Risk of Hip Fracture: The Framingham Study." *American Journal of Epidemiology* 132 (1990): 675–84.

Kromhout, D., A. Menotti, B. Bloemberg, et al. "Dietary Saturated and trans Fatty Acids and Cholesterol and 25-Year Mortality from Coronary Heart Disease: The Seven Countries Study." *Preventive Medicine* 24 (1995): 308–315.

Kushi, L.H., E.B. Lenart, and W.C. Willett. "Health Implications of Mediterranean Diets in Light of Contemporary Knowledge. 2. Meat, Wine, Fats, and Oils." *American Journal of Clinical Nutrition* 61 (suppl) (1995): 1416S–27S.

Lang, S.S. "The World's Healthiest Diet." *American Health,* Sept. (1989): 106–110.

Lappe, F.M. *Diet for a Small Planet.* (New York: Ballantine Books, 1991).

Leadbetter, J., M.J. Ball, and J.I. Mann. "Effects of Increasing Quantities of Oat Bran in Hypercholesterolemic People." *American Journal of Clinical Nutrition* 54 (1991): 841–845.

Liebman, Bonnie. "Antioxidants: Surprise, Surprise." *Nutrition Action* 21 (1994): 4.

Lindenbaum, J., I.H. Rosenberg, P.W.F. Wilson, et al. "Prevalence of Cobalamin Deficiency in the Framingham Elderly Population." *American Journal of Clinical Nutrition* 60 (1994): 2–11.

Linkswiler, H.M., M.B. Zemel, M. Hegsted, and S. Schuette. "Protein-Induced Hypercalciuria." *Federal Processings* 40 (1981): 2429–2433.

Marsh, A.G., T.V. Sanchez, O. Michelsen, et al. "Vegetarian Lifestyle and Bone Mineral Density." *American Journal of Clinical Nutrition* 48 (1988): 837–841.

Massey, Linda K. "Dietary Factors Influencing Calcium and Bone Metabolism: Introduction." *Journal of Nutrition* 123 (1993): 1609–10.

Massey, Linda K., and Susan J. Whiting. "Caffeine, Urinary Calcium, Calcium Metabolism and Bone." *Journal of Nutrition* 123 (1993): 1611–14.

McDonald, B.E., J.M. Gerrard, V.M. Bruce, et al. "Comparison of the Effect of Canola Oil and Sunflower Oil on Plasma Lipids and Lipoproteins and On in vivo Thromboxane A2 and Prostacyclin Production in Healthy Young Men." *American Journal of Clinical Nutrition* 50 (1989): 1382–1388.

McDougall, John. *McDougall's Medicine: A Challenging Second Opinion.* (Piscataway, NJ: New Century Publishers, Inc., 1985).

McIntosh, G.H., J. Whyte, R. McArthus, and P.J. Nestel. "Barley and Wheat Foods: Influence on Plasma Cholesterol Concentrations in Hypercholesterolic Men." *American Journal of Clinical Nutrition* 53 (1991): 1205–9.

Mensink, R.P., and M.B. Katan. "Effect of Monounsaturated Fatty Acids Versus Complex Carbohydrates on High-Density Lipoproteins in Healthy Men and Women." *Lancet* i (1987): 122–124.

Mensink, R.P., and M.B. Katan. "Effect of Dietary *Trans* Fatty Acids on High-density and Low-density Lipoprotein Cholesterol Levels in Healthy Subjects." *New England Journal of Medicine* 343 (1990): 439–445.

Morris, D.L., S.B. Kritchevsky, and C.E. Davis. "Serum Carotenoids and Coronary Heart Disease: The Lipid Research Clinics Coronary Primary Prevention Trial and Follow-up Study." *Journal of the American Medical Association* 272 (1994): 1439–1441.

Newman, R.K., S.E. Lewis, and C.W. Newman. "Hypocholesterolemic Effect of Barley Foods on Healthy Men." *Nutrition Reports International* 39, no. 4 (1993): 749–59.

Ornish, Dean. *Dr. Dean Ornish's Program for Reversing Heart Disease.* (New York: Random House, 1990).

Ornish, D., S.E. Brown, L.W. Scherwitz, et al. "Can Lifestyle Changes Reverse Coronary Heart Disease." *Lancet* 335 (1990): 129–133.

Oxman, T.E., D.H. Freeman, and E.D. Manheimer. "Lack of Social Participation or Religious Strength and Comfort as Risk Factors for Death After Cardiac Surgery in the Elderly." *Psychosomatic Medicine* 57 (1995): 5–15.

Pennebaker, J.W., and S.K. Beall. "Confronting a Traumatic Event: Toward an Understanding of Inhibition and Disease." *Journal of Abnormal Psychology* 95 (1986): 274–281.

Pennebaker, J.W., J.K. Kiecolt-Glaser, and R. Glaser. "Disclosure of Traumas and Immune Function: Health Implications for Psychotherapy." *Journal of Consultative Clinical Psychology* 56 (1988): 239–245.

"Position of the American Dietetic Association: Vegetarian Diets–Technical Support Paper." *Journal of the American Dietetic Association* 88 (1988): 352–355.

Potter, S.M. "Overview of the Proposed Mechanisms for the Hypocholesterolemic Effect of Soy." *Journal of Nutrition* 125 (1995): 606S

Qureshi, A.A., W.C. Burger, D.M. Peterson, and C.E. Elson. "The Structure of an Inhibitor of Cholesterol Biosynthesis Isolated From Barley." *Journal of Biolologic Chemistry* 1986 261, no. 23 (1986): 10544–10550.

Renaud, S., F. Godsey, E. Dumont, et al. "Influence of Long-term Diet Modification on Platelet Function and Composition in Moselle Farmers." *American Journal of Clinical Nutrition* 43 (1986): 136–150.

Renaud, S., M. de Lorgeril, J. Delaye, et al. "Cretan Mediterranean Diet for Prevention of Coronary Heart Disease." *American Journal of Clinical Nutrition* 61 (suppl) (1995): 1360S–7S.

Riemersma, R.A., D.A. Wood, D.D.H. Macintyre, et al. "Risk of Angina Pectoris and Plasma Concentrations of Vitamins A, C, E, and Carotene." *Lancet* 337 (1991): 1–5.

Rifkin, J. *Beyond Beef.* (New York: Dutton, 1992).

Rimm, E.B., M.J. Stampfer, A. Ascherio, et al. "Vitamin E Consumption and the Risk of Coronary Heart Disease in Men." *The New England Journal of Medicine* 328 (1993): 1450–6.

Sacks, F.M., P. Hebert, L.J. Appel, et al. "The Effect of Fish Oil on Blood Pressure and High-Density Lipoprotein-Cholesterol Levels in Phase I of the Trials of Hypertension Prevention. Trials of Hypertension Prevention Collaborative Research Group." *Journal of Hypertension* 12 Supp. (1994): 234–31.

Salonen, J.T., K. Nyyssonen, and H. Korpela. "High Stored Iron Levels are Associated with Excess Risk of Myocardial Infarction in Eastern Finnish Men." *Circulation* 86 (1992): 803–811.

Sanders, T.A., and S. Reddy. "The Influence of Rice Bran on Plasma Lipids and Lipoproteins in Human Volunteers." *European Journal of Clinical Nutrition* 46,3 (1992): 167–72.

Seppanen-Laakso, T., H. Vanhanen, H.I. Laakso, et al. "Replacement of Margarine on Bread by Rapeseed and Olive Oils: Effects on Plasma Fatty Acid Composition and Serum Cholesterol." *Annals of Nutrition Metabolism* 37 (1993): 161–174.

Sirtori, C.R., E. Tremoli, E. Gatti, et al. "Controlled Evaluation of Fat Intake in the Mediterranean Diet: Comparative Activities of Olive Oil and Corn Oil on Plasma Lipids and Platelets in High-Risk Patients." *American Journal of Clinical Nutrition* 44 (1986): 635–642.

Smith, S.C., S.N. Blair, M.H. Criqui, et al. "Preventing Heart Attack and Death in Patients with Coronary Disease." Consensus Panel Statement.

Stampfer, J.J., M.R. Malinow, W.C. Willett, et al. "A Prospective Study of Plasma Homocysteine and Risk of Myocardial Infarction in U.S. Physicians." *Journal of the American Medical Association* 268 (1992): 877–881.

Stampfer, M.J., C.H. Hennekens, J.E. Manson, et al. "Vitamin E Consumption and the Risk of Coronary Disease in Women." *The New England Journal of Medicine* 328 (1993): 1444–1449.

Street, D.A., G.W. Comstock, R.M. Salkeld, et al. "A Population Based Case-Control Study of Serum Antioxidants and Myocardial Infarction." *American Journal of Epidemiology* 134 (1991): 719–720.

The Alpha-Tocopherol, Beta Carotene Cancer Prevention Study Group. "The Effect of Vitamin E and Beta Carotene on the Incidence of Lung Cancer and Other Cancers in Male Smokers." *The New England Journal of Medicine* 330 (1994): 1029–35.

Thomas, L.H., J.A. Winter, and R.G. Scott. "Concentration of 18:1 and 16:1 *Trans*unsaturated Fatty Acids in the Adipose Body Tissue of Decedents Dying of Ischaemic Heart Disease Compared with Controls: analysis by gas liquid chromatography." *Journal of Epidemiological Community Health* 37 (1983): 16–21.

Tufts University Diet and Nutrition Letter (eds.) "Eating Less Sodium Means Retaining More Bone." *Tufts University Diet and Nutrition Letter* 14 (1996): 1–2.

Ubbink, J.B., W.J. Vermaak, A. van der Merwe, and P.J. Becker. "Vitamin B12, Vitamin B6, and Folate Nutritional Status in Men with Hyperhomocysteinemia." *American Journal of Clinical Nutrition* 57 (1993): 47–53.

Ubbink, J.B., W.J. van der Merwe, P.J. Becker, R. Delport, and H.C. Potgieter. "Vitamin Requirements for the Treatment of Hyperhomocysteinemia in Humans." *Journal of Nutrition* 124 (1994): 1927–1933.

Verschuren, W.M.M., D.R. Jacobs, B.P.M. Bloemberg, et al. "Serum Total Cholesterol and Long-term Coronary Heart Disease Mortality in Different Cultures." *Journal of American Medical Association* 274 (1995): 131–136.

Weaver, B.J., E.J. Corner, V.M. Bruce, et al. "Dietary Canola Oil: Effect on the Accumulation of Eicosapentaenoic Acid in the Alkenylacyl Fraction of Human Platelet Ethanolamine Phosphoglyceride." *American Journal of Clinical Nutrition* 51 (1990): 594–598.

White, R., and E. Frank. "Health Effects and Prevalence of Vegetarianism." *The Western Journal of Medicine* 160 (1994): 465–471.

Willett, W.C., and A. Ascherio. "*Trans* Fatty Acids: Are the Effects Only Marginal?" *American Journal of Public Health* 84 (1994): 722–724.

Willett, W.C., F. Sacks, A. Trichopoulou, et al. "Mediterranean Diet Pyramid: A Cultural Model for Healthy Eating." *American Journal of Clinical Nutrition* 61 (suppl) (1995): 1402S–6S.

Willett, W.C., M.J. Stampfer, J.E. Manson, et al. "Intake of *Trans* Fatty Acids and Risk of Coronary Heart Disease Among Women." *The Lancet* 341 (1993): 581–85.

Williams, R., and V. Williams. *Anger Kills.* (New York: Random House, 1993).

Wilson, P.W.F. "Cholesterol Screening: Once Is Not Enough." (editorial) *Archives of Internal Medicine* 155: 2146–2147.

Wolinsky, H. "Prayers Do Aid Sick, Study Finds." *Chicago Sun-Times,* January 26, 1986.

Chapter 3: Lowering Your Risk of Excess Weight and Diabetes

Acheson, K., E. Jequier, A. Burger, et al. "Thyroid hormones and thermogenesis: the metabolic cost of food and exercise." *Metabolism* 33 (1984): 262–65.

Acheson, K.J., E. Ravussin, D.A. Schoeller, et al. "Two-week stimulation or blockage of the sympathetic nervous system in man: influence on body weight, body composition, and twenty-four-hour energy expenditure." *Metabolism* 37 (1988): 91–98.

Anderson, J.W., et al. "Metabolic Effects of High-Carbohydrate, High-Fiber Diets for Insulin-Dependent Diabetic Individuals." *American Journal of Clinical Nutrition* 54 (1991): 936–43.

Barnard, R.J., T. Jung, and S.B. Inkeles. "Diet and Exercise in the Treatment of NIDDM." *Diabetes Care* 17 (1994): 1469–1472.

Cerda, J.J., et al. "The Effects of Grapefruit Pectin on Patients at Risk for Coronary Heart Disease Without Altering Diet or Lifestyle." *Clinical Cardiology* 11 (1988): 589–94.

Durstine, J.L., A. King, P.L. Painter, et al. (contributing editors). *American College of Sports Medicine's Resource Manual for Guidelines for Exercise Testing and Prescription,* 2nd Ed. (Media, Pa.: Williams & Wilkins, 1993).

Fontvieille, A.M., et al. "The Use of Low Glycaemic Index Foods Improves Metabolic Control of Diabetic Patients Over Five Weeks." *Diabetic Medicine* 9 (1992): 444–450.

Gwinup, G. "Weight Loss Without Dietary Restriction: Efficacy of Different Forms of Aerobic Exercise." *American Journal of Sports Medicine* 15 (1987): 275–279.

Hubert, Helen B., F. Manning, P.M. McNamara, and W.P. Castelli. "Obesity as an Independent Risk Factor for Cardiovascular Disease: A 26-year Follow-up of Participants in the Framingham Heart Study." *Circulation* 67 (1983): 968–977.

Liljeberg, H., Y. Granfeldt, and I. Bjorck. "Metabolic Responses to Starch in Bread Containing Intact Kernels Versus Milled Flour." *European Journal of Clinical Nutrition* 46 (1992): 561–575.

Miller, J.B., E. Pang, and L. Bramall. "Rice: A High or Low Glycemic Index Food?" *American Journal of Clinical Nutrition* 56 (1992): 1034–6.

Nuttall, F.Q. "Dietary Fiber in the Management of Diabetes." *Diabetes* 42 (1993): 503–508.

Progoff, I. *At a Journal Workshop: The Basic Text and Guide for Using the Intensive Journal Process.* (New York: Dialogue House Library, 1990).

Riccardi, G., and A. A. Rivellese. "Effects of Dietary Fiber and Carbohydrate on Glucose and Lipoprotein Metabolism in Diabetic Patients." *Diabetes Care* 14 (1991): 1115–25.

Sanders, T.A., and S. Reddy. "The influence of rice bran on plasma lipids and lipoproteins in human volunteers." *European Journal of Clinical Nutrition* 46,3 (1992): 167–72.

Shukla, K., et al. "Glycaemic Response to Maize, Bajra and Barley." *Indian Journal of Physiological Pharmacology* 35, no. 4 (1991): 249–254.

Society of Actuaries: *Build and Blood Pressure Study.* (Chicago: Society of Actuaries, 1959–1960).

Thorburn, Anne W., Jennie C. Brand, and A. Stewart Truswell. "Salt and the Glycaemic Response." *British Medical Journal* 292 (1986): 1697–1699.

Truswell, A.S. "Glycaemic Index of Foods." *European Journal of Clinical Nutrition* 46, no. 2 (1992): S91–S101.

Wolever, T.M.S. "Relationship Between Dietary Fiber Content and Composition in Foods and the Glycemic Index." *American Journal of Clinical Nutrition* 51 (1990): 725.

Chapter 4: Lowering Your Risk of High Blood Pressure

Anderson, J.W., and J. Tietyen-Clark. "Dietary Fiber: Hyperlipidemia, Hypertension, and Coronary Heart Disease." *The American Journal of Gastroenterology* 81 (1986): 907–919.

Blackburn, H., and R. Prineas. "Diet and Hypertension: Anthropology, Epidemiology, and Public-Health Implications." *Progress in Biochemical Pharmacology* 19 (1983): 31–79.

Capacchione, L. *The Power of Your Other Hand.* (North Hollywood, Ca.: Newcastle Publishing Co., Inc., 1988).

Dossey, L. *Healing Words.* (New York: Harper, 1993).

Dunbar, F. *Mind and Body: Psychosomatic Medicine.* (New York: Random House, 1947).

Foster, R. *Prayer: Finding the Heart's True Home.* (New York: Harper, 1992).

Graham, Thomas, Berton H. Kaplan, et al. "Frequency of Church Attendance and Blood Pressure Elevation." *Journal of Behavioral Medicine* 1 (1978): 37–43.

Joint National Committee on Detection, Evaluation, and Treatment of High Blood Pressure. "The Fifth Report of the Joint National Committee on Detection, Evaluation, and Treatment of High Blood Pressure (JNC V)." *Archives of Internal Medicine* 153 (1993): 154–176.

Kelsey, M.T. *Psychology, Medicine, and Christian Healing.* (San Francisco: Harper and Row, 1988).

Kempner, W. "Treatment of Hypertensive Vascular Disease with Rice Diet." *American Journal of Medicine* 4 (1948): 545–77.

Kempner, W. "Treatment of Heart and Kidney Disease and of Hypertensive and Arteriosclerotic Vascular Disease with the Rice Diet." *Annals of Internal Medicine* 31 (1949): 821–56.

Kempner, W. "Radical Dietary Treatment of Hypertensive and Arteriosclerotic Vascular Disease, Heart, and Kidney Disease, and Vascular Retinopathy." *General Practitioner* 9 (1954): 71–93.

Liebman, B. "One Nation, Under Pressure." *Nutrition Action* 22 (1995): 1–9.

Lynch, J. *The Broken Heart.* (New York: Basic Books, Inc., 1977).

National Research Council. *Recommended Dietary Allowances, 10th Edition.* Washington, D.C.: National Academy Press, 1989.

Ornish, D. *Dr. Dean Ornish's Program for Reversing Heart Disease.* (New York: Random House, 1990).

The Trials of Hypertension Prevention Collaborative Research Group. "The Effects of Nonpharmacologic Interventions on Blood Pressure of Persons with High Normal Levels: Results of the Trials of Hypertension Prevention, Phase I." *Journal of the American Medical Association* 267 (1992): 1213–1220.

Truswell, A.S., et al. "Blood Pressure of !Kung Bushmen in Northern Botswana." *American Heart Journal* 84 (1972): 5–12.

Chapter 5: Assessing Your Heart's Health
Enos, W.F., J.C. Beyer, and R.H. Holmes. "Pathogenesis of Coronary Disease in American Soldiers Killed in Korea." *Journal of the American Medical Association* 158 (1955): 912–14.

Chen, J., et al. *Diet, Life-style, and Mortality in China: A Study of the Characteristics of Sixty-Five Chinese Counties.* (Oxford: Oxford University Press, 1990).

Connor, W.E., and Sonja, L. Connor. *The New American Diet.* (New York: Simon Schuster, 1986), 21–22.

deWolfe, M.S., and H.M. Whyte. "Serum Cholesterol and Lipoproteins in Natives of New Guinea and Australians." *Australasian Annals of Medicine* 7 (1958): 51.

Hannah, J.B. "Civilization, Race, and Coronary Atheroma with Particular Reference to Its Incidence and Severity in Copperbelt Africans." *Central African Journal of Medicine* 4 (1958): 1–5.

Kagawa, Y. "Impact of Westernization on the Nutrition of Japanese: Changes in Physique, Cancer, Longevity, and Centenarians." *Preventive Medicine* 7 (1978): 205–7.

Keys, A., et al. "Lessons from Serum Cholesterol Studies in Japan, Hawaii, and Los Angeles." *Annals of Internal Medicine* 48 (1958): 83–94.

Leaf, A. "Management of Hypercholesterolemia: Are Preventive Interventions Advisable?" *New England Journal of Medicine* 321 (1989): 681.

McGill, H.C., Jr., ed. *The Geographic Pathology of Atherosclerosis.* (Baltimore: Williams and Wilkins Company, 1968).

National Cholesterol Education Program. Second Report of the Expert Panel on Detection, Evaluation, and Treatment of High Blood Cholesterol in Adults. NIH Publication No. 93-3095; September 1993.

National Research Council, Diet and Health. *Implications for Reducing Chronic Disease Risk.* (Washington, D.C.: National Academy Press, 1989), 102.

Pazzanese, D., et al. "Serum-Lipid Levels in a Brazilian Indian Population." *Lancet* Sept. (1964): 615–17.

The Trials of Hypertension Prevention Collaborative Research Group. "The Effects of Nonpharmacologic Interventions on Blood Pressure of Persons with High Normal Levels." *Journal of the American Medical Association* 267 (1992): 1213–20.

World Health Organization. *Statistics Annual,* 1988.

Chapter 6: Designing Your Personal Heal Your Heart Program

American College of Sports Medicine. *American College of Sports Medicine Fitness Book.* (Champaign, Illinois, 1992).

Blair, Steven, P. Painter, R. Pate, et al. *Manual for Guidelines for Exercise Testing and Prescription.* (Philadelphia: Lea and Febiger Resource, 1988), 288.

Borg, G.A. "Medicine and Science in Sports and Exercise." 14 (1982): 377–378.

Durstine, J.L., A.C. King, P.L. Painter, et al. *American College of Sports Medicine's Resource Manual for Guidelines for Exercise Testing and Prescription,* 2nd Ed. (Media, Pa.: Williams & Wilkins, 1993).

Gwinup, G. "Weight Loss Without Dietary Restriction: Efficacy of Different Forms of Aerobic Exercise." *American Journal of Sports Medicine* 15 (1987): 275–279.

Liebman, B., and D. Schardt. "Vitamin Smarts." *Nutrition Action* 22 (1995): 1–10.

Ornish, D. *Dr. Dean Ornish's Program for Reversing Heart Disease.* (New York: Random House, 1990).

Rooney, Earl. "Exercise for Older Patients: Why It's Worth Your Effort." *Geriatrics* 48, 11 (1993).

Chapter 7: Healing Your Heart Through Nutrition

Dwyer, J.T. "Health Aspects of Vegetarian Diets." *American Journal of Clinical Nutrition* 48 (1988): 712–738.

Freeland-Graves, J. "Mineral Adequacy of Vegetarian Diets." *American Journal of Clinical Nutrition* 48 (1988): 859–862.

Hallberg, L., M. Brune, and L. Rossander-Hulthen. "Is There a Physiological Role of Vitamin C in Iron Absorption?" *Annals of New York Academy of Sciences* 498 (1987): 324–332.

Herbert, V. "Vitamin B12: Plant Sources, Requirements, and Assay." *American Journal of Clinical Nutrition* 48 (1988): 852–858.

Chapter 8: Deciphering the New Food Labels

American Dietetic Association. "Legislative Highlights: Final Food Labeling Regulations." *Journal of the American Dietetic Association* 93, no. 2 (1993): 146–148.

Liebman, B. "Baby 'Label' Arrives." *Nutrition Action* 20, no. 2 (1993): 7–9.

Liebman, B. "Alice in Label-land." *Nutrition Action* 20, no. 2 (1993): 8–9.

Pennington, J.A.T., and V.L. Wilkening. "Nutrition Labeling of Raw Fruit, Vegetables, and Fish." *Journal of the American Dietetic Association* 92 (1993): 1250–1254, 1257.

Chapter 9: Healing Your Heart Through Exercise

American College of Sports Medicine. *American College of Sports Medicine Fitness Book.* (Champaign, Illinois: Leisure Press, 1992).

Blair, S., P. Painter, R. Pate, et al. *Manual for Guidelines for Exercise Testing and Prescription.* (Philadelphia: Lea and Febiger Resource, 1988).

Durstine, J.L., A. King, P. Painter, et al. (contributing editors) *American College of Sports Medicine's Resource Manual for Guidelines for Exercise Testing and Prescription,* 2nd Ed. (Media, Pa.: Williams & Wilkins, 1993).

Chapter 10: Healing Your Heart Through Emotional and Spiritual Renewal

Benson, Herbert. *The Relaxation Response.* (New York: Avon Books, 1975).

Benson, Herbert. *Beyond the Relaxation Response.* (New York: Berkley Publishing Corp., 1984).

Capacchione, Lucia. *The Power of Your Other Hand.* (North Hollywood, Ca: Newcastle Publishing Co., Inc., 1988).

Foster, R. J. *Celebration of Discipline: The Path to Spiritual Growth*. Revised Ed. (San Francisco: Harper and Row, 1988).

Foster, Richard J. *Prayer: Finding the Heart's True Home*. (San Francisco: Harper, 1992).

Friends in Recovery. *The Twelve Steps—A Spiritual Journey*. (San Diego, Ca.: Recovery Publications, Inc., 1988).

Friends in Recovery. *The Twelve Steps—A Way Out*. (San Diego, Ca.: Recovery Publications, Inc., 1988).

Kelsey, Morton T. *Adventure Inward*. (Minneapolis: Augsburg Publishing House, 1980).

Kelsey, Morton T. *The Other Side of Silence*. (New York: Paulist Press, 1976).

Kelsey, Morton, T. *Dreams: A Way to Listen to God*. (New York: Paulist Press, 1978).

Progoff, Ira. *At a Journal Workshop*. (New York: Dialogue House Library, 1992).

Sanford, Agnes. *The Healing Light*. (St. Paul: Macalester Park Publishing Co., 1972).

van der Post, Laurens. *Jung and the Story of Our Time*. (New York: Anchor/Doubleday, 1972), 184.

Westerhoff, J.H. *Spiritual Life: The Foundation for Preaching and Teaching*. (Louisville, Ky: Westminster John Knox Press, 1994).

Chapter 12: Cooking Heart-Healthy Rice, Grains, and Beans

Ewald, E.B. *Recipes for a Small Planet*. (New York: Ballentine Books, 1985).

Simmons, M. *Rice, the Amazing Grain*. (New York: Henry Holt and Co., 1991).

Chapter 13: Flavoring Your Heart-Healthy Foods with Herbs and Spices

Hill, M., G. Barclay, and J. Hardy. *Southern Herb Growing*. (Fredericksburg, Texas: Shearer Publishing, 1987).

Holt, G. *Geraldene Holt's Complete Book of Herbs*. (New York: Henry Holt and Company, 1991).

Michalak, Patricia S. *Rodale's Successful Organic Gardening: Herbs*. (Emmaus, Pa.: Rodale Press, 1993).

INDEX

❖

Page numbers in italics indicate figures; page numbers followed by t indicate tables.